MCAT*

success

Biological Sciences, Beryl Packer • Diane A. Ryan

Physical Sciences, Hans Minnich • Rick Needham

Dana Freeman • John W. Dooley • Kent E. Wagner

Verbal Reasoning and Writing, Patricia Burgess

Mathematics, Mark Weinfeld

PETERSON'S

THOMSON LEARNING ™

Australia • Canada • Mexico • Singapore • Spain • United Kingdom • United States

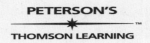

About Peterson's

Founded in 1966, Peterson's, a division of Thomson Learning, is the nation's largest and most respected provider of lifelong learning resources, both in print and online. The Education Supersite^{SM} at www.petersons.com—the Internet's most heavily traveled education resource—has searchable databases and interactive tools for contacting U.S.-accredited institutions and programs. In addition, Peterson's delivers unmatched financial aid resources and test-preparation tools. Peterson's serves more than 100 million education consumers annually.

Peterson's is a division of Thomson Learning, one of the world's largest providers of lifelong learning. Thomson Learning serves the needs of individuals, learning institutions, and corporations with products and services for both traditional and distributed learning. Headquartered in Stamford, Connecticut, with offices worldwide, Thomson Learning is a division of The Thomson Corporation (www.thomson.com), one of the world's leading e-information and solutions companies in the business, professional, and education marketplaces. For more information, visit www.thomsonlearning.com.

Acknowledgments: The authors wish to acknowledge the following individuals for their assistance in the preparation of this book: Christopher Cramer, Ph.D., University of Minnesota; Elaine Bender, M.A., El Camino College, Torrance, CA; and Elward K. Alford, Ph.D.

An American BookWorks Corporation Project

ISBN 0-7689-0733-0

Printed in the United States of America

10 9 8 7 6 5 4 3 2 1   02 01

CONTENTS

Red Alert: Introduction. 1

Red Alert: Study Plan 5

Diagnostic Test 9
    Verbal Reasoning. 9
    Physical Sciences. 26
    Writing Sample 39
    Biological Science 41
    Quick-Score Answers for the Diagnostic Test. 56
    Explanatory Answers for the Diagnostic Test 57

Unit 1: Verbal Reasoning Strategies 87

Unit 2: Writing Sample Strategies 99

Unit 3: Mathematics Review 105

Unit 4: Physical Sciences Review 141
    Chemistry. 141
    Physics 155

Unit 5: Biological Science Review 171

MCAT Practice Test 1 201
    Verbal Reasoning. 201
    Physical Sciences. 219
    Writing Sample 232
    Biological Sciences 234
    Quick-Score Answers for Practice Test 1 248
    Explanatory Answers for Practice Test 1 249

MCAT Practice Test 2 275
    Verbal Reasoning. 275
    Physical Sciences. 295
    Writing Sample 311
    Biological Science 313
    Quick-Score Answers for Practice Test 2 326
    Explanatory Answers for Practice Test 2 327

Paying for School—Financing Your Graduate Education 353

WHAT IS THE MCAT?

The Medical College Admission Test (MCAT) is one of the major parts of your medical school application process. Most institutions require that you take this exam. Unlike most of the standardized tests that you have taken earlier in your career, the MCAT requires that you be knowledgeable in the areas of biology, chemistry, and physics. In addition, you must also have good test-taking skills, as well as communications and writing skills.

At this point, as you begin to prepare for the MCAT, it is likely that you have already completed several years of college-level study, and you will undoubtedly have taken most of the applicable science courses. Additionally, you should have a solid background in mathematics, including algebra, trigonometric functions, and sine and cosine; in the use of both metric and English units, and in statistics. You will not be required to know calculus.

WHAT DOES THE TEST CONSIST OF?

There are four major sections of the MCAT: Verbal Reasoning, Physical Sciences, Writing Sample, and Biological Sciences.

VERBAL REASONING

This section is actually a reading comprehension test and consists of nine passages, each of which is followed by a series of questions. The passages will be drawn from the humanities, social sciences, and natural sciences. Unlike the questions in the specific science sections, the questions in verbal reasoning will be based solely on the passages and will not require any supplementary knowledge.

PHYSICAL SCIENCES

The Physical Sciences portion consists of both passages and discrete (individual) questions from physics and chemistry. Traditionally, there are ten sets of problems accompanied by a series of questions based on the information given. However, you will have to have some basic knowledge of both physics and chemistry in order to fully understand the material and answer the questions correctly. There will also be 15 discrete questions—a single statement followed by only one question.

WRITING SAMPLE

There are normally two topics that you will have to write about, and you will have 30 minutes to compose each essay. As part of the essay, you will be asked to explain the given statements, describe specific situations that will illustrate your approach to those statements, develop alternative approaches to the problem, and incorporate all of this into cogent essays, clearly written and well organized.

BIOLOGICAL SCIENCES

The Biological Sciences section is similar to the Physical Sciences portion of the test; there will be ten problem sets accompanied by a series of questions. In this section you will have to have a knowledge of basic biology, including everything from molecular biology, cells, various systems (circulatory, lymphatic, immune, digestive, excretory, muscular, skeletal, etc.), genetics, organic chemistry, to spectroscopy. In addition, you will also have to answer fifteen individual problem sets.

THE TIMETABLE

These four sections of the test will take approximately 5 hours and 45 minutes to complete. In addition, you will receive 1 hour for lunch and two 10-minute breaks.

Verbal Reasoning	85 minutes	65 questions
Physical Sciences	100 minutes	77 questions
Writing Sample	60 minutes	2 essay topics (30 minutes per topic)
Biological Sciences	100 minutes	77 questions

It is strongly suggested that while you study, you use this table to estimate the amount of time you have for each question. It is important to pace yourself properly during the test. If you analyze the number of questions and the amount of time you are given for each test, it works out to about 1½ minutes for each question. However, you will have to subtract time for reading the passages. It is more than likely that you will have no more than 1 minute to answer each question in the Verbal Reasoning, Physical Sciences, and Biological Sciences tests. Keep that in mind as you study.

SCORING THE TEST

Each part of the MCAT receives a separate score—four scores in all. You will receive copies of the scores, as will the medical schools you designate to receive them. Also, if you request, the scores will be sent to your undergraduate adviser.

These scores are based on *the number of questions you answered correctly*. This

means that wrong answers are scored the same as questions that are unanswered— *there is no penalty for getting wrong answers*. Thus, guessing can't hurt you, and if you don't know the answer at all, it can only help. Since all the questions are multiple-choice questions with four choices each (A–D), you have a 25 percent chance of guessing correctly.

The Writing Sample is based on the total of the scores you receive for each of the two essays you write. Each essay is read by two separate readers; therefore, each essay receives two scores, for a total of four. This total is your raw score.

A word about the raw score. Because the conversion of raw scores to scaled scores (percentile score) tends to change, it is not helpful to present a complete scoring chart here. However, as with any test, the higher your raw score, the higher your scaled score. Your report will provide all the scores to you.

PREPARING FOR THE MCAT

This book will help you prepare for the test, if you use it correctly. As you go through the book, taking the practice tests, studying the review sections, be sure to make notes about anything you don't understand. If you have enough time before the test, take the time to research material that is unfamiliar to you.

REVIEW SECTION FORMAT

The presentation of the material in this book is somewhat different from most of the other MCAT test preparation books on the market. Most books will give you a mini-review book to help you review what you don't know. We've done that in the mathematics review chapter to help you recall material that you may not have studied in school for several years. However, because you are preparing for one of the most important tests you will ever take in your career, it is important for you to understand how to answer questions, as well as understanding the material. Therefore, the review sections of this book are set up in a question-and-answer format.

What this means is that in each section you will be presented with a series of questions based on the suggested curriculum of the Association of American Medical

Colleges, the administrator of the MCAT. Immediately following each question is the answer, with an explanation. The purpose of this setup is twofold: to test you on the specific material that will be covered on the exam, and to help you practice the question-and-answer format. In addition, following the answer is the specific topic that is covered by the question. These topics are based on the syllabus for the MCAT, and we have tried to include questions from all of the categories and subtopics that will be covered on the exam.

As you go through the review sections, write your answers in the margin and then immediately check your answer and the explanation. If you got it right and you understand the answer, move on to the next question. Circle those topics that need further review, so you can come back to them later on to review them again or to consult your textbook for a more in-depth explanation.

Obviously, in a book like this, it is impossible to cover everything. However, the basics have been covered, and by using the question-and-answer format, it is more likely that you will understand and retain the material much better than by merely reading an outline of the material in another book.

TAKING THE SAMPLE TESTS

This book contains three full-length tests. The first is a diagnostic test, and you should use the results of the test to determine your knowledge of the material as well as your readiness to take the actual MCAT. When you have determined your strengths and weaknesses from this diagnostic test, you can then determine which material you need to review.

When you have completed all your review work, it will be time to take the two Practice Tests. Although it is difficult to set aside the solid block of nearly 6 hours you will need to take the test we recommend that you try so you can condition yourself to concentrate for a long period of time. Check your scores when you have completed the entire test. If you still have time left after you've taken all the exams and checked all your answers, then go back and review again.

The MCAT scores—combined with your college grades, the types of courses you have taken, extracurricular activities, the school you attended, along with other objective and subjective items—are one element of the medical school admissions process. Because the MCAT is a scored, objective test, the higher your score, the better your chances are of being accepted into the medical school of your choice. As you surely know at this point in the process, medical schools view your scores as a barometer of your future success in the basic medical curriculum. The road to successful test taking is practice, and this book is designed to give you the basic guidelines and practice for taking the MCAT.

EXPLANATORY ANSWERS

Each of the three MCAT practice tests are followed by explanatory answers to help you further understand the rationale behind each answer. Following most explanations is a reference to a section in Peterson's *Gold Standard MCAT* by Brett L. Ferdinand, M.D. (ISBN 0-7689-0192-8).

This section will give you additional in-depth instruction on the topic tested in each item. Call 800-338-3282 if you wish to order Peterson's *Gold Standard MCAT.*

THE STUDY PLANS

With the purchase of this book, you begin your preparation for the MCAT examination. Since it is likely that you are also studying for your regular college courses, this Study Plan has been designed to help you prepare for the MCAT, as well as find time to spend on your other studies. We offer you three separate study plans. The first is the **9-Week Plan,** which requires concentrated study with this book at least twice a week. The second is a somewhat more leisurely plan—the **18-Week Plan**. In actuality, it is the former study plan, but spread out over a longer period of time. This will give you more time to focus on your strengths and weaknesses and give you some extra time to study those areas that require more in-depth attention. Finally, the **Panic Plan** is for those of you who are almost ready to take the MCAT and have only a few weeks to study. Obviously, this is not the preferred plan—the more time you have to study and review, the more you are assured of learning and understanding the material in this book.

These plans are meant to be modified by your needs as well as your own study habits. Once you have taken the diagnostic test, and determined which areas need additional study, you can then change this plan to maximize your time and effort.

THE 9-WEEK PLAN—2 LESSONS PER WEEK

WEEK 1

Lesson 1: Diagnostic Test. Take the Verbal Reasoning section of the diagnostic MCAT.

Lesson 2: Diagnostic Test. Take the Physical Sciences section of the diagnostic MCAT.

WEEK 2

Lesson 1: Diagnostic Test. Take the Biological Science section of the diagnostic test. Also, check all of the answers for the entire test.

Lesson 2: Diagnostic Test. Take the Writing Sample section of the diagnostic test. After writing the two essays, check your writing against the statements to make sure you have satisfied all of the criteria.

WEEK 3

Lesson 1: Verbal Reasoning. Read through this chapter and answer all of the questions. This is essentially a reading comprehension section. Check your answers and review again if you don't understand the explanations or how you arrived at your own answers.

Lesson 2: Mathematics Review. Although there is no specific mathematics test on the MCAT, it is important to understand basic concepts in order to do well on the Biological and Physical Sciences sections of the test. Review this chapter carefully and answer all of the review questions.

WEEK 4

Lesson 1: Physical Sciences Review. Answer all of the questions in the Chemistry section. Check your answers after each question. Take notes to help you determine which topics will require more study.

Lesson 2: Physical Sciences Review. Answer all of the questions in the Physics section. Check your answers after each question. Take notes to help you determine which topics will require more study.

WEEK 5

Lesson 1: Biological Science Review. Answer the first 67 questions in the Biology section. This will cover the material through *The Nervous System*. Check your answers after each question. Take notes to help you determine which topics will require more study.

Lesson 2: Biological Science Review. Answer the balance of the questions in the Biology section. This will cover the material from *Organs of Special Senses* through *The Endocrine System*. Check your answers after each question. Take notes to help you determine which topics will require more study.

Also, read the Writing Sample section. If you have time, write one or two of the suggested essays. Do not take more than 30 minutes for each writing sample.

WEEK 6

Lesson 1: Practice Test 1. Take the Verbal Reasoning section of Practice Test 1.

Lesson 2: Practice Test 1. Take the Physical Sciences section of Practice Test 1.

WEEK 7

Lesson 1: Practice Test 1. Take the Biological Science section of Practice Test 1. Also, check your answers for the Verbal Reasoning, Physical Sciences, and Biological Sciences sections.

Lesson 2: Practice Test 1. Take the Writing Sample section of Practice Test 1. After writing the two essays, check your writing against the statements to make sure you have satisfied all of the criteria.

WEEK 8

Lesson 1: Practice Test 2. Take the Verbal Reasoning section of Practice Test 2.

Lesson 2: Practice Test 2. Take the Physical Sciences section of Practice Test 2.

WEEK 9

Lesson 1: Practice Test 2. Take the Biological Science section of Practice Test 2. Also, check your answers for the Verbal Reasoning, Physical Sciences, and Biological Sciences sections.

Lesson 2: Practice Test 2. Take the Writing Sample section of Practice Test 2. After writing the two essays, check your writing against the statements to make sure you have satisfied all of the criteria.

THE 18-WEEK PLAN—1 LESSON PER WEEK

This is the ideal plan. If you have enough time to devote 18 weeks to studying for your MCAT, you stand a much better chance of achieving higher scores than if you have to rush. Even though you can spread out each lesson over a week, you have more than enough time to go back and review each of the individual sections, retake portions of the test for additional practice, and spend more time delving into those topics that need additional study.

Each lesson in the 9-Week Plan can be done in one week. If, however, you can move through a test section or review material quickly, you surely can combine study lessons. Feel free to alter the plan at any time. If a subject needs more concentrated work, take an extra day during the week to focus on that section. You may wish to designate a specific week to studying only one subject, such as biology. You may, on the other hand, need two, or more, weeks for that subject. These plans, after all, are only general guidelines to help you develop your own study schedule.

THE PANIC PLAN

This is the part that may be difficult for you. You may not have the luxury of 18 weeks to prepare for the test. You may not even have 9 weeks. Thus, the **Panic Plan** can offer you several pointers in order to help you focus on specific areas for study.

1. Read through the official test booklet from the Association of American Medical Colleges. It probably won't tell you anything much different from what you'll find in this *MCAT Success* book, but it's worth getting another point of view.

2. Understand the directions for each section of the test. Except for the Writing section, most of the questions are reading comprehension type questions. You will have a passage and then questions to answer, based on that passage. You will, however, have to have prior scientific knowledge in order to answer most of the questions. A portion of the science questions will be based on individual statements, rather than on an entire passage.

3. Read through the introduction to this book found in the next Red Alert section. If you are not already familiar with the format of the test, this chapter will help you prepare for the different types of material that will be covered and give you an idea of how much time you will have for each question.

4. If you have time, take the Diagnostic MCAT test. If you still have enough time, take one, or both, of the Practice Tests. The results of these tests will give you a good idea of where you stand and help you determine where to spend your studying time. In addition, by taking these tests, you will become familiar with the style of the exam questions.

Despite the fact that this last section is called the **Panic Plan**—don't panic! The more you practice answering questions, the more you will learn, and more important, the more comfortable you will be when you take the actual MCAT.

Diagnostic Test

There are nine passages in the Verbal Reasoning test. Each passage is followed by several questions. After reading a passage, select the one best answer to each question. If you are not certain of an answer, eliminate the alternatives that you know to be incorrect and then select an answer from the remaining alternatives. Indicate your selection by blackening the corresponding circle on your answer sheet.

PASSAGE 1 (QUESTIONS 1-6)

Vitamins are a group of important compounds that are found in very small proportions in food. They are needed in trace amounts for the proper functioning of the body. Vitamins function along with enzymes to carry out very specific, important chemical reactions in the body. Like enzymes, vitamins act by helping a reaction take place (in some cases, enzymes and vitamins make reactions possible that could not occur in their absence), but vitamins are neither changed nor incorporated into the products of the reaction. Because of this action, vitamins are called "coenzymes."

Except for vitamins D and K, vitamins cannot be synthesized directly in the body; they must be obtained through the diet. And even though vitamins D and K are synthesized within the body, the chemicals from which they are synthesized still must come from what we eat. Consequently, they also depend on a proper diet. As shown in a vitamins table, whether a vitamin will dissolve in water or in fat (or oil) is important. This can tell you the source of a vitamin, how it is absorbed into the body, and what happens to it inside the body.

Water-soluble vitamins are not stored in the body and should be taken in each day. In general, fat-soluble vitamins are stored within body tissues and can cause toxic effects in large overdoses. Excessively high intake of fat-soluble vitamins, such as A and D, especially in infants, whose bodies are small, should be avoided. On the other hand, the absence of fat-soluble vitamins has serious consequences. An entire class of diseases, called "vitamin deficiency diseases," can result from a lack of these vital chemicals in the diet.

A number of vitamins—such as B6 (pyridoxine), C, and E—have become very controversial in the last few years. Powers have been ascribed to them that many nutritionists feel are unproven, while others insist large amounts of these vitamins are needed for good health. It will take years of continued research to completely substantiate many of the claims made for these vitamins.

9

1. The reader can infer from this article that a coenzyme is a(n):

   A. product of the marriage of an enzyme and a vitamin.

   B. pair of enzymes working together for the good of the body.

   C. vitamin that has not been changed or incorporated into its reaction.

   D. enzyme broken down into more than one part within the body.

2. The focus of this article is to:

   A. persuade the reader to use more vitamins.

   B. narrate the trip of vitamins through the body.

   C. define vitamins and their role in building strength.

   D. explain the body's need for vitamins.

3. When considering vitamins and their function within the body, one must also be aware of:

   A. whether a vitamin will dissolve in water or in fat (or oil).

   B. the proportion of contents within the vitamin.

   C. the consistency of intake.

   D. the effects of other chemicals within the body.

4. Among those vitamins that must be taken in daily are:

   A. those from citrus products.
   B. water-soluble vitamins.
   C. iron and potassium.
   D. enzymes.

5. Among those vitamins that should be taken in measured quantities is (are):

   A. fat-soluble vitamins.
   B. water-soluble vitamins.
   C. vitamins D and K.
   D. vitamin B6.

6. The reader of this selection might infer that vitamins A and D may be of:

   A. no importance in the body's daily function.

   B. questionable importance.

   C. significant importance to the body.

   D. insignificance in the body's function.

PASSAGE 2 (QUESTIONS 7-16)

Throughout the years, opium, morphine, codeine, and heroin, classed collectively as the opiates, have relieved people's physical pain and eased their mental misery. These derivatives of the poppy plant, while serving as valuable pain relievers, also have been among the most socially destructive drugs in existence. Between the Asian opium smoker of 2,000 B.C. and the American heroin addict of 1990, there stretches a long, tragic story of misuse and mishandling of these drugs.

The practice of opium smoking existed for thousands of years before humans discovered that it possessed undesirable attributes beyond those that left people humdrum, drowsy, and forgetful. It was not until the drug invaded European cities in the form of gum opium and laudanum (tincture of opium) that people realized something stronger than a mere desire for "repose" was tying them to the opium habit. Samuel Taylor Coleridge, who supposedly wrote the poem "Kubla Khan" under the influence of opium, later called it "an accursed habit, a wretched vice, a species of madness, a derangement, an utter impotence of volition"—in other words, drug addiction. Today, this condition is understood to be physical dependence upon a drug because the body cells adapt to it or build up tolerance, thus instilling a physical craving that cannot be denied without painful suffering.

This relationship between humans and the opiates was not scientifically recognized, however, until after morphine was isolated from opium resin. Called "God's own medicine" by the English surgeon Sir William Osler because of its pain-killing properties, the new drug soon became the mainstay of the medical profession. But as more doctors began to depend on it medically, their patients became dependent upon it physically.

In 1848, a new technical invention seemed to provide a safe method of prescribing morphine. The invention was the hypodermic needle. At the time, most experts believed the needle would stop addiction because direct injection prevented the drug from passing through the stomach. Unfortunately, the hypodermic syringe greatly heightened the drug's effects (60 milligrams of morphine taken by mouth is less effective in killing pain than 8 milligrams administered through injection), and the availability of both drug and needle helped spread addiction on a "do-it-yourself" basis. The addict no longer had to buy a "prepared medicine." He or she could purchase everything necessary at the drugstore. By 1898, it was estimated that 1.4 million people—or 4 percent of the American population—were addicted to some form of opium.

In 1874, a German doctor, Heinrich Dreser, discovered another "cure" for morphine addiction. Christened "heroin" after the Greek god Heros, thereby reflecting hopes that it should be of great benefit to mankind, the new drug was enthusiastically prescribed as a cure for both opium and morphine addiction. A few months later pharmacologists and doctors realized their error. Heroin not only caused addiction, it soon proved to be 2½ times stronger than morphine. And of all drug dependencies, heroin addiction is perhaps the most difficult to cure.

Because of its powerful addicting properties, heroin has been banned from medical use in the United States and is therefore available only through illicit channels. Illegal traffickers keep the price high and the quality low.

As a result, the story of heroin addiction in the United States today is perhaps typified by an ex-addict's description of his or her experience. "It's a twenty-four-hour-a-day thing. You get up in the morning, you shoot some drugs, and you go out on the street. You commit a crime to get more money. You buy some more drugs. It is a constant thing."

The positive effects of the opiate have been far overshadowed by the negative effects, such as illustrated herein.

7. The focus of this article is the:

   A. dangers of opiates.
   B. effects of codeine as a prescriptive drug.
   C. history of drugs in the United States.
   D. poppy plant and what it can become.

8. The beginning of an awareness of opium as an addictive agent:

   A. came about when opium came into Europe.
   B. comes when people realize that they are using it for more than "repose."
   C. is people's awareness of their need.
   D. all of the above.

9. People's use of opium in an addictive manner, according to this article, comes about because:

   A. of an inability to control oneself.
   B. drugs are readily available in most American cities.
   C. of a physical tolerance and physical craving.
   D. drugs are popular in today's society.

10. One can infer from this reading that:

   A. opium and its derivative, morphine, have no place in medicine today.
   B. the medical properties of opium found their way into accepted medicines.
   C. the introduction of morphine into the world was a disaster.
   D. neither opium nor morphine has legitimate uses.

11. People's dependence upon opium and its derivatives is inferred to have come from:

   A. education about drug effects.
   B. physicians' dependence upon the drug as medicine.
   C. the movement of the drug through European cities.
   D. increased availability of the drug.

12. A supposed curb to morphine addiction was the:

   A. publication of the works of Samuel Taylor Coleridge.
   B. invention of the hypodermic needle.
   C. increased use of the drug by physicians.
   D. aftereffects of the drug.

13. In order to increase the effects of the drug, addicts have learned that:

   A. mixing opium and morphine is unwise.
   B. using a doctor's suggestions about the drug is unwise.
   C. switching from opium to morphine is beneficial.
   D. the hypodermic syringe is very effective.

14. The discovery of heroin caused the medical community to:

    A. realize the hopelessness of addiction.
    B. hope for relief from opium and morphine addiction.
    C. seek another outlet for lowering the threshold of pain.
    D. prescribe the drug with great reluctance.

15. According to this article, the most difficult addiction to cure is:

    A. opium.
    B. morphine.
    C. heroin.
    D. tincture of opium.

16. The reader might infer from this passage that:

    A. the discovery of the opiates has provided no benefits to mankind.
    B. opiates have no place in modern medicine.
    C. all of the opiates are dangerous to mankind's health.
    D. there are positive uses and effects for the opiates.

PASSAGE 3 (QUESTIONS 17–26)

All food is not alike. Nor are humans able to synthesize all of those chemicals that they fail to get through eating. Supplying known physiological requirements demands eating a balance of nutrients in kind and amount. A well-fed person is not necessarily a well-nourished person. Balance is the key—balance not only in vitamins and calories, but also in protein, minerals, essential fatty acids, and water.

The quantity of energy released from a given quantity of food is measured in Calories (the capital "C" designates this unit as equaling one thousand "small" calories). One Calorie is the amount of heat energy required to raise 1 liter (approximately one quart) of water 1 degree centigrade. In nutrition, this large calorie (C) is most often not capitalized and referred to as kcal (kilocalorie).

The energy released from food, though measured in a heat energy unit, is readily converted into these forms of energy needed by the system—electrical energy (for nerve impulses), light energy (as in the glow of a firefly), mechanical energy (for movement of the body and of internal muscles such as the heart), and sound energy.

The human body is an efficient machine and, like any machine, it needs energy to function. The body converts certain types of food into the energy it needs. Such food contains "potential" energy, or energy in a form that can be set into action. The body is able to convert this potential energy into heat, movement, growth, and all of the processes that take place in the body. Energy that is being used or is working is termed "kinetic energy."

The conversion of potential energy into kinetic energy takes place through chemical reactions in every cell of the body. The term "metabolism" refers to the total of all the chemical processes that make up the functions of life. The extent of metabolic functions in the human body can be viewed as existing on two levels. The body requires energy just to stay alive; this energy is used for those processes that sustain the living system—breathing, heartbeat, and glandular secretions. This basal metabolic rate (BMR) is the total energy needed by the body for internal body functioning only. The BMR is a useful measure of the healthy functioning of the body. The basal metabolic rate is most directly under the influence of the thyroid gland, through the secretion of the hormone thyroxin.

The basal metabolic rate (BMR) is highest in childhood and drops gradually throughout life. This requires a gradual decrease in the amount of food a person should eat to avoid excess weight. The average man (late teens to early thirties) needs about 1,600 to 1,800 kcal per day for basal metabolism. A woman typically has a lower basal metabolic rate than a man and needs 1,200 to 1,450 kcal per day.

Determination of your BMR (usually measured while you are awake, but reclining and relaxed) should be added to the number of calories you use by general resting activities throughout the day (sleep, general minimal movements). This sum is an individual's "resting metabolism" (BMR plus calories used while at general rest) and is about 10 percent above the BMR. The RM (resting metabolism) ranges from 0.8 to 1.4 kcal per hour per kilogram (2.2 pounds) of body weight, depending on the amount of fat present or "lean body mass" (LBM).

An individual's energy requirements also include the degree of physical activity he or she engages in during the day. The need for kcal is proportional to the amount of daily exercise and one's RM. If one is an inactive individual, add 30 percent of your resting metabolism; add 50 percent if you engage in light activity; 75 percent for moderate activity; and, 100 percent for strenuous physical activity. Calculate your daily energy requirements and see if you are eating too much or exercising too little.

17. The focus of this selection is:

    A. how to calculate the body's need for food.
    B. explaining that food creates energy.
    C. the importance of balancing foods.
    D. defining calories and their work.

18. There is so much stress on counting calories in order to balance one's food intake. A calorie is:

    A. the amount of heat energy required to raise 1 liter (approximately one quart) of water 1 degree centigrade.
    B. abbreviated as "C."
    C. often referred to as kcal.
    D. all of the above.

19. As one's activities increase, so does one's need for energy as provided by kcal. One who is only slightly active would add about what percent of the daily energy requirement?

    A. 25 percent
    B. 30 percent
    C. 50 percent
    D. 75 percent

20. In order to achieve the balance that is required for the body, one must intake:

    A. proteins.
    B. minerals.
    C. vitamins and water.
    D. all of the above.

21. The kilocalorie is an indicator of energy and is indicated by:

    A. k
    B. C
    C. c
    D. kcal

22. The purpose of the calorie designation is to determine the:

    A. measure for the quantity of energy released in food.

    B. measure for the weight of food as it enters the body.

    C. energy one can derive from the intake of food.

    D. fat added by the intake of food.

23. Food taken into the body is converted into energy to provide:

    A. kinetic energy.

    B. lubricating of joints for movement.

    C. units of heat to create cells for growth.

    D. deposits of energy within the reservoirs of the body.

24. When the author speaks of "metabolism," the inference is:

    A. the more food taken in, the more energy created.

    B. the levels needed to take in food and not turn it into fat.

    C. the lack of necessary chemicals to utilize food taken in.

    D. the human body taking food in and converting it to useful functions by chemical reaction.

25. In order to measure the healthy functioning of the body, what is measured?

    A. kinetic energy

    B. calorie intake

    C. kcal

    D. bmr

26. The information contained in this article indicates that without the proper functioning of the thyroid gland:

    A. calorie intake would have to increase significantly.

    B. one's kcal measure would drop rapidly.

    C. one's basal metabolic rate would not be properly influenced.

    D. the influence of fatty acids would create less heat energy.

PASSAGE 4 (QUESTIONS 27–36)

It is an extraordinary paradox that while much of the world's population is fighting starvation, more than 25 percent of the people in the United States are overweight due to excessive eating. The preoccupation that captivates many people in this country is that of weight control. The magnitude of the problem is shown by the one-quarter-to one-half-billion dollars a year that Americans pay "fat doctors" to help in overcoming this problem Such concern is not only a reflection of the importance we attach to proper weight, but also a frank commentary on the failure many people encounter in their attempts to maintain a satisfactory weight.

Appetite and hunger control relate to the ability to control weight. Appetite and hunger are known to be controlled by a small area in the brain called the "appetite center" or "appestat." It is composed of two sets of nuclei. One determines your perception of a satisfied feeling; your willingness to eat is regulated by the comparison between the two. Thus, the appestat works something like a thermostat controlling the temperature of a room.

As to what activates the appestat, there is still some question. It may be the glucose level (blood-sugar level) in the blood, body temperature changes, or the level of amino acids in the blood. But it is known that the appetite center has nerve connections with the cortex of the brain and may also be consciously controlled. This means that emotional factors, as well as chemical ones, appear to control appetite. Worry, tension, frustration, and conflicts in interpersonal relations can influence a person's appetite. Other research has shown that appestats vary in different individuals. Thus, a person may inherit a "higher setting" in the appestat than another person and require more food before feeling satisfied. Consequently, we can say that appetite is regulated by emotions, body chemistry, and inheritance. All of these factors influence the ability to control weight. Most of us succeed in accomplishing things we want to accomplish; we do things that interest or motivate us. If we are to maintain a desirable weight, we must want to. Reasons for losing weight or maintaining a desirable weight that appeal to or motivate people include the following:

1. A desire to look attractive. Whether a person likes it or not, he or she must admit that clothing styles are directed toward slender figures. Of course, larger sizes are provided for those who need them, but these are not influenced by the fashion market. Then again, it's always pleasant to fit into a standard-size theater or lecture-hall seat, or to take no more than our half

or third of the car seat. The overweight person faces such dilemmas daily.

2. Longer life. According to studies, a man forty-five years of age, of medium height and frame, and weighing 170 pounds, can expect to live two to four years less than a similar man weighing 150 pounds. A man forty-five years of age, of medium height and frame, weighing 200 pounds, can expect to live four to six years less than a similar man weighing 150 pounds.

3. Fewer diseases. Cardiovascular disease, diabetes, gallbladder disease, cirrhosis of the liver, certain forms of cancer, and arthritis occur more often or can be more serious in overweight people than in those of desirable weight.

4. Fewer painful conditions. Overweight is a factor in such common conditions as varicose veins, high blood pressure, gout, pulmonary emphysema, nephritis, and toxemia in pregnancy. It is estimated that for every pound of added fat an additional two thirds of a mile of blood vessels are required to keep this pound of fat alive.

Excess fat complicates all surgery and increases surgical risks. The same is true in the delivery of a newborn. It takes extra body effort to carry body weight that is not needed; thus, the overweight person is more often tired. Fat accumulates around internal vital organs (such as the heart and lungs) and tends to crowd them. The overweight person is less agile, has more balancing problems, moves more slowly, and has more physical accidents than a person of normal weight.

27. According to this article, one of the least desirable effects of being overweight includes:

    A. the inability to find appropriate clothing.
    B. uncomfortable seating in public places.
    C. discomfort in car sizes.
    D. all of the above.

28. When a person is overweight, an additional strain is placed upon the:

    A. kidneys.
    B. bowels.
    C. bones.
    D. blood vessels.

29. One of the causes for a larger appetite than is necessary to maintain the body is:

    A. environment.
    B. genetic.
    C. age.
    D. gender.

30. In order to control the desire for food, the body is equipped with:

    A. a basic metabolic rate.
    B. energizing proteins to build up the appestat.
    C. a thermometer-type device to measure the heat intake of calories.
    D. a set of nuclei called the "appetite center."

31. Among the physical complications involved with one who is overweight are:

    A. inferior genetic legacies.
    B. decreased sex drive.
    C. extreme nervous energy levels.
    D. surgical risks and fatigue.

32. The reader may infer from this selection that:

    A. surveys of overweight people are inconclusive.

    B. loss of physical skills such as balance, caution, and agility are among the results of being overweight.
    C. the genetics of being overweight are insurmountable.
    D. the effects of being overweight do not interfere with the functioning of one's respiratory system.

33. According to the author, the appestat, or one's appetite control, may be activated by a number of factors that include:

    A. blood, glucose level, and environmental temperature.
    B. body temperature, brain waves, and emotions.
    C. blood conditions.
    D. amino acids and fat content of food.

34. Based upon the information contained in this article, the inference is that being overweight is primarily what kind of problem?

    A. worldwide
    B. national
    C. gender-specific
    D. age

35. The author enumerates the serious health problems that can be the result of being overweight, which include:

    A. blood flow problems.
    B. diseases of the internal organs.
    C. liver and heart diseases.
    D. all of the above.

36. According to the author of this article, among the advantages to those people who are not overweight are:

    A. greater self-esteem.
    B. a longer life span.
    C. an increased sex drive.
    D. increased job opportunities.

PASSAGE 5 (QUESTIONS 37-42)

For centuries, the people of the world have wondered about the floor of the oceans of the world. Relief maps intrigue us with their ranges of underwater mountains; pictures from submarines built to explore the deepest ranges of the oceans show a terrain that is often smooth as a plain but then as rugged as the highest mountains on dry land. Caves, shelves, and pockets of unknown blackness all provide material for questions.

There are a number of ocean topographic features:

CONTINENTAL SHELF—Extending from the coastal shoreline to a point at which a marked slope occurs, the point where the slope gradually increases is called the SHELF BREAK, and the steeper slope is called the CONTINENTAL SLOPE. The width of the continental shelf can vary from a few meters to 1,300 km. The broadest shelves occur off the northern Siberian coast, North American northeastern coast, West Pacific regions from Alaska to Australia, and around the Arctic regions near Canada and Greenland.

SUBMARINE CANYONS—Canyons cut into the continental slope and shelf. They exhibit steep walls and tributaries just like canyons cut from rivers on land. The canyons were one of the primary features studied by Francis P. Shepard (father of marine geology). These canyons form a basic trough through which sediments and other heavier-than-water minerals are carried toward the ocean floor and form a DEEP SEA FAN. Most submarine canyons form from the mid-ocean ridges toward the continental shelves and are presumed to cut farther toward the shore as they age.

CONTINENTAL RISE—Deep-sea fans accumulate at the mouths of submarine canyons and are partly responsible for the development of a continental rise. Other contributing factors are currents around the continental shelf, which, after the currents make the turns, they begin to slow and deposit more sedimentary elements onto the ocean floor. These currents pick up sediment from the BETHNIC NEPHELOID LAYER (BNL), which is a layer of sediment that is suspended above the ocean floor.

ABYSSAL PLAINS—Abyssal plains are composed of fairly level sediment deposits along the continental slope. These abyssal plains consist of sand, sediment, and reddish brown clays. The abyssal zones accumulate at about a rate of 1 mm/1,000 years.

OCEANIC RIDGES—Ocean ridges are usually formed where two tectonic plates come together, the most predominant being the Atlantic Ocean ridge, where the North American and Eurasian plates meet. These ridges are also where most sea floor spreading occurs, due to large amounts of magma pushing through the ocean crust from the asthenosphere through the lithosphere.

37. The focus of this article is to:

   A. explain the terrain of the oceans' floors.
   B. describe the bottom of the ocean.
   C. answer questions about the floor of the oceans.
   D. convince readers about the creation of the floor of the oceans.

38. The soil or sediment flowing canyons into the sea deposits itself on the ocean floor as:

A. dunes.
B. undersea hills.
C. the continental shelf.
D. ridges of mountains.

39. The best explanation for the formation of canyons on the floor of the oceans is that they:

A. resemble land rivers.
B. form a trough to carry the sediment into the oceans.
C. carry soil that is heavier than water.
D. all of the above.

40. The reader can infer from this passage that the Atlantic Ocean ridge:

A. was formed when two plates came together.
B. is the halfway point between North American and Europe and Asia.
C. is an opening or spreading in the floor of the oceans.
D. is formed in the lithosphere.

41. The reader can infer that growth of the plains on the floor of the oceans occurs with:

A. rapidity.
B. great slowness.
C. fluctuating magnitude.
D. intricate patterns.

42. The inference of this article is that the floor of the oceans determines the relation between the land and the sea by:

A. varying currents of the waves of the ocean.
B. creation of submarine canyons.
C. the deposits of ridges.
D. the varying deposits of sediment.

PASSAGE 6 (QUESTIONS 43–48)

A characteristic of the style of objective accuracy lies in the frequent concealment by the artist of the technique used to achieve his effects. It is as if he were trying to deny that his pictures are made of paint or his sculptures modeled in clay or carved from stone. The marks of his tools must not be visible in the final product. The artist wishes to focus the viewer's attention on his subject, not on the way the picture was put together. There is a certain artistic modesty implied by this approach, a self-effacement in the interest of heightening the illusion created by the image. Where a painter like Chaim Soutine was anxious to reveal his brushstrokes and the vigor and sureness with which he applied paint, an artist like Charles Sheeler used a smooth, thinned-out, impersonal technique that seems highly appropriate to his machine-made industrial subject matter.

The attitude of the objective artist is one of detachment. He presents himself to his audience as a person who selects, arranges, and represents reality but suppresses his own personality in the process. If we are to learn anything about the artist as a person, it is through his choice of themes and organization of subject matter, not because of his individuality of vision or intensely personal manner of execution. There is something scientific in such an attitude. As we know, the scientist takes many precautions to be sure that his private feelings will not affect the observations and measurements he must make. He hopes other investigators will come to the same conclusions that he has if they examine the same data. The artist interested in accuracy also wishes his results to have a validity independent of his personality; the work should appear to be almost anonymous; only the signature reveals the author.

The suppression of the personal in the artist's style is due to his desire to make vision, the act of seeing, the most important part of experiencing his work. In a sense, the Impressionists fit this description; they used scientific theories of color and optics, they freely exchanged technical "secrets", they painted as accurately as possible the object seen quickly in a particular light. For example, in the Rouen Cathedral series of Claude Monet (1840–1926), we have a very single-minded effort to represent the same building under varying light conditions according to a theory of color that was considered more "realistic"—that is, based on a firmer scientific foundation—than conventional techniques of applying color. It is quite correct to think of Impressionism as a style of objective accuracy, since it constituted a disciplined endeavor to use scientific discoveries about color and visual perception to present the object in its atmospheric setting with full fidelity. The genius of Impressionism lay in the realization that the object—a tree, a mountain, a still life—could not be seen or represented accurately without considering the character of the light and atmosphere around the object and the source and nature of the illumination which enables us to see the object in the first place.

43. Artists have many instruments available to establish themselves as individuals with a signature technique; however, the artist, whose style is objective accuracy, chooses:

A. the more obvious approach of a specific signature.
B. to let the illusion of art speak for itself.
C. an impersonal technique to hide the obvious and create a machine-made product.
D. to develop an individual technique that grabs the audience and makes them aware of who he is.

44. The purpose of Impressionism is to:

A. use scientific discoveries to enhance visions.
B. create objects presented accurately but objectively.
C. make color and visual awareness present a message.
D. all of the above.

45. The fact that objects that are real can be viewed as symbolic—stand for themselves and for something else—is:

A. the intent of artists.
B. a characteristic of Realism.
C. the basic use of light and atmosphere.
D. the genius of Impressionism.

46. An artist painting as an Impressionist would use the science of color and optics to paint accurately but would:

  A. seek to make the objects painted stationary and concrete.
  B. seek a technique that would be unmistakably his.
  C. rely on models and objects for technical accuracy.
  D. try to conceal a style that would interfere with the vision.

47. The focus of this passage is:

  A. the artist and his use of texture and stroke to establish himself as a master of a specific technique.
  B. an artist's desire to have his impression of his subject imparted to an audience instead of himself.
  C. the impression left by an artist when viewing a tree or other object.
  D. the use of light and texture to convey style and structure.

48. An artist with vision or appreciation might not be considered as an Impressionist if:

  A. he had no organization.
  B. there was no imaginative color in his work.
  C. he proffered his own personality.
  D. there were no themes in his work.

PASSAGE 7 (QUESTIONS 49–55)

Lead poisoning may be observed in the acute or chronic form. Most cases of acute poisoning are accidental and seldom homicidal. Acute cases result from the ingestion of large amounts of soluble salt (acetate or nitrate) or many small doses at intervals. Retention of lead is cumulative, so that a sudden acute attack may occur after a long period of administration.

The continued intake of small doses when released suddenly by the body may give rise abruptly to a type of poisoning similar to that which follows the ingestion of a large amount. Removal of old paint by workers in a closed environment or with minimal ventilation may be responsible for on-the-job lead poisoning. Ingestion of lead-containing paint and plaster by children still accounts for many cases of poisoning.

Although the symptoms of acute poisoning are varied, the patient may complain of a metallic taste, a dry burning sensation in the throat, cramps, retching, and persistent vomiting. Hematemesis (vomiting of blood) may occur.

Lead, after absorption, is carried by the blood to different organs, where it produces a multiform symptomatology. Symptoms can include weakness, anorexia, loss of weight, abdominal colic, constipation, backache, headache, hypertension, and a variety of neurological signs.

In children, absorbed lead is often deposited near the epiphyseal ends of the bones and can often be seen on X ray as a dark band near the cartilage.

In lead poisoning there are small blue particles that can be seen in some of the red blood cells (stippled cells)

The three organ areas where lead has the greatest effect are:

1. The hematopoietic system (blood and blood-producing organs), where lead affects the blood and the body's ability to produce blood. Lead is transported throughout the body by the blood from either the pulmonary system (where lead can be absorbed in a gas form) or via the digestive tract.

2. The central nervous system, where lead encephalopathy is the most prominent in acute poisoning, but may also occur in chronic lead ingestion. Widespread degeneration of the cortical and ganglionic neurons is accompanied by diffuse edema (swelling) of the gray and white matter.

   This can lead to convulsions, seizures, high levels of unconsciousness, and eventual death.

   The peripheral nerves of the body are also affected to the most active of the body's muscles. Degeneration is seen usually in the wrist and finger muscles in chronic poisoning.

3. The kidneys will eventually manifest lesions as a result of the lead being excreted from the body via the kidneys. Eventually the patient suffers kidney failure in the most severe poisoning cases.

Laws prohibiting the use of lead paint and lead in gasoline have gone a long way in helping to reduce the incidence of this preventable disease.

49. The PRIMARY focus of this article is to _____ lead poisoning.

   A. describe the reactions of
   B. warn against causes of
   C. define ways to prevent .
   D. explain the nature of

50. Lead poisoning when absorbed into the blood spreads throughout the body, creating the symptoms of:

   A. stomach pains.
   B. aches and pains in the back.
   C. loss of appetite and weight.
   D. all of the above.

51. Lead poisoning caused by the ingestion of paint containing lead can happen without the subject realizing it because:

   A. inhaling the fumes can be accidental.
   B. the poison is tasteless.
   C. lead is stored in the body.
   D. only a portion is required to be fatal.

52. Lead poisoning affects the entire body because of its effect on:

   A. the brain and nervous system.
   B. the muscular system and kidneys.
   C. the pulmonary system, nervous system, and muscular system.
   D. the kidneys, nervous system, and blood.

53. While there are many indicators of poisoning in the system, the most obvious affect is:

   A. heavy vomiting and a feeling of faintness.
   B. on the taste, the touch, and sight.
   C. dry heaving and a metallic taste, with cramps.
   D. a burning in the throat and heavy breathing.

54. Lead poisoning is dangerous because:

    A. it can cause brain damage.

    B. there is the potential in many places.

    C. it is so commonplace.

    D. small amounts are collected, held within the body, and released at one time.

55. One might infer that the absence of antidotes and cures in this article indicates:

    A. an omission by the author.

    B. an editing mistake.

    C. the seriousness of lead poisoning.

    D. the impropriety to the subject.

PASSAGE 8 (QUESTIONS 56–61)

The fear of public speaking is one of the most common fears of people. More people are afraid of public speaking than they are of spiders, snakes, death, and flying. If you are afraid of public speaking you are NOT alone. But fear is not necessarily a bad thing! There are ways that you can tone down your nervousness.

Why are people afraid? Most people are afraid that the audience will laugh at them. Most people don't want to look foolish or be humiliated. But the thing is, ALL of us have looked foolish at some time or another. We have all been embarrassed at some time. However, we ALL live through it . . . there is nothing to be afraid of if people do laugh. Things happen . . . a situation can be even more embarrassing if you make a big deal about it. People are really more friendly than you think when you are standing in front of an audience. People want you to succeed . . . they want to have a good time. So if YOU have a good time, your audience will find it very easy to join in.

The best way to have a good time with a speech is to BE PREPARED! Pick a speech topic that you are TRULY interested in . . . pick something you WANT to talk about. If YOU are interested in something, your enthusiasm will carry over to the audience. If you HAVE to give a speech about some-thing you don't like, try to figure out some way to involve yourself in the topic. If your speech is about squid, talk about your experiences with squid or use other people's experiences with squid. Don't mope around and complain about what a horrible topic squid is . . . MAKE it interesting . . . find things about squid that YOU find interesting. THAT will make it more interesting to the audience, too!

Once you have developed your speaking outline or written your speech, PRACTICE as much as you can. Give your speech to your family, your cat, your dog, your fish, your friends, your plants. Practice, practice, practice. Lots of people are afraid that they won't know what to say or they will forget their speech. If you practice as much as you can, you can tone down your nervousness that way.

The MOST IMPORTANT thing you can do is THINK POSITIVE! This is the KEY! DO NOT think about failing . . . Do NOT think about messing up. Think about doing a great job. Imagine yourself walking up to the front of the room, confidently. You feel great because you are PREPARED. You got a good night's sleep and you had a light meal. You LOOK fabulous because you dressed neatly and you brushed your teeth. You stand in front of the audience and they look at you and then you SMILE at them . . . and they SMILE back!!!! They WANT you to succeed . . . You take out your note cards and begin to speak . . . After you are done, the audience applauds because they learned something from you and they had a good time. You SMILE again and walk back to your chair, confidently! You did a FABU-LOUS job!

ACT POSITIVE . . . even if you don't feel that way . . . ACT CONFIDENT . . . even if you don't feel that way. If you keep telling yourself you are positive and confident, you will begin to really feel that way. Sports athletes call it "getting psyched up." Use your excess nervous energy by using your hands and moving around the front of the room.

Above all, REMEMBER . . . YOU are a great person with something important to say . . . even if your speech is about SQUID!

56. According to this article, the selection of a topic for a speech is important and should be accomplished by:

A. asking for a topic to be assigned.
B. selecting something controversial.
C. choosing some topic in which the teacher is interested.
D. selecting a topic with which you are familiar and which you enjoy.

57. The fear of public speaking is born, according to the author:

A. when the speaker becomes ener-vated.
B. out of the personal fear of looking foolish or humiliated.
C. when the audience is quite large.
D. when audience members share expertise in a discipline related to the speaker's topic.

58. In the face of great nervousness, a public speaker would:

A. grasp the podium and speak firmly.
B. drink water and mop the brow.
C. turn the nervousness into strength by gestures and animation.
D. check the speech notes and be sure of the continuity.

59. The focus of this article is:

A. confidence in public speaking.
B. a positive attitude for the public speaker.
C. overcoming the fear of public speaking.
D. selecting a topic for a speech.

60. An important and practical way to conquer nervousness is to:

A. breathe deeply.
B. rest before speaking.
C. tell a joke.
D. practice.

61. According to this article, positive feelings can be fostered by:

A. smiling.
B. dressing neatly.
C. being rested.
D. all of the above.

PASSAGE 9 (QUESTIONS 62-65)

Blood can be thought of as having two huge roles. First, it is the highway system of our body. It serves to transport material necessary for our body's proper functions. Second, it is responsible for providing the much-needed oxygen to the cells of the body, without which life would cease to function.

Blood is composed of a cellular component—blood cells of different types—as well as a fluid component, known as plasma. When we spin blood in a centrifuge, the two components are separated. The bottom layer, which is the cellular portion, is heavier and is red-colored, being composed mostly of red blood cells. These cells have the ability to carry oxygen that they pick up from the lungs as blood travels through them. Furthermore, these red blood cells can give up the oxygen to the cells of the body and exchange it for carbon dioxide, which is a waste product. On the next trip through the lungs, the carbon dioxide is exchanged for oxygen and the whole process repeats itself.

There are other cells that make up the blood. There are white blood cells that function to protect us from infection, and platelets that are cells that participate in clotting. Without white blood cells, we would suffer from repeated bacterial and viral illnesses, and without platelets, we would be unable to stop bleeding.

The fluid component of blood is the transport system. All the products produced by other cells such as hormones, and the products absorbed from the digestive tract such as sugars and fats, travel through our bodies via the blood. Medications that we take are transported as well. The cells that are involved in fighting off infection are brought to the site of infection in the blood. Chemicals that are produced by the body that are necessary for our normal functioning, such as antibodies against infection and clotting factors to assist the platelets in the stopping of bleeding, are carried in the blood plasma. The vitamins and minerals that we obtain from the food we eat also use the plasma as a means of getting to the cells of the body. Finally, the waste products of cells are disposed of into the blood and are brought to the liver and kidneys for disposal.

Scientists have tried for years to develop an artificial blood that can carry oxygen without blood cells and can transport all the cellular products to the rest of the body. It seems, though, that human blood is so unique in the way it puts all these functions together that this dream has yet to be realized.

62. The focus of this article is to:
    A. trace the route of blood through the body.
    B. define blood.
    C. investigate the role of blood in the body.
    D. describe the composition of blood.

63. The blood of the human body serves to transport:
    A. medications.
    B. fats.
    C. sugars.
    D. all of the above.

64. In order to combat germs, the blood carries:
    A. lymph.
    B. red blood cells.
    C. platelets.
    D. white blood cells.

65. According to this article, the function(s) of the red blood cells is/are to:
    A. carry oxygen and collect carbon dioxide.
    B. dispense plasma.
    C. fight germs.
    D. prevent clotting.

PHYSICAL SCIENCES	TIME—100 MINUTES	77 QUESTIONS

Most questions in the Physical Sciences test are organized into groups, each preceded by a descriptive passage. After studying the passage, select the one best answer to each question in the group. Some questions are not based on a descriptive passage and are also independent of each other. You must also select the one best answer to these questions. If you are not certain of an answer, eliminate the alternatives that you know to be incorrect and then select an answer from the remaining alternatives. A periodic table is provided for your use. You may consult it whenever you wish.

1 H 1.0																	2 He 4.0
3 Li 6.9	4 Be 9.0											5 B 10.8	6 C 12.0	7 N 14.0	8 O 16.0	9 F 19.0	10 Ne 20.2
11 Na 23.0	12 Mg 24.3											13 Al 27.0	14 Si 28.1	15 P 31.0	16 S 32.1	17 Cl 35.5	18 Ar 39.9
19 K 39.1	20 Ca 40.1	21 Sc 45.0	22 Ti 47.9	23 V 50.9	24 Cr 52.0	25 Mn 54.9	26 Fe 55.8	27 Co 58.9	28 Ni 58.7	29 Cu 63.5	30 Zn 65.4	31 Ga 69.7	32 Ge 72.6	33 As 74.9	34 Se 79.0	35 Br 79.9	36 Kr 83.8
37 Rb 85.5	38 Sr 87.6	39 Y 88.9	40 Zr 91.2	41 Nb 92.9	42 Mo 95.9	43 Tc (98)	44 Ru 101.1	45 Rh 102.9	46 Pd 106.4	47 Ag 107.9	48 Cd 112.4	49 In 114.8	50 Sn 118.7	51 Sb 121.8	52 Te 127.6	53 I 126.9	54 Xe 131.3
55 Cs 132.9	56 Ba 137.3	57 La* 138.9	72 Hf 178.5	73 Ta 180.9	74 W 183.9	75 Re 186.2	76 Os 190.2	77 Ir 192.2	78 Pt 195.1	79 Au 197.0	80 Hg 200.6	81 Tl 204.4	82 Pb 207.2	83 Bi 209.0	84 Po (209)	85 At (210)	86 Rn (222)
87 Fr (223)	88 Ra 226.0	89 Ac† 227.0	104 Unq (261)	105 Unp (262)	106 Unh (263)	107 Uns (262)	108 Uno (265)	109 Une (267)									

*	58 Ce 140.1	59 Pr 140.9	60 Nd 144.2	61 Pm (145)	62 Sm 150.4	63 Eu 152.0	64 Gd 157.3	65 Tb 158.9	66 Dy 162.5	67 Ho 164.9	68 Er 167.3	69 Tm 168.9	70 Yb 173.0	71 Lu 175.0
†	90 Th 232.0	91 Pa (231)	92 U 238.0	93 Np (237)	94 Pu (244)	95 Am (243)	96 Cm (247)	97 Bk (247)	98 Cf (251)	99 Es (252)	100 Fm (257)	101 Md (258)	102 No (259)	103 Lr (260)

PASSAGE 1

The modern periodic table is based essentially on the work of a Russian chemist, Dmitri Mendeleev, and a German chemist, Lothar Meyer, who independently came to the conclusion that the properties of the elements repeat regularly and are periodic functions of their atomic masses. The modern periodic table evolved from their collective observations and is arranged in vertical columns called groups or families that contain elements with similar properties, and horizontal rows known as periods that contain elements with similar valence shell electron patterns. Comparisons of elements can be made from an understanding of the general "trends" or patterns that elements exhibit within their families and/or periods.

1. Which element would be considered the most metallic?

   A. K
   B. Cr
   C. Fe
   D. Br

2. Which element will have the largest atomic radius?

   A. Mg
   B. Ca
   C. Na
   D. K

3. Which element will be the most electronegative?

   A. Li
   B. F
   C. K
   D. Br

4. Which element would exhibit the lowest first ionization energy?

   A. Na
   B. Cl
   C. Rb
   D. I

5. Which element would exhibit the lowest second ionization energy?

   A. Li
   B. Be
   C. F
   D. Mg

6. Which element is most likely to exist in nature as a diatomic molecule?

   A. Be
   B. B
   C. C
   D. N

PASSAGE 2

A force of 20 Newtons is exerted on a mass of 10 kg. Another force of 20 Newtons is exerted on a 5 kg mass as shown in the diagram.

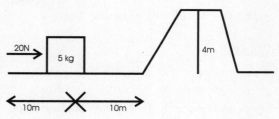

7. Compared to the acceleration on the 10 kg mass, the acceleration on the 5 kg mass will be:

   A. equal.
   B. twice as great.
   C. one half as great.
   D. neither mass undergoes an acceleration.

8. The two blocks in the above diagram collide. We can say that the force exerted by the 10 kg block on the 5 kg block, compared to the force exerted by the 5 kg block on the 10 kg block, is:

   A. twice as great.
   B. one half as great.
   C. equal and opposite.
   D. equal and in the same direction.

9. As the two blocks are colliding, we can conclude that the acceleration of the 10 kg block is:

   A. twice that of the 5 kg block.
   B. one half that of the 5 kg block.
   C. equal to that of the 5 kg block.
   D. zero.

10. If you were to observe that the two blocks are traveling at a constant velocity, then you could conclude that:

    A. there are no forces at all acting on the blocks.
    B. the blocks must be free falling.
    C. the forces acting on the blocks must add up to zero.
    D. the acceleration is constant.

PASSAGE 3

The understanding of a molecule's structure, or geometry, requires a solid mastery of a concept known as VSEPR (The Valence Shell Electron Pair Repulsion) theory. By molecular structure, we mean the geometrical arrangement of the atoms of a molecule or ion in three dimensions. According to the VSEPR theory, the electron pairs associated with the valence shell of the central atom of a molecule are present either as bonded (covalent) pairs, or as lone pairs that occupy a region in space that is shaped rather like that region that would be occupied by a bonded pair. The electrostatic (negative)

charge of either the bonded pair(s) or the lone pair forces these regions of high electron density away from each other, giving the molecule or ion a distinct geometric shape. We can examine both the geometry of the regions of high electron density (bonded electrons and lone pairs) and/or the actual geometry of the molecule or ion itself. The following questions deal with both the geometry of the regions of high electron density and molecular geometry.

11. Predict the geometry of the NH_4^{+1} ion.

    A. angular
    B. tetrahedral
    C. trigonal pyramidal
    D. trigonal bipyramidal

12. Water is described as an angular, or "bent," molecule; however, its regions of high electron density will be classified as:

    A. trigonal planar.
    B. tetrahedral.
    C. linear.
    D. trigonal bipyramidal.

13. The molecular geometry of a molecule of PF_5 would be best described as:

    A. trigonal pyramidal.
    B. tetrahedral.
    C. trigonal bipyramidal.
    D. octahedral.

14. A molecule of ICl_3 will have its regions of high electron density arranged in a trigonal bipyramidal fashion. Describe the molecular structure of this molecule within the overall trigonal bipyramidal arrangement.

    A. linear
    B. t-shaped
    C. seesaw
    D. octahedral

15. A molecule of XeF_4 will have its regions of high electron density arranged in an octahedral fashion. Describe the molecule's geometry within the confines of this octahedron.

   A. octahedral
   B. square bipyramidal
   C. square planar
   D. trigonal pyramidal

16. Which of the molecules below will have a molecular structure that would be described as trigonal bipyramidal?

   A. NH_3
   B. NH_2^{-1}
   C. PF_5
   D. SF_4

17. A molecule of the NH_2^{-1} ion will have a molecular geometry that most resembles:

   A. NH_3
   B. PCl_3
   C. NO_2^{-1}
   D. H_2O

18. The regions of high electron density of a molecule of SF_4 would be arranged in a trigonal bipyramidal fashion. Describe the molecule's overall geometry.

   A. seesaw
   B. t-shaped
   C. linear
   D. trigonal bipyramidal

Questions 19 through 23 are **NOT** based on a descriptive passage.

19. While exploring a new planet, you drop a hammer over a cliff. It falls 3 meters in 1.5 seconds. What is the acceleration due to gravity on this planet?

   A. 0.5 m/sec
   B. 1.33 m/sec
   C. 2 m/sec
   D. 2.67 m/sec

20. The train in the accompanying figure has its cars joined by ropes and is accelerating at a rate of 1.5 m/sec^2. What is the tension in the rope marked "B?" *Neglect friction in this problem.*

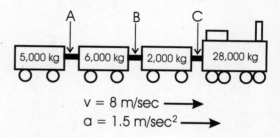

   A. 5.88×10^4 Newton
   B. 9×10^3 Newton
   C. 1.65×10^4 Newton
   D. 6.15×10^4 Newton

21. For the 5 kg box sliding downhill on the inclined plane in the figure, the coefficient of kinetic friction is mk = 0.4. In the coordinate system shown, the x component of the force of gravity is +13.5 Newtons and the y component of the force of gravity is −47 Newtons. At the instant shown, the velocity of the box is 3 m/sec. What is the acceleration of the box?

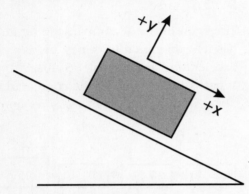

- A. 1.1 m/sec², uphill
- B. 5.2 m/sec², uphill
- C. 1.2 m/sec², downhill
- D. 3.75 m/sec², downhill

22. You throw a 10 kg bag of birdseed into a 25 kg stationary shopping cart. The cart moves away with a speed of 1.2 m/sec. What was the horizontal speed of the bag of birdseed before it hit the cart? (Ignore friction.)

- A. 3.0 m/sec
- B. 4.2 m/sec
- C. 36 m/sec
- D. 42 m/sec

23. A small satellite weighs 4,000 Newtons as it sits in the nose of a rocket awaiting launch. The rocket puts the satellite in orbit a distance of 6,000 km above the surface of the earth. What is the force of gravity upon the satellite when it is in orbit? (Take the radius of the earth to be 6,000 km.)

- A. 500 Newtons
- B. 1,000 Newtons
- C. 2,000 Newtons
- D. 4,000 Newtons

PASSAGE 4

Examine the organic compounds drawn below:

24. Drawing A represents a molecule of:

- A. methane.
- B. ethane.
- C. propane.
- D. butane.

25. There are several ways of naming the chemical represented in drawing B. One accepted name is 1,2 dichlorobenzene. Another correct name is :

- A. cis-dichlorobenzene.
- B. ortho-dichlorobenzene.
- C. meta-dichlorobenzene.
- D. paradichlorobenzene.

26. Changing the locations of the chlorine atoms in drawing B above to the 1,4 positions would change the name of the compound to:

    A. trans-dichlorobenzene.
    B. orthodichlorobenzene.
    C. metadichlorobenzene.
    D. paradichlorobenzene.

27. The correct name of the alcohol represented in drawing C is:

    A. butanol.
    B. ethanol.
    C. 3-butanol.
    D. 2-butanol.

28. A common name for the chemical represented by drawing D is acetylene; however the correct IUPAC name for this chemical is:

    A. ethyne.
    B. ethene.
    C. ethane.
    D. ether.

29. Organic chemicals known as saturated hydrocarbons contain only atoms of carbon and hydrogen and have only single covalent bonds linking carbon atoms to carbon atoms in a chain. Consider a saturated hydrocarbon that contains 15 carbon atoms in a single chain (it would be called pentadecane). This chemical would contain how many hydrogen atoms?

    A. 15
    B. 17
    C. 30
    D. 32

PASSAGE 5

Two masses—m1 and m2—are connected on a frictionless horizontal surface. A rope is attached to m2 and a force is exerted toward the right, as shown in the diagram.

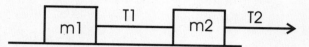

30. In the figure above, as the force increases from zero, the acceleration of the system will be:

    A. directly proportional to the force.
    B. inversely proportional to the force.
    C. independent of the force.
    D. zero.

31. As compared with the tension in the rope T2, the tension in the rope T1 will:

    A. always be greater.
    B. always be less.
    C. be the same.
    D. depend on the masses m1 and m2.

32. There is now a frictional force between the masses and the surface. As the force F acts toward the right, the frictional force will be directed:

    A. toward the right.
    B. toward the left.
    C. up, perpendicular to the surface.
    D. down, perpendicular to the surface.

33. As the force now increases from zero, the frictional force will:

    A. be directly proportional to the force.
    B. be inversely proportional to the force.
    C. increase in direct proportion to the force, then suddenly decrease as the masses start moving.
    D. remain the same.

34. Suppose the masses m1 and m2 were doubled. Then the frictional force would:

    A. remain the same.
    B. double.
    C. be four times as great.
    D. be halved.

35. Starting from rest, another force in addition to force F and with equal magnitude to force F but in the opposite direction, acts upon the two masses m1 and m2. The frictional force on this system is:

    A. proportional to the velocity of the system.
    B. proportional to the square of the velocity.
    C. constant as long as it's not moving.
    D. zero.

PASSAGE 6

The gravitational acceleration near the surface of the earth is 9.8 m/s^2. The radius of the earth is 6.4×10^6 meters. A man standing on the surface of the earth has a mass of 100 kg. The universal gravitational constant $G = 6.67 \times 10^{-11} N* \frac{m^2}{kg^2}$.

36. What is the weight, in Newtons, of this man standing on the surface of the earth?

    A. 9.8 N
    B. 98.0 N
    C. 980.0 N
    D. 98,000 N

37. Suppose this man went to a position 12.8×10^6 m from the center of the earth. His weight at this point would be:

    A. the same as on the surface.
    B. ½ his weight on the surface.
    C. ¼ his weight on the surface.
    D. ¾ his weight on the surface.

38. Suppose the mass of the earth doubled and its radius remained the same. Then the weight of the man would:

    A. double and his mass would double.
    B. double and his mass would remain the same.
    C. quadruple and his mass would remain the same.
    D. decrease and his mass would increase.

39. The 100 kg man and his 50 kg friend both jump off a building at the same time. You can say that:

    A. they both accelerate at the same rate.
    B. the 100 kg man accelerates at twice the rate of the 50 kg man.
    C. the gravitational force is the same for both of them.
    D. both B and C.

40. The man and his friend travel to a planet with 3 times the mass of the earth and twice the radius of the earth. You can say that the:

    A. gravitational acceleration on the planet is ¾ that of the earth.
    B. gravitational acceleration is ½ that of the earth.
    C. gravitational acceleration is the same as that of the earth.
    D. gravitational acceleration is greater for the 100 kg man than for the 50 kg man.

41. Based on the information given, what is the mass of the earth in kilograms?

   A. 4×10^{24}

   B. 5×10^{24}

   C. 6×10^{24}

   D. 2×10^{30}

Questions 42 through 46 are **NOT** based on a descriptive passage.

42. Which of the following has the electron configuration: $1s^2, 2s^2, 2p^6, 3s^2, 3p^6, 4s^2, 3d^{10}, 4p^6$?

   A. argon atoms

   B. bromide ions

   C. potassium atoms

   D. magnesium ions

43. Which of the following is the ending typical of a binary compound?

   A. -ide

   B. -ic

   C. -ate

   D. -ous

44. Mendeleev's periodic table was based on his findings having to do with:

   A. atomic radii.

   B. electronegativity.

   C. atomic mass.

   D. atomic number.

45. When a liquid solidifies, all of the following happen except the:

   A. average kinetic energy decreases.

   B. particles move slower.

   C. motion of particles is restricted to vibration.

   D. temperature is raised.

46. The ideal gas is defined as having no:

   A. molecular volume.

   B. mass.

   C. boiling point.

   D. temperature.

PASSAGE 7

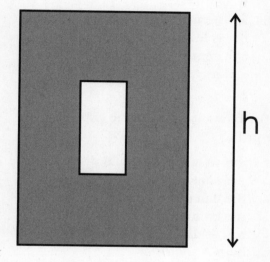

A uniform cube is immersed in a liquid of uniform density in a container with height h.

47. As the cube drops farther down the liquid, we can say that the pressure on the bottom of the cube:

   A. is always equal to the pressure on the top of the cube.

   B. remains constant as the cube drops to the bottom.

   C. increases as the cube drops.

   D. is always less that the pressure on the top of the cube.

48. If one were to weigh the cube as it descends, one would notice that its:

A. apparent weight increases as it descends, but is less than its weight in air.
B. apparent weight increases as it descends, but is greater than its weight in air.
C. apparent weight remains the same, but is less than its weight in air.
D. apparent weight remains the same, and it weighs more than it does in air.

49. The buoyant force on the cube is equal to:

A. the weight of the fluid displaced by the cube.
B. the difference between the force on the bottom and the force on the top of the cube.
C. both A and B.
D. neither A nor B.

50. The block is placed in a liquid of slightly higher density in which it still sinks. One will notice that the block will sink:

A. but at a slightly slower rate.
B. but at a slightly higher rate.
C. at the same rate.
D. It cannot be determined from the information provided.

51. Suppose the cube has a specific gravity less than 1. This would mean that the:

A. block will float on any liquid.
B. block will float on water only.
C. block will float on any fluid with a specific gravity greater than 1.
D. block will float on any fluid with a specific gravity less than 1.

52. The reason a wooden sailing ship floats is because:

A. wood is less dense than water.
B. the buoyant force of the water is greater than the ship's weight.
C. the wind exerts an upward force on the ship.
D. the density of the ship as a whole is less than that of water.

53. As one descends into a freshwater lake, one would notice that the pressure:

A. increases in direct proportion to the depth.
B. increases in direct proportion to the square of the depth.
C. decreases in direct proportion to the depth.
D. remains constant.

54. One descends to the bottom of a saltwater lake with an equal depth to the freshwater lake. One would notice that:

A. the pressure would be greater.
B. the pressure would be less.
C. the pressure would be the same.
D. There is insufficient information to know the answer.

PASSAGE 8

Many chemical reactions can be classified as *oxidation-reduction* types. These reactions involve the loss or gain of electrons by an atom, molecule, or ion. When one of these species loses electrons, it is *oxidized*; conversely, when electrons are gained, the species is said to be *reduced*. Oxidation and reduction always occur simultaneously, and their reactions are referred to as *redox*. Examine the following redox reactions. (Some are balanced, others are unbalanced.)

A. $Na + Cl_2 \Rightarrow 2\ NaCl$
B. $Zn + H_2SO_4 \Rightarrow ZnSO_4 + H_2$
C. $SnCl_2 + PbCl_4 \Rightarrow SnCl_4 + PbCl_2$
D. $CO + NO \Rightarrow CO_2 + N_2$
E. $Zn + NO_3^{-1} + H^{+1} \Rightarrow Zn^{+2} + NH_4^{+1} + H_2O$

55. In equation A above, elemental chlorine is:

A. both reduced and is the reducing agent.
B. both oxidized and is the oxidizing agent.
C. being reduced and is the oxidizing agent.
D. being oxidized and is the reducing agent.

56. In equation B above, the oxidation number that would be assigned to the sulfur atom in a molecule of sulfuric acid would be:

A. +2
B. +4
C. +6
D. +8

57. In equation B above, which species is being oxidized?

A. Zn
B. H
C. S
D. O

58. In equation C above:

A. lead is being reduced, and lead IV chloride is the oxidizing agent.
B. lead is being oxidized, and lead IV chloride is the reducing agent.
C. tin is being reduced, and tin II chloride is the oxidizing agent.
D. tin is being oxidized, and tin II chloride is the oxidizing agent.

59. In equation D above, the correct set of "balancing coefficients" in this equation would be:

A. 1 1 1 1
B. 2 2 2 2
C. 2 2 2 1
D. 1 2 2 1

60. In equation D above, the value of the oxidation number assigned to an atom of carbon in carbon monoxide is:

A. 0
B. +1
C. +2
D. +3

PASSAGE 9

The use of chemical reactions to determine the concentrations of solutions (to standardize solutions) and the determination of the amount of a substance present in a sample using a known concentration (a standard solution) make up the branch of quantitative analysis called volumetric analysis. A solution of reactant is added to a solution of a sample drop by drop from a burette in a process called titration. An indicator that is also added will change color when the reaction is completed or the end point is reached. Such procedures are helpful in determining the concentrations of unknown solutions and also for determining the pH of unknown solutions.

61. A liter of aqueous HCl is prepared by diluting 17 ml of concentrated HCl solution to about 1 liter. The solution is standardized by titrating a 0.5015 gram sample of pure, dry Na_2CO_3. The balanced equation for this reaction is:

$$Na_2CO_3 + 2\ HCl \rightarrow 2\ NaCl + H_2O + CO_2$$

What is the exact concentration of the HCl solution if the titration requires 48.47 ml of acid to reach the end point?

A. 0.0976 M
B. 0.1952 M
C. 0.3904M
D. 0.7808 M

62. What is the pH of the HCl solution used for titration?

A. 0.108
B. 2.08
C. 0.709
D. 1.10

63. The same HCl solution is also tested using three indicators: litmus, phenolphthalein, and an experimental indicator known as "RioRed," which changes from green to red when a solution's pH is *below* 2.00. Predict the final colors of the three indicators.

A. litmus = red; phenolphthalein = colorless; RioRed = green
B. litmus = red; phenolphthalein = red; RioRed = red
C. litmus = red; phenolphthalein = colorless; RioRed = red
D. litmus = blue; phenolphthalein = red; RioRed = red

64. Titration of a 40.0 ml sample of H_2SO_4 requires 35.00 ml of 0.1500 M KOH to reach the end point. Determine the molar concentration of the sulfuric acid if the balanced equation representing this reaction is:

$$2KOH + H_2SO_4 \rightarrow K_2SO_4 + 2HOH$$

A. 0.150 M
B. 0.300 M
C. 0.2625 M
D. 0.066 M

65. Determine the pH of the sulfuric acid solution prior to titration:

A. 0.44
B. 0.88
C. 2.36
D. 1.18

66. Using the same three indicators described in question 63 above, predict the final colors.

   A. litmus = blue; phenolphthalein = red; RioRed = green
   B. litmus = red; phenolphthalein = colorless; RioRed = red
   C. litmus = red; phenolphthalein = colorless; RioRed = green
   D. litmus = red; phenolphthalein = red; RioRed = red

PASSAGE 10

An object 1 cm high is placed 20 cm to the left of a convex lens with a focal length of f = +10 cm.

67. Where is the image formed by this lens?

   A. 20 cm to the right of the lens, and it is a real image
   B. 20 cm to the right of the lens, and it is a virtual image
   C. 20 cm to the left of the lens, and it is a real image
   D. 20 cm to the left of the lens, and it is a virtual image

68. As the object distance approaches the focal length of 10 cm, what happens to the image distance?

   A. it approaches $+\infty$
   B. it approaches $-\infty$
   C. it approaches +10 cm.
   D. it approaches −10 cm.

69. An object is placed to the left of the lens at a distance less than the focal length of +10 cm.

   The image formed by the lens will be:

   A. real and inverted.
   B. real and erect.
   C. virtual and inverted.
   D. virtual and erect.

70. An object is placed 20 cm to the left of a concave lens with a focal length −10 cm. The image formed by this lens will be:

   A. inverted and to the left of the lens.
   B. real and to the right of the lens.
   C. erect and to the left of the lens.
   D. virtual and to the right of the lens.

71. The magnification produced by the concave lens will:

   A. always be + and less than 1.
   B. always be − and less than 1.
   C. always be + and greater than 1.
   D. depend on the object distance.

72. An object is placed 30 cm to the left of a lens. An image is formed by this lens 15 cm to the right of this lens. You can say that this lens is:

   A. concave with a focal length of −10 cm.
   B. convex with a focal length of +45 cm.
   C. concave with a focal length of −15 cm.
   D. convex with a focal length of +10 cm.

Questions 73 through 77 are **NOT** based on a descriptive passage.

73. The ideal gas in an engine expands at a constant temperature, pushing a piston ahead of it. The graph shows a plot of the pressure of the gas versus the volume which it occupies. As the volume increases from point A to point B, how much heat must be added to the gas to maintain constant temperature?

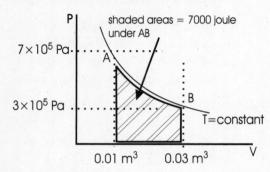

A. 7×10^3 Joules
B. 8×10^3 Joules
C. 9×10^3 Joules
D. 21×10^3 Joules

74. Which circuit has the highest resistance?

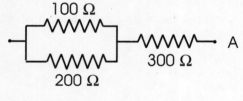

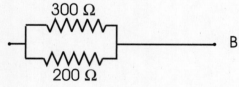

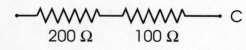

A. A
B. B
C. C
D. A and B are the same.

75. You use a system of pulleys and ropes to raise a 1,000 kg safe to the second floor of a bank. The theoretical mechanical advantage of the system is 15. (Suppose that the system is ideal, so the actual mechanical advantage is also 15.) The work done on the safe to raise it was 90,000 Joules. How much work did you do?

A. 6,000 Joules
B. 9,000 Joules
C. 10,000 Joules
D. 90,000 Joules

76. A siren sounds a single note, which you hear when your car sits at a stoplight. You drive your car towards the siren at 80 mph. What do you hear?

A. The pitch is higher because your ear collects more sound wave crests per second as it travels into the sound wave.
B. The pitch is higher because distances shrink at high speeds and this makes the wavelength shorter.
C. The pitch is lower because meter sticks shrink at high speeds and this makes the wavelength appear longer.
D. The pitch is unchanged.

77. A microscope lens with a focal length of 0.2 cm forms an image of an object, which is 0.25 cm away from the lens. The object is 0.03 cm in diameter. Describe the image.

A. inverted real image 0.0075 cm in diameter
B. erect real image 0.0075 cm in diameter
C. erect virtual image 0.12 cm in diameter
D. inverted real image 0.12 cm in diameter

WRITING SAMPLE 1

Americans today are living longer than ever, which gives rise to a need for some type of genocide.

Write a unified essay in which you perform the following tasks: explain what you think the statement means; describe one or more specific situations in which genocide is necessary in this country; discuss ways which indicate that genocide is not the most viable alternative as you provide at least one other; provide evidence of what this means to today's society; conclude with a justification of the positive or negative implications.

WRITING SAMPLE 2

Moving into the twenty-first century, the demands upon education will change dramatically.

Write a unified essay in which you perform the following tasks: explain what you think the statement means; describe one or more specific situations in which you foresee a dramatic change in the way we educate our young people in the coming century; discuss ways that the statement may not be totally true when compared to the traditional twentieth-century education philosophy; provide evidence of what this means to today's society; conclude with a justification of the positive or negative implications.

Most questions in the Biological Sciences test are organized into groups, each preceded by a descriptive passage. After studying the passage, select the one best answer to each question in the group. Some questions are not based on a descriptive passage and are also independent of each other. You must also select the one best answer to these questions. If you are not certain of an answer, eliminate the alternatives that you know to be incorrect and then select an answer from the remaining alternatives.

PASSAGE 1 (QUESTIONS 1–7)

The primary function of the respiratory system is the exchange of oxygen and carbon dioxide. Oxygen is carried primarily by the red blood cells, while carbon dioxide reacts with water, and is thus carried primarily as carbonic acid in the blood plasma. This weak acid acts as a biological buffer. In addition, other gases in the air may also diffuse into the blood through the capillaries in the lungs. Nitrogen, a major component of air, can diffuse along a partial pressure gradient to enter the bloodstream, where gaseous nitrogen is dissolved in the plasma. This can occur under conditions of greater-than-atmospheric pressure, such as when people scubadive. Although nitrogen gas is essentially inert in this form, the nitrogen can diffuse out of the plasma as the diver ascends to the surface, due to the decrease in pressure during ascent. When divers ascend too rapidly, this process causes a painful and potentially deadly condition called "the bends." This rapid decompression can cause nitrogen bubbles to form, clogging capillaries, which prevents blood from reaching the brain, heart, and muscles. This painful condition can cause permanent brain damage, and it can be fatal in some cases.

1. When the thoracic cavity is at rest, the pressure inside the lungs equals the pressure of the atmosphere (atm), which is approximately 1 atm or 760 mm Hg. In order for air to flow into the lungs:

    A. the volume of the thoracic cavity must be reduced.
    B. pressure in the lungs must be increased.
    C. pressure in the lungs must be greater than the pressure of the atmosphere.
    D. lung volume must increase and lung pressure must decrease.

2. When people acclimated to sea-level atmospheric pressure travel to areas of high altitude, such as the Rocky Mountains, they may experience respiratory stress. Which of the following would apply to this situation?

A. The change in altitude results in greater arterial O_2 pressure, increasing the chances of "the bends."

B. Lower pressure in the arterial oxygen stimulates peripheral chemoreceptors to increase alveolar ventilation.

C. The more rapid the ascent, the less respiratory distress that would be experienced.

D. A long-term adaptation to the higher altitude would be a decrease in hematocrit.

3. When divers experience exposure to great pressure, they can minimize a rapid increase in pressure and the resultant pain and danger by:

A. ascending at a fairly rapid pace so that the lungs can quickly equilibrate under normal atmospheric pressure.

B. consuming a solution of sodium bicarbonate immediately after surfacing.

C. ascending very slowly to prevent formation of bubbles as the nitrogen gas diffuses out of solution.

D. descending and ascending as rapidly as possible at all times.

4. Venous blood is darker than arterial blood because it contains more:

A. oxyhemoglobin.
B. deoxyhemoglobin.
C. CO_2.
D. bicarbonate.

5. Normal alveolar PO_2 is 100 mm Hg, and PO_2 in the extracellular fluid surrounding the tissues is about 40 mm Hg. When arterial blood enters tissue capillaries and encounters the lower PO_2, it:

A. absorbs O_2 from the tissues by active transport.

B. contains O_2 bound to hemoglobin that remains in equilibrium with dissolved O_2 in the tissues.

C. unloads or gives up some of its bound O_2 to the surrounding tissue through simple diffusion.

D. absorbs O_2 from the tissues through simple diffusion.

6. In human beings, a decrease in plasma pH from 7.4 to 7.2 increases the P_{50} from 26 mm Hg to 30 mm Hg. The increase in P_{50}:

A. results in a greater loading of oxygen.

B. results in a greater unloading of oxygen.

C. causes no change in loading of oxygen.

D. is irrelevant to loading of oxygen.

7. Most CO_2 that enters the capillaries reacts with water to form carbonic acid, which dissociates to form a bicarbonate ion and a hydrogen ion, H^+. As the hydrogen ion concentration increases, this would cause:

   A. an increase in pH and increased oxygen unloading.
   B. a decrease in pH and decreased oxygen unloading.
   C. an increase in pH and decreased oxygen unloading.
   D. a decrease in pH and increased oxygen unloading.

Passage 2 (Questions 8–13)

A scientist was conducting research on a new drug, Alpha-10, to determine it's efficacy in controlling high blood pressure. During the course of study, she noticed that a high number of mice had developed tumors, and she was concerned that the new drug might have some carcinogenic properties. Subsequent studies were undertaken to evaluate the effect of Alpha-10 on tumor development. Groups of mice were given varied doses of the drug daily over a three month period. All environmental variables were carefully controlled.

The results were as follows:

Group	# Mice Treated	Dosage (mg/day)	# Mice w/Tumors
A	10	0	0
B	10	20	2
C	10	40	3
D	10	50	6
E	10	75	8
F	10	100	10

8. Which of the following served as the experimental control(s)?

   A. Groups A and F
   B. Group F
   C. Group A
   D. Groups B, D, E, and F

9. The hypothesis that Alpha-10 was carcinogenic was developed by the scientist based on observations made during a study on hypertension. She predicted that if the hypothesis were correct, then the mice would develop tumors when treated with the drug, and that this could be dose-dependent. This type of reasoning is called:

   A. inductive.
   B. conclusive.
   C. logical.
   D. deductive.

10. Based on the results of the study, which of the following conclusions would be appropriate?

   A. No definite conclusion could be drawn.
   B. Alpha-10 is carcinogenic, and its effect increases in a dose-dependent manner.
   C. Alpha-10 is carcinogenic but there is no dose effect.
   D. Alpha-10 is probably not carcinogenic.

43

11. What is the value of the control group in this experiment?

 A. It shows that the results were due to the treatment with the drug and not due to environmental or physical factors.
 B. It shows that the study was invalid.
 C. It shows that some environmental or physiologic factor other than the treatment caused the tumors.
 D. It shows that the strain of mouse used was prone to spontaneous tumor development.

12. Assume that none of the mice in Groups A, B, or C developed tumors. Groups D, E, and F remain the same. Which of the following could be concluded?

 A. The control group was not a valid control.
 B. The drug is not carcinogenic.
 C. The drug is carcinogenic in a dose-dependent manner.
 D. The drug is safe if used only at low levels.

13. Assume that the above experiment was conducted as described, but that five mice in Group A developed tumors. Which of the following could then be concluded from the study?

 A. Alpha-10 is not carcinogenic.
 B. Alpha-10 may increase the incidence of tumors caused by some other factor when used at high doses, but may actually help prevent tumors when used at low doses.
 C. It is impossible to draw any conclusion from the data because there was no experimental control.
 D. Alpha-10 is very carcinogenic even at extremely low doses.

PASSAGE 3 (QUESTIONS 14–21)

A scientist, Dr. Buckeye, has observed differences in tomato yield when different types of fertilizer are used. Based on her observations, Dr. Buckeye thinks that Cyclone fertilizer is superior to Hawkeye fertilizer. In order to test this hypothesis, she grows three groups of genetically identical hybrids of tomato plants, with the groups designated as groups X, Y, and Z. They are grown in the same greenhouses and receive identical amounts of heat, light, water, and ventilation. Plants in group X received 2 mg of Cyclone fertilizer once a week for two months. Plants in group Y received 2 mg of Hawkeye fertilizer once a week for two months. Plants in group Z received no fertilizer. The tomato yield was then evaluated over a two-week period. Plants in group X produced an average of 38 lbs. of tomatoes per plant, group Y produced an average of 21 lbs. per plant, and group Z produced an average of 20.5 lbs. per plant. This experiment was conducted in the same manner three separate times with identical results.

14. Which of the following is the appropriate hypothesis for this experiment?

 A. Hawkeye fertilizer is superior to Cyclone fertilizer.
 B. There is no difference between Cyclone and Hawkeye fertilizers.
 C. Treatment with fertilizer will not affect yield.
 D. Cyclone fertilizer is superior to Hawkeye fertilizer.

15. Which of the following is the dependent variable?

 A. fertilizer
 B. tomato yield
 C. 2 mg/week for 2 months
 D. light, heat, hybrids used, water

16. Which of the following is the independent variable?

A. fertilizer
B. tomato yield
C. 2 mg/week for 2 months
D. light, heat, hybrids used, water

17. Which of the following is the level of treatment?

A. fertilizer
B. tomato yield
C. 2 mg/week for 2 months
D. light, heat, hybrids used, water

18. The controlled variable(s) in this experiment was/were:

A. light, heat, hybrids used, and water.
B. Group Z, with no treatment.
C. Group X, receiving Cyclone fertilizer.
D. Group Y, receiving Hawkeye fertilizer.

19. The experimental control(s) in this experiment was/were:

A. light, heat, hybrids used, and water.
B. Group Z, with no treatment.
C. Group X, receiving Cyclone fertilizer.
D. Group Z, receiving Hawkeye fertilizer.

20. Why was this experiment designed to include three plants per treatment group, and why was it conducted in its entirety at three different times?

A. to vary the treatment levels
B. to change the controlled variables
C. to correct errors made the first time the experiment was conducted
D. to determine whether the results were reproducible

21. What would be a valid conclusion from this experiment?

A. There is no difference between the two fertilizers.
B. Hawkeye fertilizer is superior to Cyclone fertilizer.
C. Statistical analysis will be required to determine if significant differences exist between the groups.
D. Cyclone fertilizer is inferior to Hawkeye fertilizer.

Questions 22–26 are **NOT** based on a descriptive passage.

22. Trabecular or spongy bone is subject to thinning in osteoporosis because:

A. It is more metabolically active.
B. It is thinner.
C. There is more of it.
D. None of the above is true.

23. Energy, in the form of ATP, is required during skeletal muscle:

A. contraction.
B. relaxation.
C. Both A and B are correct.
D. Neither A nor B are correct.

24. Which of the following is not associated with continued strenuous muscle activity?

A. creatine phosphate
B. aerobic glycolysis
C. anaerobic glycolysis
D. lactate

25. The correct associations of vein anatomy are:

A. aorta, thick intima, thick media, thick adventitia with vasa vasorum.

B. large artery, thin intima, more smooth muscle than elastin, thick adventitia.

C. large vein, thin intima, thin media, thick adventitia with vasa vasorum.

D. arteriole, thin intima, thick media, thick adventitia.

26. The incorrect association of the lymphatic system is:

A. thoracic duct to venous circulation.

B. right lymphatic duct to venous circulation.

C. red marrow stem cell, germinal center, lymphocyte.

D. All of the above are correct.

PASSAGE 4 (QUESTIONS 27–32)

White blood cells are produced in the bone marrow, initially in the form of a pluripotential stem cell (PPSC). The PPSC then goes on to differentiate into a variety of cell types, varying in both function and morphology. White blood cells (WBCs), red blood cells, and platelets are among the products of this process. The major functions of the white blood cells include the specific immune response as well as mediation of inflammation. The following questions deal with the role of the white blood cells, as well as their specific characteristics.

27. Which of the following WBCs typically respond first to tissue injury and contribute to the process of inflammation?

A. macrophages

B. neutrophils

C. T lymphocytes

D. B lymphocytes

28. Which of the following WBCs are the effector cells for a cellular immune response, such as direct destruction of tumor cells or virus-infected cells?

A. monocytes

B. T lymphocytes

C. B lymphocytes

D. neutrophils

29. A differential WBC count is used to determine:

A. the relative percentage of each type of leukocyte in blood.

B. the diagnosis of sickle cell anemia.

C. the packed volume of red blood cells.

D. whether specific antibodies are being produced.

30. Leukemia is a disorder in which there is/are:

A. sickle-shaped red blood cells in circulation.

B. less than normal numbers of leukocytes in the blood.

C. a greater than normal number of leukocytes in the blood.

D. a complete absence of leukocytes and a reduction in red blood cells.

31. B lymphocytes mature into plasma cells upon proper stimulation with antigens and certain cytokines. This results in the production of:

    A. cytotoxic T lymphocytes and Interleukin 1.
    B. antibodies as part of the humoral response.
    C. additional red blood cells.
    D. monocytes.

32. Which of the following is not one of the granulocytic WBCs?

    A. eosinophils
    B. neutrophils
    C. T lymphocytes
    D. basophils

PASSAGE 5 (QUESTIONS 33–40)

Many organisms produce ATP through the metabolic pathways of glycolysis, Krebs cycle, and the Electron Transport Chain (ETC). Carbohydrates such as glucose, in addition to other organic compounds, may be metabolized during these processes. While glycolysis may occur whether or not oxygen is present, the Krebs cycle and the ETC are aerobic processes. These pathways involve a variety of redox reactions that result in the production of ATP. Under anaerobic conditions, the end product of glycolysis may enter fermentation rather than the Krebs cycle.

33. What are the end products of glycolysis?

    A. ATP, lactic acid, and NADH
    B. pyruvate, ATP, and NADH
    C. pyruvate, lactic acid, and ATP
    D. pyruvate, lactic acid, ATP, and NADH

34. When pyruvate enters the Krebs cycle, it goes through a transition reaction. What is produced during this reaction?

    A. citric acid and CO_2
    B. acetyl-coenzyme A and CO_2
    C. citric acid and O_2
    D. acetyl-coenzyme A and O_2

35. Where does glycolysis occur in animal cells?

    A. in the matrix of the mitochondria
    B. in the cristae
    C. in the cytosol
    D. in the intermembrane space of the mitochondria

36. Substrate-level phosphorylation takes place in both glycolysis and the Krebs cycle. Which of the following best explains the significance of this process?

    A. This is a sequence of substrate reduction reactions that produces a wide variety of organic compounds of great value commercially, such as ethanol, acetone, and organic acids.
    B. These are enzyme-substrate reactions that both produce $FADH_2$ for production of ATP in the electron transport system.
    C. This is the enzyme-catalyzed transfer of inorganic phosphate from ATP to a substrate molecule.
    D. This process transfers inorganic phosphate from a substrate in these metabolic pathways to ADP to form ATP.

37. Chemiosmosis involves production of ATP inside the mitochondria. Which of the following is most closely linked to this process?

   A. the substrate-level phosphorylation of the Krebs cycle in the inner mitochondrial membrane
   B. the substrate-level phosphorylation of the Krebs cycle in the mitochondrial matrix
   C. the oxidative phosphorylation involving the ETC and ATP-synthase in the inner mitochondrial membrane
   D. the oxidative phosphorylation involving the ETC and ATP-synthase in the mitochondrial matrix

38. The electron carriers in these metabolic pathways are:

   A. NAD^+ and FAD.
   B. NAD^+ and FMN.
   C. FAD and FMN.
   D. NAD^+, FAD, and FMN.

39. Under conditions of aerobic respiration, oxygen serves as:

   A. a reducing agent.
   B. the final electron acceptor.
   C. an electron donor.
   D. an electron carrier.

40. In bacteria, the complete oxidative breakdown of one molecule of glucose produces:

   A. 2 ATP.
   B. 38 ATP.
   C. 34 ATP.
   D. 4 ATP.

PASSAGE 6 (QUESTIONS 41–46)

Osmoregulation involves the balancing of salt and water. The kidneys serve as the master organs for controlling excretion of wastes, water recycling, and salt balance. They cleanse the blood and maintain homeostatic balance by means of filtration, tubular reabsorption, and tubular secretion. Thirst helps maintain intracellular and cardiovascular homeostasis by regulating fluid intake, and a variety of hormones regulate the amount of water and salt the body retains.

41. Alcohol causes an increase in urine output primarily because it:

   A. inhibits ADH secretion.
   B. stimulates aldosterone.
   C. increases tubular absorption.
   D. increases the efficiency of filtration.

42. Diuretic drugs are commonly used to prevent fluid retention in hypertension. Alcohol and caffeine also act as diuretics. One possible explanation for their mechanisms of action in certain sites is that they:

   A. increase tubular reabsorption of sodium and decrease the glomerular filtration rate.
   B. increase osmotic pressure in kidney filtrate and cause water to be excreted instead of reabsorbed.
   C. promote reabsorption of Na^+ and Cl^- in distal tubules and increase osmotic pressure in interstitial fluids.
   D. increase the action of ADH on collecting ducts.

43. A person with Addison's disease does not produce sufficient aldosterone. Such an individual produces a larger volume of urine because:

   A. renin is not produced.
   B. the thirst reflex cannot work.
   C. sodium is not reabsorbed.
   D. ADH is inhibited.

44. The loop of Henle:

   A. creates a salt gradient so water is removed from the collecting duct.
   B. makes it possible for water to enter the collecting duct.
   C. makes it possible for salt to enter the nephron.
   D. makes it possible for salt to leave the collecting duct across a gradient.

45. Blood and filtrate differ in concentration of:

   A. water.
   B. salts.
   C. glucose.
   D. amino acids.

46. The blood is filtered in Bowman's capsule, but in the rest of the nephron, the filtrate:

   A. becomes less concentrated.
   B. becomes the reservoir for excess metabolites.
   C. There is no receipt of protein molecules by active secretion from the blood.
   D. All of the above are correct.

Questions 47–51 are **NOT** based on a descriptive passage.

47. All of the following are true of cardiac muscle *except*:

   A. striated branching cells, several centrally placed nuclei.
   B. branching cells, joined together at intercalated disks.
   C. intercalated disk, folded ends of adjoining cell membrane at Z lines.
   D. gap junctions, less electrical barrier for the passage of impulses, syncytium.

48. All of the following are true of the electrical activity of the heart *except*:

   A. pacemaker tissue initiates repetitive action potentials.
   B. leading pacemaker tissue is located in the right atrium.
   C. AV node is the cardiac pacemaker because it depolarizes most rapidly.
   D. extrinsic control is through the autonomic nervous system.

49. A true statement or association about platelets is:

   A. Release of granules in platelets causes vasoconstriction.
   B. Platelets adhere to collagen in vessel endothelium injury.
   C. Vessel wall adhesion results in activation of the platelets.
   D. All of the above.

50. The incorrect immunological associations are:

A. inflammatory response, granulocytes, monocytes, lymphocytes.
B. cellular immunity, red marrow stem cell, T lymphocyte.
C. Helper T, cellular immunity, humoral immunity, T4.
D. All of the above are true associations.

51. The incorrect association with the kidney structure is:

A. distal convoluted tubule, macula densa.
B. proximal convoluted tubule, brush border.
C. juxtaglomerular apparatus, loop of Henle, thick, and thin.
D. macula densa, juxtaglomerular apparatus.

PASSAGE 7 (QUESTIONS 52–57)

Large multicellular animals have highly specialized tissues that are organized to form organ systems. These organ systems are involved in the maintenance of homeostasis. Many of the physiological functions that regulate homeostasis utilize metabolic pathways that are fundamentally the same among all animals. A variety of positive and negative feedback mechanisms enable organisms to maintain a dynamic balance.

52. Which of the following is an example of negative feedback?

A. When room temperature exceeds the thermostat setting, the furnace turns off.
B. When room temperature exceeds the thermostat setting, the furnace turns on.
C. When the pressure gauge drops below a certain level, the pump turns on to fill the reservoir.
D. When sensors detect low blood pressure, they send a chemical signal to increase heart activity and decrease the diameter of arteries.

53. Which of the following best describes the nature of homeostasis?

A. chemical reactions reaching equilibrium
B. physiological conditions maintained around a constant value despite environmental changes
C. After reaching equilibrium, no further reactions occur.
D. Homeostasis is the sum of negative plus positive feedback.

54. Which of the following statements is false?

A. Epithelial tissue rests on a tightly knit basement membrane.
B. Connective tissue has many extracellular fibers.
C. Epithelial tissue has many intracellular and extracellular fibers.
D. Some connective tissues are liquid.

55. When you have a fever, what is the effect of shivering?

    A. Sweating and cooling occur.
    B. Body temperature falls.
    C. The hypothalamus is reset.
    D. Muscle action elevates body temperature.

56. Which agent acts directly on the hypothalamus to raise the temperature set point?

    A. pyrogens
    B. prostaglandins
    C. white blood cells
    D. aspirin

57. The sliding-filament theory explains events that occur at the molecular level that account for:

    A. the assembly and disassembly of microtubules.
    B. the contraction of the sarcomeres of skeletal muscle cells.
    C. the separation of chromosomes during mitosis.
    D. the reduction in dental caries when proper flossing procedures are followed.

PASSAGE 8 (QUESTIONS 58–62)

In terms of mass alone, skeletal muscles make up one of the most important tissues in the body. For instance, a 61 kg man will have about 31 kg of skeletal muscle. Weibel (*The Pathway for Oxygen*, Harvard University Press, 1984) distinguishes three major groups of skeletal muscle fibers:

    SO: slow-twitch-oxidative fibers

    FOG: fast-twitch-oxidative-glycolytic fibers

    FG: fast-twitch-glycolytic fibers

The three fiber types are distinguished based on physiological and histological characteristics, especially: (1) the speed of response to stimulation (slow- or fast-twitch) and (2) their major metabolic source of ATP (the oxidative processes of cell respiration, oxidative/glycolytic, and glycolytic). Based on this information and a general knowledge of physiology, other characteristics of each fiber type may be predicted.

58. Based on the above information, the relative concentration of mitochondria (from highest to lowest) in cells of each type of fiber can be predicted. Which of the following statements are true?

    I.   SO > FOG
    II. FG > SO
    III. FOG > FG
    IV. FG > FOG

    A. I and III
    B. II and IV
    C. I and II
    D. II and III

59. Which fibers would likely have the highest myoglobin content and why?

   A. FG fibers would need a high myoglobin content to help provide sufficient oxygen for glycolysis to be carried out.
   B. SO and FOG fibers would need a high myoglobin content to help provide sufficient oxygen for glycolysis to be carried out.
   C. SO and FOG fibers would need a high myoglobin content to help provide sufficient oxygen for oxidative processes to be carried out.
   D. FG fibers would need a high myoglobin content to help provide sufficient oxygen for oxidative processes to be carried out.

60. How would the physiology of each fiber affect its appearance? Based on your answer to the above question, which fibers are expected to be red in color and which white?

   A. FG fibers would be red due to high myoglobin content.
   B. SO and FOG fibers would be white due to low myoglobin content.
   C. SO and FOG fibers would be white due to high myoglobin content.
   D. SO and FOG fibers would be red due to high myoglobin content.

61. Which fiber(s) would predominate in skeletal muscles needed for short, intensive work?

   A. FG fibers
   B. SO fibers
   C. FOG fibers
   D. SO and FOG fibers

62. The three types of fiber differ in the size of individual fibers. Based upon an estimation of the oxygen requirements of each fiber type, list the relative sizes of the fibers from largest to smallest.

   A. FG > FOG > SO
   B. SO > FOG > FG
   C. FOG > SO > FG
   D. FG > SO > FOG

PASSAGE 9 (QUESTIONS 63–67)

Control of the internal and external environments of the human body comes partially through the nervous system. This system contains two kinds of cells: neurons, which conduct messages throughout the body, and supporting cells, which protect, assist, and insulate the neurons as well as provide structural reinforcement to the system. Transmission of the messages in the nervous system depends on electrical currents along the neurons and chemical exchanges between the neurons.

63. Since the membrane of the neuron is mostly lipid, the presence of the myelin sheath:

   A. helps conduct the electrical impulse faster.
   B. impedes the electrical impulse.
   C. is critical as a source of neurotransmitters.
   D. breaks down acetylcholine.

64. Only neurons can:

   A. reverse diffusion.
   B. carry on osmosis.
   C. increase active transport.
   D. change their action potential.

65. Which of the following is NOT true of the chemical synapses?

    A. Within the cytoplasm of the presynaptic cell are numerous synaptic vesicles.

    B. The vesicles exchange neurotransmitters by membrane fusion with the postsynaptic cell.

    C. The neurotransmitter molecules are quickly degraded by enzymes.

    D. Receptors for neurotransmitters are located only on the postsynaptic cell.

66. Which of the following is not true of the nervous system?

    A. It has a role in homeostasis.

    B. Motor neurons serve solely to control the external environment.

    C. Sensory neurons serve to control both the internal and the external environment.

    D. It carries out both the conscious and the unconscious activities of the body.

67. In the brain:

    A. only white (myelinated cells) matter exists.

    B. only gray matter exists.

    C. gray matter is in the outer regions and white matter is in the inner regions.

    D. white matter is in the outer regions and gray matter is in the inner regions.

PASSAGE 10 (QUESTIONS 68–72)

The respiratory system is responsible for the exchange of two critical gases, oxygen and carbon dioxide, with the external environment. Oxygen is a vital nutrient, which is required and utilized so rapidly that a near continuous supply is required in our tissues. Unlike most of our nutrients, even a few minutes without a supply of oxygen gathered from the external environment is deadly. Carbon dioxide is produced as a waste product of our cellular respiration and must constantly be removed, developing a deadly toxicity if a build-up of only a few minutes occurs.

68. When inspiratory muscles contract, the:

    A. volume of the thoracic cavity is decreased.

    B. volume of the thoracic cavity is increased.

    C. pressure within the lungs is increased.

    D. pressure within the lungs remains unchanged.

69. Which of the following best describes how oxygen is carried in the blood?

    A. The majority of oxygen is carried freely dissolved in the plasma.

    B. The majority of oxygen is carried attached to myoglobin.

    C. The majority of oxygen is carried attached to hemoglobin.

    D. Roughly equal amounts of oxygen are carried freely dissolved in the plasma and attached to hemoglobin.

70. Three ideal gas laws are critical to comprehension of gas exchange in the respiratory system. The concept that "when a mixture of gases is in contact with a liquid, each gas will dissolve in the liquid in proportion to its partial pressure" is a description of which of the ideal gas laws?

A. Boyle's Law
B. Henry's Law
C. Dalton's Law of partial pressures
D. None of the above is correct.

71. The bulk of carbon dioxide in the blood is carried:

A. as the ion HCO_3^- after conversion in the red blood cell.
B. combined to amino acids of hemoglobin as carbaminohemoglobin.
C. as carbonic acid in the plasma.
D. combined to the heme portion of hemoglobin.

72. The release of oxygen from the blood to the tissues is largely driven by the dissociation of oxyhemoglobin. Which of the following characteristics of working tissue enhances the release of oxygen from the blood to the tissue?

I. Working tissues release heat increasing the temperature of the blood in that area.
II. Working tissues release carbon dioxide which increases the acidity of the blood in that area.
III. Working tissues release 2,3-diphosphoglycerate, increasing its concentration in the blood in that area.
IV. Working tissues release carbon monoxide, which has a higher affinity for hemoglobin than oxygen.

A. II only
B. I and II
C. III and IV
D. All of the above are correct.

Questions 73–77 are **NOT** based on a descriptive passage.

73. The countercurrent multiplier of the kidney is explained by the statement:

A. Fluids flowing in opposite directions in the loop of Henle increase the efficiency of solute exchange.
B. Fluids flowing in the same direction in the loop of Henle increase the efficiency of solute exchange.
C. Fluids flowing in opposite directions in the proximal convoluted tubule and the efferent arteriole increase the efficiency of solute exchange.
D. Fluids flowing in the same direction in the proximal convoluted tubule and the efferent arteriole increase the efficiency of solute exchange.

74. Renin and aldosterone control of sodium concentration involves:

   A. the macula densa.
   B. the adrenal cortex.
   C. angiotensin II.
   D. All of the above.

75. True associations of the dermis layer include all but:

   A. melanin granules and clear cells.
   B. blood vessels, lymphatic channels, and nerves.
   C. sensory nerve endings, hair follicles, and sweat glands.
   D. All of the above are in the dermis layer.

76. True associations with sebaceous glands are:

   A. Meibomian glands.
   B. holocrine glands, arrector pili muscle, and sebum.
   C. Moll glands and Zeis glands.
   D. All of the above are true.

77. All but one of the following is involved in healing of the skin:

   A. fibrin
   B. hair follicle
   C. sweat gland
   D. All of the above are involved in healing the skin.

ANSWERS FOR THE DIAGNOSTIC MCAT

Verbal Reasoning			Physical Sciences			Biological Sciences		
1. C	23. A	45. D	1. A	27. D	53. A	1. D	27. B	53. B
2. D	24. D	46. D	2. B	28. A	54. A	2. B	28. B	54. C
3. A	25. D	47. B	3. B	29. D	55. C	3. C	29. A	55. D
4. B	26. C	48. C	4. C	30. A	56. C	4. B	30. C	56. B
5. A	27. D	49. D	5. D	31. B	57. A	5. B	31. B	57. B
6. B	28. D	50. D	6. D	32. B	58. A	6. C	32. C	58. A
7. A	29. B	51. C	7. B	33. C	59. C	7. D	33. B	59. C
8. D	30. D	52. D	8. C	34. B	60. C	8. C	34. B	60. D
9. C	31. D	53. C	9. B	35. D	61. B	9. D	35. C	61. A
10. B	32. B	54. D	10. C	36. C	62. C	10. B	36. D	62. A
11. B	33. C	55. C	11. B	37. C	63. C	11. A	37. C	63. A
12. B	34. B	56. D	12. B	38. B	64. D	12. C	38. A	64. D
13. D	35. D	57. B	13. C	39. A	65. B	13. B	39. B	65. B
14. B	36. B	58. C	14. B	40. A	66. B	14. D	40. B	66. B
15. C	37. C	59. C	15. C	41. C	67. A	15. B	41. A	67. C
16. D	38. C	60. D	16. C	42. B	68. A	16. A	42. B	68. B
17. C	39. D	61. D	17. D	43. A	69. D	17. C	43. C	69. C
18. D	40. A	62. C	18. A	44. C	70. C	18. A	44. A	70. B
19. C	41. B	63. D	19. D	45. D	71. A	19. B	45. C	71. A
20. D	42. D	64. D	20. C	46. A	72. D	20. D	46. C	72. B
21. D	43. B	65. A	21. A	47. C	73. A	21. C	47. A	73. A
22. A	44. D		22. B	48. C	74. A	22. A	48. C	74. D
			23. B	49. C	75. D	23. C	49. D	75. A
			24. C	50. A	76. A	24. B	50. D	76. D
			25. B	51. C	77. D	25. C	51. C	77. D
			26. D	52. D		26. D	52. A	

EXPLANATORY ANSWERS FOR THE DIAGNOSTIC TEST

VERBAL REASONING

PASSAGE 1

1. The correct answer is (C). The author writes, "Like enzymes, vitamins act by helping a reaction take place (in some cases, enzymes and vitamins make reactions possible that could not occur in their absence), but vitamins are neither changed nor incorporated into the products of the reaction. Because of this action, vitamins are called 'coenzymes.'" Answer (A) is incorrect. There is no evidence in this article that the vitamin and enzyme join for their work. Answer (B) is incorrect. There is no mention in this selection of a pair of enzymes working together for the good of the body. Answer (D) is incorrect. This selection provides no evidence that an enzyme is broken down into more than one part within the body.

2. The correct answer is (D). At the beginning of the article, the author states: "Vitamins are a group of important compounds that are found in very small proportions in food. They are needed in trace amounts for the proper functioning of the body." Answer (A) is incorrect. There is no effort to persuade the reader to use more vitamins; you can recognize this because there are no alternate arguments presented. Answer (B) is incorrect; to narrate means to tell a story. There is no effort to follow the vitamin through the body. Answer (C) is incorrect. This answer appears correct; however, there is no mention of strength as a focus.

3. The correct choice is (A). The author states: "As shown in a vitamins table, whether a vitamin will dissolve in water or in fat (or oil) is important." Answer (B) is incorrect. While this may be a valid statement, there is no mention of this within the article in question. Answer (C) is incorrect. Again, while this may be a legitimate concern, this is not mentioned in the article. Answer (D) is incorrect. This article does not mention the effects of other chemicals within the body. Remember, you must not choose answers based upon what you know or believe, but upon what is clearly stated or implied within the selection given.

4. Answer (B) is the correct choice. The author writes: "Water-soluble vitamins are not stored in the body and should be taken in each day." Answer (A) is incorrect. While this may be true, there is no mention of this in this article. Answer (C) is incorrect. Iron and potassium are not mentioned as such in this article. Answer (D) is incorrect. Enzymes are not vitamins.

5. The correct choice is (A). The author states: "In general, fat-soluble vitamins are stored within body tissues and can cause toxic effects in large overdoses." Answer (B) is incorrect. Water-soluble vitamins are not stored within the body and therefore are not as suspect as fat-soluble vitamins. Answer (C) is incorrect. Vitamins D and K are synthesized within the body and therefore not suspect. Answer (D) is incorrect. Vitamin B6 is one of the vitamins still under study.

6. Answer (B) is correct. The writer states; "Powers have been ascribed to them that many nutritionists feel are unproven." Answer (A) is incorrect. There is no evidence in the article to indicate that there is no importance to these vitamins within the body. Answers (C) and (D) are incorrect. While there may be truth in these statements, the inference is that the importance is unproven.

PASSAGE 2

7. The correct answer is (A). While the article does mention some positive effects, the content emphasizes negative effects. Answer (B) is incorrect. The article does make this description; however, this is not the primary focus. Answer (C) is incorrect; while the history is covered briefly, this is not the primary focus. Answer (D) is incorrect; the poppy plant and what it can become are only one portion of the article.

8. The correct answer is (D). In paragraph 2, the author states: "The realization that it was not until the drug invaded European cities in the form of gum opium and laudanum (tincture of opium) [Answer (A)] that man realized something stronger than a mere desire for 'repose' [Answer B)] was tying him to the opium habit." Answer (D) is implied in the forgoing statements.

9. The correct answer is (C). Answer (A), while seemingly a correct statement, is not the correct choice since that is not covered in this article. Answer (B) is incorrect. There is no real evidence of this fact in the article, though it may be true. Answer (D) may be a true statement, but it is not the correct choice according to the information stated in paragraph 3.

10. The correct answer is (B). The author describes the discovery of morphine and its "pain-killing" properties with this statement: "This relationship between humans and the opiates was not scientifically recognized, however, until after morphine was isolated from opium resin. Called 'God's own medicine' by the English surgeon Sir William Osler because of its pain-killing properties, the new drug soon became the mainstay of the medical profession." Answer (A) is incorrect; the author specifically says; " . . . the new drug soon became the mainstay of the medical profession." Answer (C) is incorrect. The introduction of morphine into the world is described as a "mainstay" of the medical profession. The implication is that it was not a disaster. Answer (D) is incorrect. Both opium and morphine have legitimate uses according to this article.

11. The correct answer is (B). The author states: "But as more doctors began to depend on it medically, their patients became dependent upon it physically." Answer (A) is incorrect. That education about drug effects has increased dependence is contraindicated. In fact, when man realizes the effects, dependence should decrease. Answer (C) is incorrect. The movement of the drug through European cities increased the awareness of the effects, but not the awareness of addiction. Answer (D) is incorrect. While there is truth in the fact that increased availability of the drug promotes addiction, this is not the indication of this article. Remember, you are not going by what you know or believe, but by what the article states.

12. The correct answer is (B). The author states that: "In 1848, a new technical invention seemed to provide a safe method of prescribing morphine. The invention was the hypodermic needle. At the time, most experts believed the needle would stop addiction because direct injection prevented the drug from passing through the stomach." Answer (A) is incorrect. Coleridge and his works are mentioned in connection with his own use of the drug. Answer (C) is incorrect. The increased use of the drug by physicians did lead to it addictive popularity; however, this is NOT a deterrent, or curb, to the addictive use. Answer (D) is incorrect. The aftereffects of the drug are not discussed.

13. The correct answer is (D). The author states that using the " . . .hypodermic syringe greatly heightened the drug's effects (60 milligrams of morphine taken by mouth is less effective in killing pain than 8 milligrams administered through injection)." Answer (A) is incorrect. The article does not mention that mixing opium and morphine is unwise. Answer (B) is incorrect. The inference of the article is that doctors advise against conditions leading to addiction. Answer (C) is incorrect. There is no mention in the article of switching from opium to morphine.

14. The correct answer is (B). The author writes: "A German doctor, Heinrich Dreser, discovered another 'cure' for morphine addiction. Christened 'heroin' after the Greek god Heros, thereby reflecting hopes that it should be of great benefit to mankind, the new drug was enthusiastically prescribed as a cure for both opium and morphine addiction." Answer (A) is incorrect; the author states ". . . the new drug was enthusiastically prescribed as a cure for both opium and morphine addiction." Answer (C) is incorrect. While heroin may have been used for pain relief, this is not the best answer to the question. Answer (D) is incorrect. The author indicates that the physicians were enthusiastic about the drug.

15. The correct answer is (C). The 5th paragraph states; ". . . heroin addiction is perhaps the most difficult to cure." Answers (A), (B), and (D) are incorrect. There is no basis for any of these answers, based upon the author's statement.

16. The correct choice is (D). The author states in the conclusion: "The positive effects of the opiate have been far overshadowed by the negative effects." Answer (A) is incorrect. The author's statement indicates that there are benefits. Answer (B) is incorrect. The author indicates the positive uses. Answer (C) is incorrect. While the statement is true if the opiates are used to excess, they do have benefits and are not necessarily dangerous.

PASSAGE 3

17. The correct answer is (C). The author says in the opening paragraph; "Supplying known physiological requirements demands eating a balance of nutrients in kind and amount." Answer (A) is incorrect; while there is the mention of such a calculation, this is not the focus. Answer (B) is incorrect; this explanation is included, but is not the focus. Answer (D) is incorrect; while calories and their work are mentioned, their definition is not the focus; instead it is a means of illustrating the importance of balance.

18. The correct answer is (D). The author states: "One Calorie is the amount of heat energy required to raise 1 liter (approximately one quart) of water 1 degree centigrade [Answer (A)]. In nutrition, this large calorie (C) [Answer (B)] is most often not capitalized and referred to as kcal (kilocalorie) [Answer (C)]." Answer (D) is correct as explained throughout the article.

19. Answer (C) is the correct choice. The author states: ". . . add 50 percent of your resting metabolism." Answer (A) is incorrect. This figure is not mentioned in this article. Answer (B) refers to inactive people. Answer (D) refers to moderate activity.

20. The correct answer is (D). The author states: "Balance is the key—balance not only in vitamins [Answer (C)] and calories, but also in protein [Answer (A)], minerals [Answer (B)], essential fatty acids, and water [Answer (C)]."

21. The correct answer is (D). The author writes: "In nutrition, this large calorie (C) is most often not capitalized and referred to as kcal (kilocalorie)." Answer (A) is incorrect; the abbreviation "k" is not used in this article. Answer (B) is incorrect; the abbreviation "C" is for Calorie. Answer (C) is incorrect; the abbreviation "c" is not used in this article.

22. The correct answer is (A). The quantity of energy released from a given quantity of food is measured in Calories. Answer (B) is incorrect. There is no indicator of measuring the weight of food. Answer (C) is incorrect. A calorie measures heat energy required, or not obtained. Answer (D) is incorrect. This selection does not mention fat at all.

23. The correct answer is (A). The author states: ". . . food contains 'potential' energy, or energy in a form that can be set into action. The body is able to convert this potential energy into heat, movement, growth, and all of the processes that take place in the body. Energy that is being used or is working is termed 'kinetic energy.'" Answer (B) is incorrect. While the author does mention energy for movement, there is no mention of lubricating of joints. Answer (C) is incorrect. While growth is mentioned, there is no mention of the creation of cells. Answer (D) is incorrect. There is no mention of deposits of energy.

24. The correct answer is (D). The author states: "The conversion of potential energy into kinetic energy takes place through chemical reactions in every cell of the body. The term "metabolism" refers to the total of all the chemical processes that make up the functions of life." Answer (A) is incorrect. This article contains no evidence to support that the more food taken in, the more energy created. Answer (B) is incorrect; there is no mention of taking in food without turning it into fat. Answer (C) is incorrect; there is no indicator of a lack of necessary chemicals.

25. The correct choice is (D). The author states: "The BMR is a useful measure of the healthy functioning of the body." Basal metabolic rate is abbreviated as BMR. Answer (A) is incorrect. Energy that is being used or is working is termed "kinetic energy." Answer (B) is incorrect; the quantity of energy released from a given quantity of food is measured in Calories, not in healthy functioning. Answer (C) is incorrect; kcal is the term for a large calorie, according to this article, and not an indicator of healthy functioning.

26. Answer (C) is correct. The author states: "The basal metabolic rate is most directly under the influence of the thyroid gland, through the secretion of the hormone thyroxin." Answer (A) is incorrect; calorie intake would not be influenced by improper functioning of the thyroid. See the statement of the author above. Answer (B) is incorrect. The kcal is not directly influenced by the thyroid, only the BMR. Answer (D) is incorrect. There is no mention of fatty acids in relation to the thyroid.

PASSAGE 4

27. The correct answer is (D). The author states: "Among the reasons for not being overweight are: Whether a person likes it or not, he or she must admit that clothing styles are directed toward slender figures [Answer (A)]. Of course, larger sizes are provided for those who need them, but these are not influenced by the fashion market. Then again, it's always pleasant to fit into a standard-size theater or lecture-hall seat [Answer (B)], or to take no more than our half or third of the car seat [Answer (C)]." Because all of the choices are found within this statement, Answer (D) is correct.

28. The correct answer is (D). The author states that "It is estimated that for every pound of added fat an additional two thirds of a mile of blood vessels are required to keep this pound of fat alive." Answers (A), (B), and (C) are incorrect. There is no mention of kidneys, bowels, or bones, in this article.

29. The correct answer is (B). The author states: ". . . appetite is regulated by emotions, body chemistry, and inheritance." Answers (A), (C), and (D) are incorrect. There is no mention of these as causes for increased appetite.

30. The correct answer is (D). The author states: "Appetite and hunger are known to be controlled by a small area in the brain called the "appetite center" or "appestat." It is composed of two sets of nuclei." Answer (A) is incorrect; the basic metabolic rate concerns the use of calories and not the control of appetite. Answer (C) is incorrect; the appetite is controlled by the appestat which is a type of thermometer. Answer (D) is correct; the appestat is the appetite control center.

31. The correct answer is (D). The author states: "Excess fat complicates all surgery and increases surgical risks." Answer (A) is incorrect; while there is a possible genetic cause for overweight, there is no mention of the creation of inferior genetic legacies. Answer (B) is incorrect; a decreased sex drive is not mentioned. Answer (C) is incorrect; while there may be nervous reasons for being overweight, there is no mention of the creation of extreme nervous energy levels.

32. The correct answer is (B). The author states: "The overweight person is less agile, has more balancing problems, moves more slowly, and has more physical accidents than a person of normal weight." Answer (A) is incorrect. This article begins with the statistics of those who are overweight in America. Answer (C) is incorrect; the inherent effects of being overweight are not insurmountable; indeed, they are not even a surety, according to the research cited. Answer (D) is incorrect; this article states: "Fat accumulates around internal vital organs (such as the heart and lungs) and tends to crowd them."

33. The correct answer is (C). According to the author, "As to what activates the appestat, there is still some question. It may be the glucose level (blood-sugar level) in the blood, body temperature changes, or the level of amino acids in the blood." Therefore, since blood sugar or glucose and amino acids are both in the blood, this is the correct choice. Answer (A) is incorrect. There is no mention of environmental temperature as an appetite control. Answer (B) is incorrect; there is no indicator that the brain waves may be a factor. Answer (D) is incorrect; there is no mention of fat content of food.

34. The correct answer is (B). The author states: "It is an extraordinary paradox that while much of the world's population is fighting starvation, more than 25 percent of the people in the United States are overweight due to excessive eating." The inference here is that the problem is more ordinary in this country. Answer (A) is incorrect; the same sentence infers that this is not a worldwide problem. Answer (C) is incorrect. There is no evidence in the article of gender inferences for over-weight. Answer (D) is incorrect. There is no indicator of age as an inference.

35. The correct choice is (D). The author states: "Cardiovascular disease [Answer (A)], diabetes, gallbladder disease [Answer (B)], cirrhosis of the liver [Answer (C)] occur more often or can be more serious in overweight people than in those of desirable weight."

36. The correct answer is (B). According to the author of this article, among the advantages to those people who are not overweight are: "A man forty-five years of age, of medium height and frame, weighing 200 pounds, can expect to live four to six years less than a similar man weighing 150 pounds." Answers (A), (C), and (D) are incorrect. There is no evidence given in the article of self-esteem, increased sex drive, or increased job opportunities.

PASSAGE 5

37. The correct answer is (C). The last sentence of the first paragraph states: "Caves, shelves, and pockets of unknown blackness all provide material for questions." Answer (A) is incorrect. After reading the entire article, the reader is better able to determine that there is no effort made to explain, but rather to inform. An explanation would involve telling why, when, where, and how. That is not done in this article. Answer (B) is incorrect; while there are certain areas of description, that is not the intent. A true description would have involved detailed information of heights and widths as well as colors and texture. Answer (D) is incorrect; there is no mention of the creation of the floor of the oceans.

38. The correct answer is (C). The author states: "Deep-sea fans accumulate at the mouths of submarine canyons and are partly responsible for the development of a continental rise. Other contributing factors are currents around the continental shelf." Answer (A) is incorrect; while there may be the small hills of dunes, this is not included in this article. Answer (B) is incorrect; the article indicates that there are hills but these are not at the submarine canyon mouth. Answer (D) is incorrect for the same reason.

39. The correct answer is (D). The author states: "They [canyons] exhibit steep walls and tributaries just like canyons cut from rivers on land [Answer (A)] . . . These canyons form a basic trough through which sediments [Answer (B)] and other heavier-than-water minerals [Answer (C)] are carried toward the ocean floor and form a DEEP SEA FAN. With all of the choices indicated in this statement, (D) is the correct choice.

40. The correct answer is (A). The author states: "Ocean ridges are usually formed where two tectonic plates come together, the most predominant being the Atlantic Ocean ridge, where the North American and Eurasian plates meet." Answer (B) is incorrect. There is no indication of the location of the Atlantic ridge. Answer (C) is incorrect. The author states: "These ridges are also where most sea-floor spreading occurs due to large amounts of magma pushing through the ocean crust." The reader can infer that a ridge is not a spreading but a rising. Answer (D) is incorrect; there is no indicator that the lithosphere is the origin of the ridge.

41. The correct answer is (B). The author writes: "The abyssal zones accumulate at about a rate of 1 mm/1,000 years." This indeed is great slowness. Answer (A) is incorrect. The statement above contradicts this answer. Answer (C) is incorrect; the word magnitude, in light of the foregoing, would be incorrect. Answer (D) is incorrect; while this may be true, this is not indicated in this selection.

42. The correct answer is (D). The author writes: "Extending from the coastal shoreline to a point at which a marked slope occurs, the point where the slope gradually increases is called the SHELF BREAK, and the steeper slope is called the CONTINENTAL SLOPE." Answer (A) is incorrect. The currents do not contribute to the varying meeting of the land and sea, but to the patterns created. Answer (B) is incorrect. The submarine canyons would not affect the meeting of the land and water. Answer (C) is incorrect; the ridges do not occur where the land and sea meet.

Passage 6

43. The correct answer is (B). The author says: "There is a certain artistic modesty implied by this approach, a self-effacement in the interest of heightening the illusion created by the image." Answer (A) is incorrect. The first paragraph countermands this. Answer (C) is incorrect. Artists strive for a product that is not machine-made. Answer (D) is incorrect. Again, the artist does not want to make the audience aware.

44. The correct answer is (D). Impression-ism is "as a style of objective accuracy [Answer (B)], since it constituted a disciplined endeavor to use scientific discoveries [Answer (A)] about color and visual perception [Answer (C)]". Because all of the choices are repre-sented in this sentence, Answer (D) is the correct choice.

45. The correct answer is (D). The author writes: "The genius of Impressionism lay in the realization that the object—a tree, a mountain, a still life—could not be seen or represented accurately without considering the character of the light and atmosphere around the object and the source and nature of the illumination that enables us to see the object in the first place." Answer (A) is incorrect. While this may be true, this is not indicated in this article. Answer (B) is incorrect; Realism would not require symbolism according to this article. Answer (C) is incorrect; light and atmosphere are important; however, their illumination is not the intent of the artist.

46. The correct answer is (D). The writer states: "The suppression of the personal in the artist's style is due to his desire to make vision the most important part of experiencing his work. Answer (A) is incorrect. This is counter to the focus of this article. Answer (B) is incorrect; the author of this article indicates in the sentence above that the artist tries to suppress his style. Answer (C) is incorrect; models are used, not for technical accuracy but to begin a vision.

47. The correct answer is (B). In the first paragraph the author establishes this message. Answer (A) is incorrect. The exact opposite is illustrated throughout the article. Answer (C) is incorrect. While this is an illustration used, it is not the focus because it is mentioned only in passing. Answer (D) is incor-rect. Again the use of light and texture to convey style and structure is men-tioned, but it is not the focus.

48. The correct answer is (C). The author writes: "If we are to learn anything about the artist as a person, it is through his choice of themes and organization of subject matter, not because of his individuality of vision or intensely personal manner of execution. There is something scientific in such an attitude." The artist as a person must be discovered because it is not obvious. Answer (A) is incorrect; the author indicates that an Impressionist must have "organization of subject matter." Answer (B) is incorrect; the author indicates that the artist is an individual and that the products are reflections that require imagination. Answer (D) is incorrect. The writer indicates that "through his choice of themes" the author establishes his individuality.

Passage 7

49. The correct answer is (D). In order to explain, one must give the causes, the effects, and the outcomes in an organized manner. The author begins with and continues with the reality of lead poisoning and continues to explain in an orderly form all of the implications. Answer (A) is incorrect; the reactions are a part of the article but not the primary focus. Answer (B) is incorrect. Warnings implied are not the primary focus. Answer (C) is incorrect; defining the ways to prevent lead poisoning, while implied, are not the primary focus.

50. The correct answer is (D). The author writes: "Lead, after absorption, is carried by the blood to different organs, where it produces a multiform symptomatology. Symptoms can include weakness, anorexia, loss of weight [Answer (C)], abdominal colic [Answer (A)], constipation, back ache [Answer (B)]." Because all of the answers are found in this quote, (D) is the correct choice.

51. The correct answer is (C). The author writes: "The continued intake of small doses when released suddenly by the body stores, may give rise abruptly to a type of poisoning similar to that which follows the ingestion of a large amount." Answers (A), (B), and (D) are incorrect. While these may be true, there is no mention of them in this article.

52. The correct answer is (D). The author outlines these three within the article: "1. The hematopoietic system (blood and blood producing organs). . . . 2. The central nervous system. . . . 3. The kidneys. . . ." Seeing these three areas, answer (A) is incorrect; the brain, while affected, is not listed. Answer (B) is incorrect, the muscular system is not listed.

53. The correct answer is (C). The author writes: "Although the symptoms of acute poisoning are varied, the patient may complain of a metallic taste, a dry burning sensation in the throat, cramps, retching, and persistent vomiting. Hematemesis (vomiting of blood) may occur." With this statement in mind, answer (A) is incorrect; faintness is not mentioned. Answer (B) is incorrect; sight is not mentioned. Answer (D) is incorrect; heavy breathing is not mentioned.

54. The correct answer is (D). The author writes: "Retention of lead is cumulative, so that a sudden acute attack may occur after a long period of administration." Answer (A) is incorrect. There is no indicator of brain damage in this selection. Answer (B) is incorrect; while the statement may be true, this is not the answer to this question. Answer (C) is incorrect; while again, this may be true, this is not indicated in this selection.

55. The correct answer is (C). The selection given is the one with which we must deal. Remember, you cannot bring in what you do not see here. Authorial omission would not be a factor, so answer (A) is incorrect. Answer (B) is incorrect; remember, again, all you have is what is before you. Answer (D) is incorrect; an antidote to poison would never be improper.

PASSAGE 8

56. The correct answer is (D). The author writes: "Pick a speech topic that you are TRULY interested in . . . pick something you WANT to talk about." Answer (A) is incorrect in light of the foregoing sentence. Answer (B) is incorrect; there is no mention of the importance of selecting a controversial subject. Answer (C) is incorrect; there is no indication of the need to please the teacher.

57. The correct answer is (B). The author writes: "Most people are afraid that the audience will laugh at them. Most people don't want to look foolish or be humiliated." Answer (A) is incorrect; there is no indication of the speaker becoming weakened. Answer (C) is incorrect; this article mentions nothing about the size of an audience. Answer (D) is incorrect; this article does not mention the discipline of the audience.

58. The correct answer is (C). The author writes: "Use your excess nervous energy by using your hands and moving around the front of the room." Answer (A) is incorrect. The article has no reference to grasping the podium even though this might be an accepted technique. Answer (B) is incorrect; while this might be a legitimate choice, this is not mentioned in the article. Answer (D) is incorrect; while this might be appropriate, this is not mentioned in the article.

59. The correct answer is (C). The author states: "The fear of public speaking is the most common fear for people." Answer (A) is incorrect; confidence is only a part of the focus of this article. Answer (B) is incorrect; a positive attitude is a part of this article. Answer (D) is incorrect; selecting a topic is part of the emphasis of this article.

60. The correct answer is (D). The author writes: "If you practice as much as you can, you can tone down your nervousness that way." Answers (A), (B), and (C) are incorrect; while these may be good techniques, none are featured in this article.

61. The correct answer is (D). The author writes: "The MOST IMPORTANT thing you can do is THINK POSITIVE! You got a good night's sleep [Answer (C)]. . . . You LOOK fabulous because you dressed neatly [Answer (B)]. . . . you SMILE [Answer (A)] at them. . . .

Passage 9

62. The correct answer is (C). The author states: "Blood can be thought of as having two huge roles. First, it is the highway system of our body. It serves to transport material necessary for our body's proper functions. Second, it is responsible for providing the much-needed oxygen to the cells of the body, without which life would cease to function." Answer (A) is incorrect; the focus is not the route of blood, which is only a part of the selection. Note: "First, it is the highway system of our body." Answer (B) is incorrect; in order to define blood, there would have to be composition and function discussion. Answer (D) is incorrect; the sentence above does not indicate the focus on composition.

63. The correct answer is (D). The author writes: "The products absorbed from the digestive tract, such as sugars [Answer (C)] and fats [Answer (B)], travel through our bodies via the blood. Medications [Answer (A)] that we take are transported as well."

64. The correct answer is (D). The author writes: "Without white blood cells, we would suffer from repeated bacterial and viral illnesses . . ." Answer (A) is incorrect; there is no mention of lymph being carried in the blood to combat germs. Answer (B) is incorrect; red blood cells are not mentioned in this connection. Answer (C) is incorrect; platelets are mentioned to prevent clotting.

65. The correct answer is (A). The author writes: ". . . red blood cells can give up the oxygen to the cells of the body and exchange it for carbon dioxide, which is a waste product." Answer (B) is incorrect. "Blood is composed of a cellular component—blood cells of different types—as well as a fluid component, known as plasma." Answer (C) is incorrect; the article states that white blood cells fight germs. Answer (D) is incorrect; platelets prevent clotting.

PHYSICAL SCIENCE

PASSAGE 1

1. The correct answer is (A). Metallic properties show a trend that *decreases* as you compare across a period. Therefore, K (potassium), which is to the extreme left of the periodic table, is chemically the most metallic.
   General Chemistry 2.3

2. The correct answer is (D). Atomic radius increases from right to left across a period and from top to bottom in a family; therefore, Ka will have the largest atomic radius.
   General Chemistry 2.3

3. The correct answer is (B). Electronegativity is described as the ability to attract electrons and become a negative ion. Electronegativity *increases* from left to right across a period and from bottom to top in a family; therefore, F will be the most electronegative.
   General Chemistry 2.3

4. The correct answer is (C). 1st ionization energy is defined as the energy required for a neutral atom to lose an electron and become a +1 ion. This energy decreases from right to left across the table and also decreases from top to bottom in a family. Therefore, Rb has the lowest 1st ionization energy.
   General Chemistry 2.3

5. The correct answer is (D). 2nd ionization energy is defined as the energy needed for a neutral atom to lose 2 electrons and become a +2 ion. This trend is slightly more complex than the 1st ionization energy. Elements in column II have low second ionization energies, and this energy trend increases from left to right beginning in column II. Elements in column I have an extremely high 2nd ionization energy. The 2nd ionization energy also decreases from top to bottom in a family. Therefore, the lowest 2nd ionization energy would be represented by magnesium (Mg).
   General Chemistry 2.3

6. The correct answer is (D). There are seven elements that naturally exist as diatomic molecules, including nitrogen (N_2).   *General Chemistry 2.3*

PASSAGE 2

7. The correct answer is (B). F = ma. For equal forces if the mass is smaller the acceleration must be greater.
   Physics 2.2

8. The correct answer is (C). From Newton's third law the forces between two colliding masses are always equal and opposite.   *Physics 2.3*

9. The correct answer is (B). Although the forces are equal and opposite, the accelerations depend on Newton's second law, F = ma. The block with the greater mass will have the smaller acceleration.   *Physics 2.2*

10. The correct answer is (C). If an object is moving at a constant velocity, it is not accelerating and its acceleration equals zero. From Newton's second law, if a=0, then F=0.
    Physics 2.2, 4.2

---

* For more information, refer to this section in Peterson's *Gold Standard MCAT*.

PASSAGE 3

To answer the molecular geometry questions successfully, these steps should be followed.

A. Draw a "Lewis Diagram" for the molecule, indicating bonded electron pairs with solid lines and lone electron pairs with "dots" (··).

B. Count the regions of high electron density (a solid line or bond and a lone pair each count as 1 region of high electron density) about the central atom.

C. The following table will help you determine how these regions of high electron density determine their geometric arrangement; however, the molecule's actual geometry will be a "subset" of this arrangement. Since only the atoms, and not the lone pairs, dictate the geometry. (The abbreviation H.E.D. = High Electron Density.)

Regions of H.E.D.	Arrangement of Regions
3	Trigonal Planar
4	Tetrahedral
5	Trigonal bipyramidal
6	Octahedral

11. The correct answer is (B). This molecule has 4 regions of high electron density resulting from 4 covalent bonds and no "lone pairs," which creates a tetrahedron. See diagram below.
Physics 3.2, 3.5

12. The correct answer is (B). Water has 4 regions of high electron density created from 2 "lone pairs" and 2 bonds; hence, its H.E.D. arrangement will be tetrahedral. *Physics 3.2, 3.5*

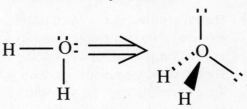

13. The correct response is (C). This molecule has 5 H.E.D. regions formed exclusively from covalent bonds. There are no "lone pairs" of electrons, so the molecular geometry is the same as the H.E.D. geometry. *Physics 3.2, 3.5*

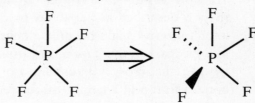

14. The correct answer is (B). With 5 H.E.D. regions, the H.E.D. shape is trigonal bipyramidal; however, the 2 "lone pairs" force the atoms into the "t-shape" geometry. *Physics 3.2, 3.5*

---

* For more information, refer to this section in Peterson's *Gold Standard MCAT.*

15. The correct answer is (C). Square planar is the result of having an octahedral arrangement created by 6 H.E.D. regions that are formed from 2 "lone pairs" and 4 covalent bonds.
Physics 3.2, 3.5

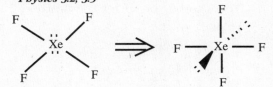

16. The correct answer is (C). PF_5 has 5 H.E.D. regions. See the solution to question 13 above.   *Physics 3.2, 3.5*

17. The correct answer is (D). This ion and water both have 4 H.E.D. regions formed from 2 "lone pairs" and 2 covalent bonds, which creates the angular geometry within the tetrahedral shape.   *Physics 3.2, 3.5*

18. The correct answer is (A). "Seesaw" is a molecule's geometry within the trigonal bipyramidal shape created when 5 H.E.D. regions are formed from 1 "lone pair" and 4 covalent bonds.
Physics 3.2, 3.5

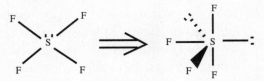

19. The correct answer is (D). For constant acceleration downward, the vertical position as a function of time is given by:

$$y = \frac{1}{2}at^2 + v_0t + y_0$$

If we take up to be the + direction, and the initial position to be zero, this becomes:

$$y = \frac{1}{2}(-g)t^2 + v_0t$$

Since the hammer was dropped, the initial velocity is zero, so that:

$$y = \frac{1}{2}(-g)t^2$$

We know a particular case for this motion: When t = 1.5 sec, y = −3 meters. Thus we know that:

$$-3m = \frac{-g}{2}(1.5 \text{ sec})^2$$

This can be solved for g, with a solution:

$$g = 2.67\frac{m}{\text{sec}^2}$$

Physics 1.4, 1.5

20. The correct answer is (C). Newton's second law tells us about the motion of an object, in terms of the sum of the forces on the object. We have the freedom (and the obligation) to decide what object to study. To answer this question most easily, choose the object to be the last two cars, as sketched in the figure. The only horizontal force on this object is the force by the rope "B." Since there is no friction considered, the sum of the horizontal forces is simple: It is just the force by the rope at B, directed to the right.

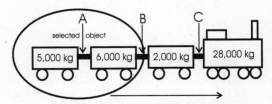

Force on selected object is the force by the rope at B, pulling to the right.

---

* For more information, refer to this section in Peterson's *Gold Standard MCAT*.

Taking the rightward direction as positive, Newton's second law is:

$$+F_{rope} = (5000kg + 6000kg)\left(1.5\frac{m}{sec^2}\right)$$
$$= 16,500 \; Newton$$

The tension in the rope is 1.65×10^4 Newton.   *Physics 2.2*

21. The correct answer is (A). The y component of Newton's second law is:

$$N - 47 Newton = ma_y = 0$$

where N is the normal force by the plane on the box. (Since the box remains on the inclined plane, it must not accelerate in the y direction.) Thus $N = 47 \; Newton$, and the magnitude of the friction force is:

$$|\vec{F}_{friction}| = \mu N$$
$$= .4 \times 47 \; Newton$$
$$= 18.8 \; Newton$$

Since the direction of the velocity is downhill, the direction of the friction force is uphill. The x component of Newton's second law is $(F_{friction})_x + F_{gravity} = (5kg)a_x$

Since uphill is in the −x direction here, this is $-18.8 \; Newton + 13.5 \; Newton = (5kg)a_x$

Solving for ax gives $a_x = -1.07\frac{m}{sec^2}$. The minus sign indicates that the direction of the acceleration is uphill; the box is slowing down.   *Physics 2.2, 3.2.1, 3.2*

22. The correct answer is (B). If we ignore friction and consider the cart-plus-bag system, the horizontal force on the system is zero. This means that the horizontal momentum of the system is constant. In particular, the momentum

before the bag hits the cart equals the momentum after the bag hits the cart:

$$(m_{bag})(v_{before}) + (m_{cart})(0)$$
$$= (m_{bag})(v_{after}) + (m_{cart})(v_{after})$$
$$= (m_{bag} + m_{cart})(v_{after})$$

This can be solved for the initial velocity of the bag:

$$(v_{before}) =$$
$$\frac{(10kg+25kg)(1.2m/sec)}{10kg} = 4.2m/sec$$

Physics 4.4.1, 4.3, 4.4

23. The correct answer is (B). The weight of the satellite is equal to the force of gravity upon it. The force of gravity is proportional to $\frac{1}{R^2}$ where R is the distance to the center of the earth. When the satellite is raised to 6,000 km above the surface of the earth, its distance from the center of the earth is twice what it was on the ground. Thus the force of gravity is diminished by a factor of $2^2 = 4$. The force of gravity of the satellite in orbit is 1,000 Newton.
Physics 2.4, 9.1.2

PASSAGE 4

24. The correct answer is (C). Understanding organic chemistry nomenclature requires a command of Greek prefixes, which signify the number of carbon atoms found in a chain. Some common prefixes are meth (1), eth (2), prop (3), but (4), pent (5), hex (6), etc. Suffixes, representing types of covalent bonds found in the chemical, are then added to complete a name. "Ane" represents single covalent bonds; "ene" represents the presence of a double covalent bond; and "yne" represents a triple covalent bond. In drawing A we have 3 carbons and a single carbon covalent bond, thus the name is prop(3)ane(single) = propane.   *Organic Chemistry 3.1*

---

* For more information, refer to this section in Peterson's *Gold Standard MCAT*.

25. The correct answer is (B). The hexagonal "ring" is an abbreviation for benzene. Attaching "side chains" (in this case chlorine) to adjacent carbons (the 1,2 position) produces an *ortho* benzene compound.
  * *Organic Chemistry 5.1*

26. The correct answer is (D). Side chains on the 1,3 benzene positions are known as *meta* benzenes, and on the 1,4 positions they are known as *para* benzenes.   * *Organic Chemistry 5.1*

27. The correct answer is (D). In naming alcohols, it is imperative that the location of the hydroxyl (OH) side chain is included in the name of the chemical. There are 4 carbons in the chain, which gives the compound a "butane base," and the addition of the OH side chain to the second carbon gives the compound the name 2-butanol. *Note*: When "counting" carbons in a chain, begin from the side that gives the *lowest* value to the location. In this case, counting from right to left puts the OH side chain on the second carbon; counting from left to right would incorrectly put the OH side chain on the third carbon.
  * *Organic Chemistry 6.1*

28. The correct answer is (A). (See prefix and suffix explanation in answer 24.)
  * *Organic Chemistry 3.1, 4.3*

29. The correct answer is (D). The formula would be $C_{15}H_{32}$. Saturated hydrocarbons follow the algebraic formula C_nH_{2n+2} (C_n = the number of carbon atoms in the compound); therefore, to calculate the number of hydrogen atoms, one multiplies the number of carbon atoms by 2, and then adds 2 to the total.
  * *Organic Chemistry 3.1, 4.2.3*

PASSAGE 5

30. The correct answer is (A). There is only one force producing an acceleration. The acceleration is given by F = ma.
  * *Physics 2.2*

31. The correct answer is (B). Newton's 2nd law applies to each part of the system. Both masses have equal accelerations. T2 must accelerate both masses m1 and m2. T1 must accelerate only m1.   * *Physics 2.2*

32. The correct answer is (B). The frictional force is always opposite to the velocity. As the applied force accelerates the system to the right, the frictional force acts toward the left.   * *Physics 2.2*

33. The correct answer is (C). Static friction applies when the system is not moving. It always acts equal and opposite to the net force up to some maximum value. Once this value is exceeded, the system begins to move and kinetic friction takes over. Kinetic friction is always lower than static friction.   * *Physics 3.2*

34. The correct answer is (B). The frictional force is directly proportional to the normal (or perpendicular) force. For a horizontal surface, the normal force equals the weight of the object.
  * *Physics 3.2*

35. The correct answer is (D). Since the net force on the system is zero, the net acceleration of the system is zero. Starting from rest, the system does not move at all. Since the system is not moving, static friction applies. Static friction is always equal and opposite to the net force on the system, which in this case is zero.   * *Physics 2.2, 3.2*

---

* For more information, refer to this section in Peterson's *Gold Standard MCAT*.

PASSAGE 6

36. The correct answer is (C). Weight is a force.

W = mass × gravitational acceleration

W = 100kg × 9.8 m/s^2

* Physics 2.1

37. The correct answer is (C). The weight of an object is given by Newton's law of gravity:

$$F = \frac{Gm_1m_2}{r^2}$$

The man is now double the distance he was at the earth's surface; therefore, the denominator will be $(2)^2$ or four times greater, and his weight will only be ¼ as great.   ** Physics 2.4*

38. The correct answer is (B). By Newton's law of gravity, if the mass of the earth was doubled, then the numerator would be twice as great and the weight would be twice as great. The man's mass does not change in any event.
* Physics 2.1, 2.4

39. The correct answer is (A). Ignoring air resistance, all things in the earth's gravitational field accelerate at the same rate.   ** Physics 2.5*

40. The correct answer is (A). By Newton's law of gravity, the numerator is three times greater, and the denominator is $(2)^2$ or four times greater.
* Physics 2.4

41. The correct answer is (C). By Newton's law of gravity,

$$F = \frac{Gm_1m_2}{r^2}$$

We have, from the answer to the first question, that the force F acting on the man is 980 N. Since we also know the mass of the man (100kg), the radius of the earth (6.4×10^6 m), and the gravitational constant, we can solve for the mass of the earth.   ** Physics 2.4*

42. The correct answer is (B). The use of the words "atoms" and "ions" suggests that this configuration could be applied to an atom that has lost or gained electrons in order to achieve the $4s^2$, $4p^6$ status of stability. Only bromide ions fit the configuration listed above.
* General Chemistry 2.1, 2.2

43. The correct answer is (A). The *-ide* ending is associated with the naming of a binary compound.
* General Chemistry 3.3

44. The correct answer is (C). Mendeleev pioneered work in the organizing of matter in chart form, but he used the atomic mass, which later was shown to be flawed.   ** General Chemistry 2.3*

45. The correct answer is (D). This is the only choice associated with the addition of energy. The other three choices are associated with the removal of energy, which is what happens when a liquid solidifies.   ** General Chemistry 4.1.2, 8.7*

46. The correct answer is (A). The definition of an ideal gas is that it has no molecular volume and is used to theoretically explore temperature/pressure relationships.
* General Chemistry 4.1.8

---

* For more information, refer to this section in Peterson's *Gold Standard MCAT.*

PASSAGE 7

47. The correct answer is (C). As the cube drops, the force of the liquid increases with depth so that the pressure on all sides of the cube increases as it sinks.
  * Physics 6.1.2

48. The correct answer is (C). The apparent weight of the cube is equal to its weight in air minus the buoyant force, which is equal to the weight of the fluid displaced by the cube. The volume of liquid displaced does not change as the cube descends, so its apparent weight is constant and smaller than it was in air.   ** Physics 6.1.2*

49. The correct answer is (C). The buoyant force is the upward force of the fluid on the immersed cube. The bottom of the cube being at a lower depth will experience an upward force that will be greater than the downward force exerted on the top of the cube.
  * Physics 6.1.2

50. The correct answer is (A). Since the density of the liquid is greater, the buoyant force will be greater. Since the liquid is only slightly more dense, the increased buoyant force will not be so great as to cause it to rise and float.
  * Physics 6.1.2

51. The correct answer is (C). Any object will float in a fluid that has a higher specific gravity.   ** Physics 6.1.1, 6.1.2*

52. The correct answer is (D). Objects float if they have a lower density than the fluid in which they are floating.
  * Physics 6.1.1, 6.1.2

53. The correct answer is (A). The pressure in an incompressible fluid such as water is equal to the (density) × (gravity) × (depth). It is directly proportional to the depth below the surface.
  * Physics 6.1.2

54. The correct answer is (A). The pressure exerted by a fluid is given by

$$P = rgh;$$

r is the density of the fluid in mass/volume; *g* is the gravitational acceleration; and *h* is the depth below the surface. Salt water has a greater density than fresh water. At the same depth, the pressure would be greater for salt water than for fresh water.
  * Physics 6.1.2

PASSAGE 8

55. The correct answer is (C). Chlorine has an oxidation number of 0 on the left side of the equation ("free" elements always have an oxidation number of 0) and has an oxidation number of −1 on the right side. The change from $0 \Rightarrow -1$ indicates a *gain* of 1 electron; hence, chlorine is being *reduced*. It is also serving as the *oxidation agent* (bringing on the oxidation of sodium, which is losing an electron to chlorine).
  * General Chemistry 1.6

56. The correct answer is (C). In a compound, the sum of the individual oxidation numbers must total *zero*. Certain elements have "fixed" oxidation numbers in molecules. Hydrogen has an oxidation number of +1 (there are 2 hydrogen atoms in the molecule, giving a total of +2), and oxygen has a fixed value of −2 (there are 4 oxygen atoms in the molecule, producing a total of −8). Therefore, sulfur must be assigned a value, which, combined with the +2 contributed by the hydrogen and the −8 contributed by the oxygen, will produce a total of *zero* (+6).
  * General Chemistry 1.6

---

* For more information, refer to this section in Peterson's *Gold Standard MCAT*.

57. The correct answer is (A). Zinc is changing from an oxidation number of 0 as a free element on the left side of the equation to a value of +2 on the right side of the equation. This is the result of a loss of electrons, which means that elemental Zn is being oxidized. *General Chemistry 1.6*

58. The correct answer is (A). Lead is changing from an oxidation number of +4 on the left side of the equation to a value of +2 on the right side of the equation. This change is the result of a gain of 2 electrons; thus, lead is being reduced. The chemical that contains the species that is reduced ($PbCl_4$) is also called the oxidizing agent, because it is accepting the electrons from the species that is being oxidized in this reaction (Sn). *General Chemistry 1.6*

59. The correct answer is (C). The equation would be correctly balanced as:

$$2CO + 2NO \Rightarrow 2CO_2 + N_2$$
General Chemistry 1.5

60. The correct answer is (C). The individual oxidation numbers assigned to atoms in compounds must total *zero*. Since oxygen has a fixed value of −2 in compounds, carbon must then be assigned a value of +2 to make the total *zero*. *General Chemistry 1.6*

PASSAGE 9

61. The correct answer is (B). In a titration problem, the key concept is that moles of acid neutralize moles of base (or vice-versa). Dividing 0.5015 grams of sodium carbonate by the molecular mass (106 grams/mole) yields the number of moles of sodium carbonate being neutralized (.0047). From the balanced equation, we see that 2 moles of HCl are needed to neutralize each mole of sodium carbonate. Multiplying by 2 yields the number of HCl moles used. Substituting this into the molarity formula (molarity = moles/liter) will give the concentration (.00946 moles /0.04847 liters) = the concentration of 0.1952M. *General Chemistry 1.5.1, 5.3.1, 6.9*

62. The correct answer is (C). pH is defined as the $-\log_{10}$ of the hydrogen (hydronium) ion concentration. HCl is a strong acid that dissociates 100 percent into H^{+1} ions and Cl^{-1} ions. Since the dissociation is in a 1:1 ratio, the 0.1952M concentration will produce an equal concentration of H^{+1} ions, and the correct answer is the −log of this number. *General Chemistry 6.1, 6.5, 6.6.1*

63. The correct answer is (C). Commonly used indicators include litmus that turns from blue to red in an acid solution and red to blue in a basic solution; and phenolphthalein which is colorless in an acidic solution and turns red when the solution becomes basic. Since the solution is an acid with a pH < 2.0, litmus will be red, phenolphthalein will be colorless, and RioRed will be red (as described in the question). *General Chemistry 6.5, 6.9*

---

* For more information, refer to this section in Peterson's *Gold Standard MCAT.*

64. The correct answer is (D). Once again, we have the titration concept of moles of acid (sulfuric) being neutralized by moles of base (potassium hydroxide). The first step is to use the molarity equation to solve for moles of base. Moles = molarity (0.15) × liters (0.035), which equals 0.00525 moles. Now, from the balanced equation we see that 1 mole of acid requires 2 moles of base for neutralization: $\frac{0.00525}{2}$ = 0.00265 moles of acid neutralized. Dividing this by the volume of acid used (0.040 liters) results in the correct concentration (0.066M).
  General Chemistry 1.5.1, 5.3.1, 6.9

65. The correct answer is (B). The concentration of the H_2SO_4 was found to be 0.066 in the last problem. However, sulfuric acid is known as a *diprotic acid*, which means that 2 moles of H^{+1} ions are produced for every 1 mole of acid that dissociates. Therefore, the concentration of H^{+1} ion following dissociation is (2) × (0.066) or (0.132). The pH is the −log of this number (.88).   *General Chemistry 6.1, 6.5, 6.6.1*

66. The correct answer is (B). See the explanation for answer 63. The colors will be exactly the same, as the pH of the initial sample of sulfuric acid was < 2.0.   *General Chemistry 6.5, 6.9*

PASSAGE 10

67. The correct answer is (A). The lens equation is:

$$\frac{1}{D_O} + \frac{1}{D_I} = \frac{1}{f}.$$

Where D_O is the object distance, D_I is the image distance, and f is the focal length. The object distance is measured from the object to the lens and is positive if in the same direction as light rays traveling from the object to the lens, and negative if in the opposite direction. The image distance is measured from the lens to the image and is positive if in the same direction as light rays traveling from the lens to the image, and negative if in the opposite direction. The focal length is positive for convex lenses and negative for concave lenses.
  Physics 11.3, 11.4, 11.5

68. The correct answer is (A). When the object is on the focal point, light will emerge as parallel rays from the lens.
  Physics 11.3, 11.4, 11.5

69. The correct answer is (D). When the lens equation is used the image distance is negative. This is a virtual and erect image.   *Physics 11.3, 11.4, 11.5*

70. The correct answer is (C). A concave lens can form a virtual image only with a real object. The image distance is negative and is found to the left of the lens and is erect.   *Physics 11.3, 11.4, 11.5*

71. The correct answer is (A). Magnification is −(D_I/D_O). The image distance will always be negative and smaller than the object distance.   *Physics 11.3, 11.4, 11.5*

---

* For more information, refer to this section in Peterson's *Gold Standard MCAT.*

72. The correct answer is (D). By solving the lens equation, the focal length is +10 cm, which means it is a convex lens.   *Physics 11.3, 11.4, 11.5*

73. The correct answer is (A). For an ideal gas the internal energy is proportional to the temperature. Thus if the temperature stays constant, the internal energy of the gas, U, remains constant also. In this case, the first law of thermodynamics: $\Delta U = \Delta Q - W^{\text{by gas}}$ (where DU is the change in internal energy, DQ is the heat added to the system, and W is the work done by the system) becomes $0 = \Delta Q - W^{\text{by gas}}$ or $\Delta Q = W$.

Since the work done from A to B is equal to the area under the PV curve, we see that $\Delta Q = 7,000$ *Joules*.
   Physics 7.2, 7.6

74. The correct answer is (A). The effective resistance of a parallel combination of resistors R_1 and R_2 is:

$$\frac{1}{R_{effective}} = \frac{1}{R_1} + \frac{1}{R_2}$$

For circuit A, you can calculate the effective resistance of the parallel combination first. Then calculate the effective resistance of the parallel combination in series with the 300 Ω resistor. The parallel combination will be less than 100 Ω. The final series combination will be between 300 Ω and 400 Ω for A.

For circuit B, the effective resistance is less than 200 Ω.

For circuit C, the effective resistance is 300 Ω.   *Physics 10.2, 10.2.1*

75. The correct answer is (D). The mechanical advantage is a comparison of the force output of a machine to the force input by you. In an ideal machine, the work in is equal to the work out, no matter what the mechanical advantage. In a real machine, the work in is greater than the work out, because some work must also be done against friction. In the problem above, the work in is simply 90,000 Joules.
   Physics 5.1

76. The correct answer is (A). The pitch of the sound is high if the ear detects pressure maxima at a high rate.
   Physics 8.3, 8.5

77. The correct answer is (D). The lens formula relates the object distance, o; the image distance, i; and the focal length, f:

$$\frac{1}{f} = \frac{1}{i} + \frac{1}{o}$$

In this case, $\frac{1}{0.2cm} = \frac{1}{0.25cm} + \frac{1}{i}$

and i = 1 cm. The size of the image, D_i, is related to the size of the object, D_o, by:

$$\frac{D_i}{D_o} = (-)\frac{i}{o}$$

where the (−) sign indicates that if both i and o are positive, the image is inverted. In this case:

$$D_i = (-)D_o\frac{1cm}{0.25cm}$$

$$= (-)0.03cm\frac{1cm}{0.25cm}$$

$$= (-)0.12cm$$

so the image is inverted, and 0.12 cm in diameter.   *Physics 11.3, 11.4, 11.5*

---

* For more information, refer to this section in Peterson's *Gold Standard MCAT*.

Biological Science

Passage 1

1. The correct answer is (D). The pressure in the lungs must reach a value lower than that of the atmosphere. Lung volume increases due to contraction of the primary inspiratory muscles, the diaphragm, and the external intercostals.   *Biology 12.4*

2. The correct answer is (B). At high altitudes the atmospheric pressure is lower, causing increased ventilation, which decreases arterial CO_2 pressure. Conflicting chemical signals may actually result in short oscillating periods of both apnea and hyperventilation. The decrease in atmospheric pressure causes a longer-term adaptation, including a higher hematocrit and a decrease in pH of the cerebrospinal fluid.   *Biology 12.4.1; Physics 6.1.2; General Chemistry 4.1.7*

3. The correct answer is (C). A slow ascent prevents a rapid decrease in pressure, thus minimizing the release of bubbles of nitrogen gas into the bloodstream. If a slow ascent is not possible, divers may be placed in a hyperbaric chamber.

4. The correct answer is (B). Oxygenated blood (with oxyhemoglobin) is a bright red color and is carried away from the lungs by the arteries, to deliver oxygen to deoxygenated tissues. Venous blood carries deoxygenated blood back to the lungs to exchange CO_2 for O_2 in the capillaries.   *Biology 7.5.1*

5. The correct answer is (B). The driving force for diffusion of oxygen from arterial blood into tissues at the arteriolar end of the pulmonary capillaries is the difference between the PO_2 of alveolar air and that of the pulmonary arterial blood.   *Biology 1.1.1, 7.5.1*

6. The correct answer is (C). The increased pressure in plasma will help force O_2 into the surrounding tissues until equilibrium is reached.   *Biology 7.5.1*

7. The correct answer is (D). An increase in $[H^+]$ decreases pH. In addition, some H^+ binds to hemoglobin, reducing the affinity of hemoglobin for O_2. As shown in the preceding question, this decrease in pH results in a change in PO_2 and a subsequent increase in oxygen unloading.   *Biology 7.5.1, 12.4.1; General Chemistry 6.5*

Passage 2

8. The correct answer is (C). The group not given the experimental treatment but subjected to all other environmental variables serves as the control.   *Appendix C1, C2*

9. The correct answer is (D). A general observation was used to draw a specific conclusion or to make a specific prediction.   *Appendix C1*

10. The correct answer is (B). Since the control, Group A, developed no tumors, the tumor development appears to be due to the drug. Since more tumors developed as the dosage was increased, the effect appears to be dose-dependent.

---

* For more information, refer to this section in Peterson's *Gold Standard MCAT*.

11. The correct answer is (A). Since the control group did not receive the drug, and none of the mice developed tumors, while some mice in each of the treatment groups did, the drug appears to be causing the tumors.   *Appendix C1*

12. The correct answer is (C). The dose-effect is very clear under these circumstances, as well.

13. The correct answer is (B). This could be a possible conclusion because the control group had a higher incidence of tumors than Group B, which received the lowest dosage of Alpha-10.

PASSAGE 3

14. The correct answer is (D). Based on the given opinion of Dr. Buckeye, it is logical to assume that the hypothesis would reflect her opinion, based on what she had observed.   *Appendix C1*

15. The correct answer is (B). Yield is dependent upon treatment.
 Appendix C1

16. The correct answer is (A). The treatment is the independent variable.
 Appendix C1

17. The correct answer is (C). The experimenter chooses both the independent variable and the levels of treatment by manipulating that variable in a controlled manner.   *Appendix C1*

18. The correct answer is (A). All environmental factors were controlled so they would have an equal effect on all treatment groups.   *Appendix C1*

19. The correct answer is (B). Evaluating yield obtained with all controlled variables present, but with no fertilizer treatment, serves as a negative control.   *Appendix C1*

20. The correct answer is (D). Repetition and reproducibility of results are essential when evaluating and validating experimental results.   *Appendix C1*

21. The correct answer is (C). Less than a 5% difference in yield may not be statistically significant. This would have to be determined by running many more repetitions and conducting statistical analysis of the data.
 Appendix C1

22. The correct answer is (A). At birth, red bone marrow fills the marrow cavity of all bones, and all red blood cells are produced here. By puberty, red marrow is found only in spongy bone, and much is gradually replaced by yellow fatty, inactive, marrow, except in the sternum, femur, humerus, ribs, and vertebrae.
 Biology 5.4.4, 11.3, 11.3.1

23. The correct answer is (C). Both contraction and relaxation require energy supplied by ATP.   *Biology 5.2*

24. The correct answer is (B). During heavy activity, ATP is used up rapidly and skeletal muscle aerobic activity, (oxidative phosphorylation), cannot meet the demand because soon the circulatory system cannot supply enough oxygen.
 Biology 4.5

---

* For more information, refer to this section in Peterson's *Gold Standard MCAT*.

25. The correct answer is (C). The veins are low pressure vessels which carry blood back to the heart, against gravity much of the time. The intima of the limb veins is folded at intervals to form venous valves to prevent backflow. Vein walls are thin and easily distended, the media smooth muscle content is much less and even absent in some protected areas such as within the skull. The adventitia contains arterial vasa vasorum which penetrate to the intima.
* *Biology 7.3*

26. The correct answer is (D).   * *Biology 7.5, 7.6, 11.3*

PASSAGE 4

27. The correct answer is (B). These cells are part of the nonspecific host defenses. The inflammatory reaction is mediated by a large number of chemicals, some of which are released by the neutrophils (also called polymorpho-nuclear cells, or PMN's).
* *Biology 7.5, 7.6, 8.2*

28. The correct answer is (B). The subset of T lymphocytes sometimes referred to as cytotoxic T cells is responsible for type of activity. However, not all T lymphocytes engage in this type of activity.
* *Biology 7.5, 7.6, 8.2*

29. The correct answer is (A). A differential WBC count is routinely used to determine the percentage of each type of WBC present in order to make a comparison to a normal range of values. It may also be used as an indicator of certain infections and diseases such as leukemia.

30. The correct answer is (C). Lymphocytes proliferate in lymphoid leukemia, and PMNs proliferate in myeloid leukemia. Despite proliferation, these cells fail to function normally.

31. The correct answer is (B). Plasma cells are the effector stage of B-lymphocyte development, and in this stage of activation they produce antibodies. This is known as a humoral (or antibody-mediated) immune response.
* *Biology 8.2*

32. The correct answer is (C). The lymphocytes are agranulocytes, because of their lack of granules in their cytoplasm, as can be seen after a differential WBC staining procedure.   * *Biology 7.5*

PASSAGE 5

33. The correct answer is (B). Lactic acid is one of the products of fermentation.
* *Biology 4.5*

34. The correct answer is (B). The three-carbon pyruvate gets converted to a two-carbon acetyl group, which bonds to coenzyme A. The carbon lost from pyruvate leaves the cell in the form of CO_2.   * *Biology 4.5*

35. The correct answer is (C). Glycolysis takes place in the cytosol of eukaryotic cells and in the protoplasm of bacterial cells.   * *Biology 4.5*

36. The correct answer is (D). Each step in both pathways involves enzyme-substrate reactions. Those that form ATP involve substrate-level phosphorylation.
* *Biology 4.6, 4.7*

---

* For more information, refer to this section in Peterson's *Gold Standard MCAT.*

37. The correct answer is (C). Electrons move through the ETS in a series of oxidation-reduction reactions, and H^+ ions pass through the ATP-synthase complex to form ATP.   *Biology 1.2.1, 4.8*

38. The correct answer is (A). The NAD^+ carries electrons from both glycolysis and the Krebs cycle to the ETS. FAD carries electrons from the Krebs cycle. *Biology 4.5, 4.7, 4.8, 4.9*

39. The correct answer is (B). Oxygen is reduced after the electrons pass through ETS, forming water as a by-product of respiration. *Biology 4.10*

40. The correct answer is (B). The net production from all three metabolic pathways is 38 ATP. In eukaryotes, 2 ATP may be used to transport NADH into the mitochondria after glycolysis, for a net production of 36 ATP. *Biology 2.2, 4.10*

PASSAGE 6

41. The correct answer is (A). Antidiuretic hormone helps the body retain water. Alcohol inhibits its production. *Biology 6.3.1, 6.3.2, 10.3*

42. The correct answer is (B). The other answer choices are exactly the reverse of what occurs.   *Biology 10.3*

43. The correct answer is (C). Aldosterone regulates sodium and potassium levels as well as fluid volumes. It causes sodium absorption and potassium secretion in kidney tubules. *Biology 6.3.2*

44. The correct answer is (A). The loop of Henle helps concentrate NaCl in extracellular fluids so that water will be reabsorbed by the body.   *Biology 10.3*

45. The correct answer is (C). Glucose is not normally found in urine. Its presence may indicate diabetes mellitus, pancreatitis, lowered renal glucose threshhold, or coronary thrombosis. *Biology 10.3*

46. The correct answer is (C). Filtration occurs in the glomerulus as the blood plasma and most of its contents pass through tiny pores into Bowman's capsule. Blood cells and the plasma proteins remain in the blood vessels and do not filter into the tubules of the nephron. Tubular reabsorption returns most of the water, dissolved salt, and the nutrients back to the blood.   *Biology 10.3*

47. The correct answer is (A). Cardiac muscle consists of elongated round striated branching cells, each with a single centrally placed nucleus. These branching cells are joined together at intercalated disks to function as a unit (a syncytium).   *Biology 5.2*

48. The correct answer is (C). The SA node is the cardiac pacemaker because it depolarizes most rapidly. Impulses starting in the SA node pass to the atrial internodal pathways, then to the AV node or atrioventricular node. *Biology 11.2*

49. The correct answer is (D).   *Biology 7.5*

50. The correct answer is (D). *Biology 7.5, 8.1, 8.2*

51. The correct answer is (C). The distal convoluted tubule begins with this modified structure, the macula densa, which is a part of the juxtaglomerular apparatus; has low epithelium and a few microvilli, but no brush border. *Biology 6.3.5, 10.3*

---

* For more information, refer to this section in Peterson's *Gold Standard MCAT*.

PASSAGE 7

52. The correct answer is (A). Negative feedback, whether mechanical or biological, is a mechanism that turns off an active process by the end product of the process. The other answers are examples of positive feedback to turn on or activate the system.
Biology 6.3.6

53. The correct answer is (B). Most body functions occur within a narrow range of conditions such as pH, temperature, and osmolarity. *Biology 6.3.1, 6.3.6*

54. The correct answer is (C). Blood is a liquid connective tissue.
Biology 5.4, 5.4.1, 5.4.2, 5.4.3

55. The correct answer is (D). Muscle action generates heat.
Biology 13.1

56. The correct answer is (B). Prostaglandins, derived from arachadonic acid, are a diverse group of molecules that regulate cellular and physiologic function.
Biology 6.1

57. The correct answer is (B). According to this theory, thin filaments slide over thick filaments. The increased overlap of filaments shortens sarcomeres without changing the length of the individual filaments. *Biology 5.2*

PASSAGE 8

58. The correct answer is (A). The concentration of mitochondria is (from highest to lowest) SO > FOG > FG. The cells in the fiber most dependent on oxidative processes for ATP production require the greatest number of mitochondria, since the oxidative and aerobic processes are located in these organelles. As the name implies, the SO fibers are most dependent on mitochondrial functions, while FG fibers primarily use glycolysis as a source of ATP. The FOG fibers also use glycolysis (which is carried out in the cytosol), as well as cellular respiration, as major sources of ATP and therefore constitute an intermediate type. *Biology 4.4*

59. The correct answer is (C). Oxygen is required to produce ATP by oxidative processes, a major source of ATP for FOG fibers and the major source of ATP for SO fibers as the fiber names imply.
Biology 4.4, 7.5.1

60. The correct answer is (D). SO and FOG fibers are rich in myoglobin, the oxygen-carrying pigment that gives red muscle its color. This is why duck is mainly dark meat and chicken white— ducks are adapted for the rigors of long-distance flight and have many SO fibers. Chickens have descended from birds adapted to making short, fast flights to escape predators and have more FG fibers as a result.
Biology 4.4, 7.5.1

61. The correct answer is (A). Muscles used in short, intensive tasks (fast-twitch) require ATP from glycolysis since the oxygen demand quickly outstrips the oxygen supply in the muscle, and ATP must be supplied by an anaerobic means. Longer, less intensive tasks require steady supplies of ATP over a time, and these needs can be met aerobically through cellular respiration in FOG and SO tissues. SO fibers have the highest oxygen demand, with FOG fibers being intermediate between SO and FG fibers. *Biology 4.4, 4.5*

---

* For more information, refer to this section in Peterson's *Gold Standard MCAT.*

62. The correct answer is (A). The SO fiber is the smallest, a fact that helps by making oxygen more available to cells and by making it easier to get rid of carbon dioxide by diffusion into the blood.

PASSAGE 9

63. The correct answer is (A). Lipids are poor conductors of electricity, and so the myelin coating serves to help conduct the electrical impulses. It contains no neurotransmitters and so does not contain nor even serve to break them down.   ** Biology 5.1, 5.1.2*

64. The correct answer is (D). While all cells possess an action potential—an electrical difference across their membranes—the unique ability of the neuron is to be able to change the action potential. Like the neurons, all other cells can change the rate of diffusion as the concentration of molecules changes, carry on osmosis, and change the rate of active transport, given sufficient ATP.   ** Biology 5.1.2*

65. The correct answer is (B). There is no contact between presynaptic and postsynaptic cells. The space between them [the synapse] never closes during the normal release of neurotransmitters. The other three statements are true of the passing of the so-called "nerve impulse" from one neuron to the other.   ** Biology 5.1*

66. The correct answer is (B). Motor neurons serve to control the outer environment by being invested in skeletal muscles, but also control the inner environment by a similar investment in the visceral musculature. By

responding to both internal and external changes, the nervous system also plays a vital role in homeostasis, through sensory and motor neuron involvement, helping to carry out both conscious and unconscious [or subconscious] activities of the body.   ** Biology 6.1, 6.1.1, 6.1.2, 6.1.3, 6.1.4, 6.2*

67. The correct answer is (C). The brain contains both types of cells: The myelinated cells are in the inner regions and the unmyelinated cells are in the outer regions.   ** Biology 6.1*

PASSAGE 10

68. The correct answer is (B). The contraction of the inspiratory muscles (primarily of the dome-shaped diaphragm) results in an overall increase in the volume of the lungs, decreasing the pressure.   ** Biology 12.4*

69. The correct answer is (C). Myoglobin is not found within the blood and only about 1.5% of oxygen is freely dissolved in the plasma.   ** Biology 7.5.1*

70. The correct answer is (B). Boyle's Law states that when temperature is constant, the pressure of a gas varies inversely with its volume. Dalton's Law of partial pressures states that the total pressure exerted by a mixture of gases is the sum of the pressures exerted independently by each gas in the mixture which will be proportional to its percentage in the total gas mixture.   ** General Chemistry 4.1.4, 4.1.7*

---

* For more information, refer to this section in Peterson's *Gold Standard MCAT.*

71. The correct answer is (A). Carbonic acid is particularly unstable in the blood and rapidly dissociates to form HCO_3^-. Although carbon dioxide is freely dissolved and carried as carbaminohemoglobin, together they account for only 30–40% of the total transported.
  * Biology 12.4.1

72. The correct answer is (B). Both increases in acidity (the Bohr Effect) and temperature, promote the dissociation of oxyhemoglobin. Working muscles do not release carbon monoxide nor 2,3-DPG.   ** Biology 7.5.1*

73. The correct answer is (A). The descending limb of the loop of Henle and the ascending limb set up a countercurrent multiplier mechanism in the medulla where the fluids flowing in opposite directions increase the efficiency of solute exchange.   ** Biology 10.3*

74. The correct answer is (D). The macula densa senses if the level of sodium is low and renin is secreted. Angiotensin II is formed, which acts on the adrenal cortex to increase the secretion of the hormone aldosterone, which regulates the conservation of sodium.
  * Biology 6.3.2, 6.3.5, 10.3

75. The correct answer is (A). The dermis or corium contains blood vessels, lymphatic channels, nerves, sensory nerve endings, hair follicles, sweat glands, sebaceous glands, cellular elements, a small amount of fat, and smooth muscles. Melanin is in the epidermis.   ** Biology 13.2*

76. The correct answer is (D). The sebaceous glands are holocrine glands (holos is Greek for "all"), which are not common in the body. A holocrine gland accumulates secretory products in its cytoplasm and then dies and degenerates. The dead cell, all of it, is the secretion. Sebaceous glands of the inner eyelid are called Meibomian glands and those of the eyelashes are Moll glands and Zeis glands.   ** Biology 13.2, 13.3*

77. The correct answer is (D). Hair is not important in man for retaining body warmth, but the hair follicle is important in skin repair. Cuts and surgical incisions through the three layers of the skin heal in a uniform manner. Fibrin forms in the bottom of the V-shaped slit in the dermis of tissue held together by sutures, and the epidermis on each side begins to bend down into the slit.
  * Biology 13.1, 13.2, 13.3

---

* For more information, refer to this section in Peterson's *Gold Standard MCAT.*

Unit 1

VERBAL REASONING STRATEGIES

The Verbal Reasoning portion of the MCAT closely resembles reading comprehension tests that you have taken in the past. The passage selections may come from the sciences, social sciences, or humanities. You are not expected to be familiar with the content of all of these passages, since you are reading for comprehension, inference, and evaluation rather than for content. Therefore, prior knowledge of the subject matter is irrelevant, although you may be familiar with most of the material. There are a number of strategies for approaching the Verbal Reasoning selections.

Basically, the selections with their questions require a close reading. The questions will fall into four primary categories:

1. COMPREHENSION: Questions of this type test your ability to read and understand a given selection on any topic. In order to comprehend, you may bring your own knowledge and/or experience to the reading of the selection; however, comprehension demands that you read and understand the given selection without ancillary suggestions. Comprehension questions call for your synthesis of the material, as well as your recall of specific information.

2. EVALUATION: Questions of this type test your ability to look at presented material and evaluate (measure) the reliability of the information contained therein to relate to the position being proffered. Evaluation questions demand that you read for understanding in order to draw upon the presented information to support certain other premises or statements. Such questions test your ability to analyze and utilize the material presented.

3. APPLICATION: Questions of this type test your ability to utilize the information presented in different situations and for different purposes. Often, these questions require you to reach an independent conclusion based upon the material presented as well as the authorial tone and intent. Occasionally, these questions will contain unfamiliar vocabulary words that will require your reading in context in order to apply the theories and/or ideas presented.

4. INCORPORATION OF NEW INFORMATION: Questions of this type require that you apply new and different information to the given situation in the selection in order to reevaluate the conclusions and/or ideas presented. In order to incorporate new information successfully, you must read for content, evaluate material presented, and apply the new premise to that material in order to support or deny a presented argument or idea.

Your success on the Verbal Reasoning portion of this examination will be determined by your ability to read given selections in the sciences, social sciences, and humanities and to comprehend, evaluate, apply, and incorporate new information. Prior knowledge of the material covered is neither required nor expected. In fact, deliberate efforts have been made to locate and present obscure passages in order to test your abilities specifically in verbal reasoning.

Nine passages of reading material will be presented to you, and each will average between 500 and 600 words. Sixty-five questions total will be asked from these passages. Your time for this section is 85 minutes. This means that you should practice your reading skills in order to complete the selections in the least amount of time. Normally, an adult can read such a passage in three minutes. This means that you will spend about 27 minutes in reading time alone. That will leave you with 58 minutes to answer 65 questions. So each question must be handled in less than 1 minute. You should practice your reading for meaning in order to cut down on the time required specifically for reading the passage and have more time with which to answer the questions involved.

There are a number of suggestions for improving reading speed. However, you must keep in mind that skimming an article is not going to give you the necessary information for making certain evaluations and applications; you may indeed even find it necessary under these circumstances to reread sections or whole passages, which will be time-consuming and counterproductive. There are two primary suggestions for you to consider in practicing your reading with speed.

First, consider reading the questions BEFORE you read the actual passage itself. Notice, the suggestion is to read the QUESTION before reading the selection, not the answers. Many readers find that reading the questions AND the answers prior to reading the selection sets certain ideas or phrases in the subconscious, which can result in preformed opinions. By reading the question first, you are able to formulate some idea of what to look for as you read the passage. Utilize the practice tests here to read the question and then the passage and determine if you do not have a better focus when you read.

Second, consider approaching long selections by reading ONLY the first sentence in each paragraph of the selection to determine if the topics you are seeking would be discussed within that paragraph. Most paragraphs have a topic sentence, which will reveal the contents of the paragraph. As you practice, utilize this technique and determine its desirability as a tool to improve your reading speed. After you read the first sentence, you may ignore the rest of the paragraph if you feel that the topic you are seeking is NOT contained in that paragraph. This saves a wealth of time.

Third, if you are uncomfortable reading ONLY the first sentence, you might try skimming the paragraph for relevance. Skimming a paragraph, unlike skimming an entire selection, allows you to determine if there is information of value in your search. If you pick up a key word or idea in your skimming, then you can read the entire paragraph for meaning.

You should realize quickly that this method will not work for everyone. The suggestion is made that you try it on the practice tests as a time-saving technique. If you find you are spending more time rereading after skimming or searching the first sentence, then you should not employ these suggestions; instead, read the entire selection for meaning.

Fourth, practice so that you can learn how to read a selection for information only and not become involved with the material presented. In your studies to this point, you have read both for information and retention knowing that the material would become a part of your knowledge base for future use; therefore, you have read with the idea of remembering and utilizing the information. That is not the case with these readings. Remember that you are reading for the four purposes presented—comprehension, evaluation, application, and incorporation of new material. The more you become involved with the material presented, the slower your rate of reading will become. Hopefully, the articles presented will be interesting enough to hold your attention; however, you should avoid pausing to think about the material or to react to it personally. Remember, you are not reading for enjoyment or for residual utilization of the material, but you are reading for information. The more you practice reading for information ONLY, the better your reading speed will become.

As you detach yourself from the reading for meaning, you must remember to discipline yourself to look ONLY for the answers to the questions you have already read. A good idea is to practice reading for information only, and if you find yourself becoming involved or your mind wandering, then force yourself to stop and start over. After you do this a number of times, you will train yourself to read ONLY for the information presented and not for any implication beyond that.

Your success with the Verbal Reasoning portion of the MCAT is largely dependent upon your good reading habits. Remember

that you learned to read a very long time ago and have utilized that skill in a number of ways for learning as well as for enjoyment. You may not enjoy reading and never do it for pleasure; however, you may be an insatiable reader who enjoys and becomes involved with every work you encounter. Whichever description fits you, you must divorce your thinking from either disliking or enjoying reading and concentrate only on the understanding and utilization of the information presented.

Practice focusing on the main idea, or theme, of each passage presented. Most readers can determine the main idea of the article after a cursory reading. You may assume that almost every passage will be followed with a question concerning the main idea, or theme, of the work. As you practice, also pay attention to details. Usually there will be questions that require you to focus on small details presented. Be aware of this as you read. Unusual words, unique emphasis, or other clues can reveal to you that this is a detail upon which you should focus.

Of great importance in reading for speed and information is your ability to determine the differences among inferred, implied, and stated facts. Each selection will present you with the need to determine an inferred fact, an implied conclusion, and/or stated facts. One of the favorite questioning techniques is to ask for what is inferred and what is not, or to differentiate between what is implied and what is not implied. You will likely be called upon to insert new information into an inference or implication and determine "if this is true, then the outcome will be that." You should be prepared to make that application.

Some of the selections with which you are presented will call upon you to follow the logical path the author sets for you, whether you agree with it or not. In addition, you will be called upon to judge arguments made by the author with which you may or may not agree. Again, you are reading the selection for the material presented ONLY, not for accuracy or coordination with your own ideas and or knowledge.

As you read, you should make certain that you do not misinterpret any of the author's statements. Remember, this author is writing from a point of view that you can determine by your reading, but which you may misinterpret if your are not aware of the author's purpose for writing. Your own point of view is not a matter of consideration in these selections. Focus upon what the author thinks, believes, and presents, and the order in which this is done.

Having focused upon the technique of reading first sentences of paragraphs, you should be aware that some questions will call upon you to determine differences between the ideas presented in different paragraphs. This is where your ability to focus upon the topics presented in different paragraphs becomes very important. Remember that each paragraph, just like the selection itself, has a main idea, or theme. The paragraphs work together to make the central idea, or theme. You will be required to make these applications in some of the selections.

Now that you have improved your speed and comprehension in reading, you should focus upon the types of questions with which you will be presented. There are several types of questions used by the preparers of this test; each of them examines a different aspect of your ability to read for information, draw conclusions, and analyze. The following list should be examined closely, since it explains the various types of questions you will encounter.

MAIN-IDEA questions call upon you to comprehend and select the central idea, or theme, of each selection. Remember, you have focused upon this as you have read.

You should begin the reading with the following question in mind: "What is this author trying to say to me?" That one idea you glean as you read becomes the main idea upon which you focus to answer the main-idea question, which will inevitably be presented in some form. Focus upon, "What is the author's purpose?" That purpose becomes the main idea.

PURPOSE questions are those that require you to understand the author's reason for writing this selection. Remember, this may have been written to describe an incident or item, to narrate an anecdote or situation, to explain a proposition or procedure, or to persuade the reader about the author's point of view. There is a purpose, and your ability to understand that will provide you with answers to several types of questions. Be sure that you can determine purpose in your practice readings.

INFERENCE questions require you to understand the author's logic and to follow the purpose for which the article is being written. Remember you may be asked to determine what types of inferences may and may NOT be made from the reading of a different selection. Be very careful not to let your own thoughts and/or ideas intrude into your ability to make inferences. A good tip to remember is that inferences are NOT spelled out for you in the selection, but rather call upon you to take facts and decide what is meant or what reasonable inference can be assumed.

EVIDENCE questions require you to examine the supporting facts the author presents for the argument of the selection. Some questions will ask you to identify that evidence as it is utilized by the author. Some questions will call upon you to evaluate the evidence for its appropriateness to the main idea as it is presented. Some of the articles presented in this examination will be persuasive in nature; therefore, you must practice using and examining supporting evidence as it is given to you by the author. One of the abilities you should train yourself for in the practice is to examine evidence AS it is presented and determine its relevance to the article presented.

ANALYSIS questions call upon you to look at the information presented and determine relationships. These relationships may be between what is presented and what is implied in the article. Basically, you are being asked to understand the method by which the author presents the material and then to evaluate for yourself whether or not the argument or situation presented is valid or invalid. Your ability to analyze will allow you to discard certain information as you read and to focus ONLY upon that which is appropriate to the argument presented. Be advised that when one analyzes a selection, one must remember to avoid the pitfall of allowing personal knowledge and/or opinion to intrude. Again, remember, you are reading for information ONLY.

NEW INFORMATION questions call upon you to insert information that may be contradictory, extraneous, or appropriate into the given situation in order to predict the effect upon the case presented. Again, you will be called upon to put aside your own ideas and opinions and to focus ONLY upon the facts at hand. The new information should be inserted into the dynamics of the situation as presented so that you can draw conclusions based upon that situation only.

SYNTHESIS or CONCEPT questions will call upon you to take the author's ideas and then determine the author's validity of conclusion or argument. Most readers find these questions to be the most difficult and time-consuming to consider. The reason for the difficulty is that your own basic knowledge and opinion may be a matter at hand, and you have to avoid using that. The word synthesis calls upon you to take what is given, apply to it what is implied or inferred, and reach a logical conclusion based ONLY upon the evidence at hand. Once you understand that definition and make the effort to do just that, you will be successful with this type of question.

IMPLICATION questions require that you make judgments about what would follow if the author's premise is correct and is exercised. In your reading, you have often met with "if this is true then that must be true or would follow." This is a judgment call in your everyday life as you make decisions that affect minute issues and life-changing situations. The key to your success in handling these questions is to remember the author's main idea, evidence, and what will be the outcome within the parameters of the answers offered. You may not personally agree with any of the outcomes; however, you must again discard your own knowledge of the situation and react from the author's standpoint alone.

Now, with this background, the following section will present two passages that have been selected because they are the kind of items that might appear on the examination itself. The questions that follow each selection have been deliberately formulated as examples of the TYPES of questions you will be asked on the test itself. The correct answers appear at the end of this section, with each answer explained in order to help you to reason for answers when you are taking the examination itself. As you practice with these sessions, note the time it takes you to read the selection and determine if you need more practice on reading speed. Also, practice a cursory reading of the questions BEFORE reading the selections and/or the reading of topic sentences only. This will give you a good idea of which technique works best for you.

PASSAGE 1

Unfortunately, there are heroes who do not always act the part. Such a man was Dan Sickles, who won military fame in the Civil War; however, that fame was overshadowed by his personal lust for love and power. Unable to avoid the controversy in his life, Sickles seemed attracted by it. Though a politician, diplomat, friend of presidents, and a one-time presidential aspirant himself, he seemed to attract controversy in his life. From his mid-thirties until his death at the age of 94, his life was one of which fiction writers dream.

Born into wealth, Sickles was famous long before the beginning of the Civil War and even accompanied the U.S. ambassador to England as secretary of the American legation in London. He returned from this trip with a lovely 19-year-old bride to resume his political career and advance his standing in the U.S. House of Representatives. Sickles's friendship with James Buchanan, then President of the United States, caused his confidence to continue to grow.

Because Sickles was a notorious womanizer, his constant ignoring of his young and beautiful bride opened the door for her to have her own affair. She chose Philip Barton Key, the United States attorney for the District of Columbia and the son of the composer of the national anthem. Sickles learned of the affair, stalked Key, and shot him to death within sight of the White House.

Tried for the murder, Sickles was imprisoned for a short stint in a ''jailer's apartment,'' after which he became the first man acquitted of a crime because of the defense called ''temporary insanity.'' He publicly forgave his wife, an act with which society did not agree, but he never lived with her again. Shunned by his former friends, he was banished to his New York home.

Recognizing the preoccupation of society with the imminent war, Sickles seized the chance for a return to the mainstream political scene by becoming a fervent anti-secessionist. Sickles was responsible for advising Buchanan to keep the garrison at Fort Sumter in Charleston, a move that led to the outbreak of the Civil War in April 1861.

The war between the states of the United States of America raged. Barely had the last cannon fallen silent at Charleston when Sickles, in New York, began seeking volunteers to restore the Union by violent means. His small group with patriotic zeal seemed to overshadow the fact that the country was being torn asunder, and mending it would take more than a day and a dollar. Though he had been involved in scandals prior to the war, his popularity was renewed with the renewal of the conflict, and his efforts met with success. Authorized to raise a corps of 1,000, Sickles was far more successful than that. Within a month, enough recruits had been enlisted to fill a large brigade, which was sent into camp on Staten Island and sheltered under a circus tent purchased for the cause.

At first there was a controversy because the five regiments of volunteers had been raised by a democrat, Sickles, and the leader of the campaign was a republican. The issue was settled however, when Sickles was refused an appointment as a brigadier general when the nomination was tabled until March 1862 at which time it was rejected. Eventually, Sickles was given his appointment by the attorney general and President Lincoln, who were able to date the appointment from the time of its earlier rejection.

Even in uniform, this soldier found it difficult to live down his past. Politicians and editors decried his military appointment and branded his troops as disreputable as their commander. In camp in Washington and on the march in northeastern Virginia, the brigade was given a wide berth by other troops, some of whom put their derision into a little song that began, "Johnny Stole a Ham, and Sickles Killed a Man."

1. The tone of this excerpt from the life of Dan Sickles is:

    A. sympathetic.
    B. derisive.
    C. conciliatory.
    D. contradictory.

2. How might one describe the leadership of the Union army based upon the information in this article?

    A. There is evidence of capabilities to organize a standing army.
    B. The Union Army leadership was unreliable because of crimes in the past.
    C. Leadership of the Union army was vested in democrats.
    D. There is not enough evidence to draw a conclusion.

3. The example concerning the song of the soldiers is designed to demonstrate that:

    A. singing was used to break the tension of the war.
    B. the culture of the time was reflected in the words of the songs.
    C. the soldiers knew of the background of their leader.
    D. crime was rampant during the war.

4. Based upon information contained in this passage, one might believe that Sickles felt himself:

    A. a servant of the people of the United States.
    B. a reliable adviser to the President of the United States.
    C. beyond the law because of his personal and public positions.
    D. capable of leading the Union Army into the Civil War.

5. The author attempts to portray Sickles as a man who thought that:

    A. "the end justifies the mean."
    B. "all's fair in love and war."
    C. "don't do as I do, do as I say do."
    D. all of the above.

6. One might infer from information in this passage that Sickles's amazing ability to raise a regiment so quickly reflected his:

    A. commitment to the cause of America.
    B. desire to become a leader of men with a high rank.
    C. education in the art of war.
    D. abilities to speak fluently and fervently.

7. The lover taken by Sickles's wife is pictured as having notable:

   A. ancestry.
   B. valor.
   C. musicianship.
   D. patriotism.

8. A brigadier general, according to this article, is an officer who:

   A. commands at least 1,000 men.
   B. is appointed to the position.
   C. has authority over 5 regiments.
   D. all of the above.

ANSWERS TO PASSAGE 1

1. The correct answer is (D). The author of the article presents the subject, Dan Sickles, in a contradictory fashion—recognizing his potential but realizing his lack of control. Answer (A) is incorrect. There is no evidence of sympathy for Sickles. Answer (B) is incorrect; in order to be derisive, the tone would have to treat Sickles without respect and his contributions as meaningless. Answer (C) is incorrect; there is no effort on the part of the author to forgive Sickles for his lack of control.

2. The correct answer is (D). There is not enough evidence to make a conclusion about the overall leadership of the Union army. Answer (A) is incorrect.; While the efforts in New York seem successful, there is no evidence for other areas. Answer (B) is incorrect. One cannot base a judgment of an entire group on the actions of one man. Answer (C) is incorrect. The author makes the point of the efforts of both democrats and republicans.

3. The correct answer is (C). Though there had been a passage of time, the soldiers obviously knew of Sickles's crime. Answers (A) and (B) are incorrect. Although both may be true, there is no evidence in the article to support either theory. Answer (D) is incorrect. There is no evidence that others than Sickle committed crimes.

4. The correct answer is (C). Because he killed Key within sight of the White House and in front of many witnesses, apparently Sickles did feel himself above the law. Answer (A) is incorrect. There is no evidence that Sickles ever thought of himself as a servant of the people of the United States. Answer (B) is incorrect. Although he was an informal adviser to the President, there is no evidence of how he perceived himself in this position. Answer (D) is incorrect. While this may be true, the article only presents Sickles's opinion of himself as capable of being a general.

5. The correct answer is (D). All statements reflect the attitude of Dan Sickles. Answers (A), (B), and (C) are all correct. In murdering his wife's lover, Sickles was defending his home without regard to his own actions.

6. The correct answer is (B). The author states that Sickles was "stumping for volunteers to restore the Union by violent means" indicating his intent to fight. Answer (A) is not correct. There is no real evidence of patriotism in this selection, even though Sickles may have been a real patriot. Answer (C) is incorrect. While Sickles was eager to fight, there is no indication that he was schooled in war. Answer (D) is incorrect. While the statement may be true, there is no evidence to reflect it.

7. The correct answer is (A). The point is made that Sickles's victim was the son of Francis Scott Key. Answers (B), (C), and (D) are all incorrect. There is no evidence to support any of these attributes to Barton Key.

8. The correct answer is (D). All of the answers given are found in the article.

PASSAGE 2

Experiments with animals often give scientists valuable clues to the effect of drugs on human beings. In a recent study, an outstanding expert in the field of mental health hit upon the idea of using spiders, long known for their extraordinary sense of balance and direction as expressed by the nearly perfect symmetry of the webs they weave. In an effort to determine the effect of drugs, he "invited" thousands of spiders to a most unusual drug party. There they were supplied with amphetamines, tranquilizers, and barbiturates, and then they were watched to see how the drugged solution they had sipped from a syringe would affect their nervous and muscular systems. The results were amazingly graphic and easily analyzed, even for the layman.

The most common result could be seen quite easily in the irregular pattern of the webs woven by the spiders. The most "disturbed" patterns were caused by high doses of barbiturates. Two photographs were taken of the webs spun by each of the spiders in the experiment—one before the dosage was administered, and one after the drug had taken effect. The results were amazing and very obvious even to the untrained eye.

One of the spiders studied was a female cross spider (weight, 89.4 mg). Her first web was a normal pattern, woven under normal conditions. There was nothing exceptional in the pattern other than the amazing delicacy and symmetry long noted in the webs spun by spiders all over the world. There was a central area closely woven with spokes originating from a common source and extending to the outer rim of the web, each one carefully anchored on the outer radial of the web, from which there were connectors to the stabilizing supports of branches or other fixed material. From the cohesive center to the outer radial, there were parallel lines in ever-widening circles to form the web itself. The balance of the completed project was amazingly strong; the delicacy of the handiwork was incredibly precise. The stability of the web had been carefully calculated and the proper supports found. The finished product was typical of the toiling spider. Photographs were taken while the web was being spun, and several photographs were taken after the completion of the web.

The drug solution was administered to the spider for two days. When the spider had been stoned on Phenobarbital, another web was spun. The result was amazing. There were large gaps in the web, destroying the symmetry. Efforts had been made by the spider to keep the delicacy and to attempt the symmetry; however, the entire web was off center and not properly anchored. The center held together in a lopsided manner; however, as the radial connecting bands were strung there was little effort to maintain the spokes in an orderly manner. Indeed, two of the spokes were woven so that they were parallel and even connected at certain meeting points with the radial bands. Three of the areas were so weak that they all but disintegrated. One area totally collapsed after the fourth band. Two of the areas at the top of the web were so heavy that the rest of the web was given to supporting these two areas. The overall effect was a hodgepodge and certainly not in keeping with the orderly and delicate symmetry of the spider's first web.

1. The example of the spider's web is designed to demonstrate that:

   A. spiders have an extraordinary capacity for working even in unusual circumstances.
   B. a spider, like a human, performs in a diminished capacity when subjected to barbiturates.
   C. most spiders know how to anchor a web carefully in order to stabilize its parts.
   D. spiders are aware of the need for order in their lives and use the web as a means of attracting food.

2. Based upon the information contained in this passage, one might assume that the introduction of barbiturates into an animal would cause:

   A. diminished sex drive or impotence.
   B. occasional difficulty in swallowing.
   C. inability to do common tasks properly.
   D. the making of poor choices.

3. Because a female spider is used in this experiment, one might infer that a male spider would:

   A. spin a more substantial web of increased size and strength.
   B. react to the introduction of the chemicals negatively, spinning no web.
   C. demonstrate an increased capacity for productivity and potency.
   D. have a similar reaction to the introduction of the barbiturates.

4. Based upon the information given, one can determine that the web of the spider resembles:

   A. a wheel with a rim, spoke, and hub.
   B. the delicate lace of a tablecloth.
   C. the intricate design of a geometric figure.
   D. all of the above.

5. The author's use of the word "disturbed" indicates that:

   A. dramatic differences were observed.
   B. the spider was erratic in behavior.
   C. there was a failure to react.
   D. the spider's web was irregular in pattern.

6. The BEST title for this selection would be:

   A. When Spiders Take to Drugs.
   B. Insects and the Effect of Barbiturates.
   C. Webs Can Be Beautiful.
   D. Disturbed Spiders.

ANSWERS TO PASSAGE 2

1. The correct answer is (B). The point is carefully made that prior to the introduction of the drugs there were outstanding qualities, some of which diminished with the dosage of drugs. Answer (A) is incorrect. While it may be a true statement, it is not the main idea of this article. Answer (C) is incorrect: the stability of the web is stated; however, it is not the main idea. Answer (D) is incorrect. There is no mention of the uses of the web in this article.

2. The correct answer is(C). The point is made that the spinning of the web is a task spiders do regularly. The introduction of drugs caused it to be done improperly. Answer (A) is incorrect. There is no mention of the spider's sex drive or potency. Answer (B) is incorrect. The ability to swallow is not mentioned. Answer (D) is incorrect. There is no mention of choices except in selection the stabilizers; however, the spider's choice or lack thereof is not mentioned.

3. The correct answer is (D). There is no information given upon which to base an opinion that gender had an effect on this study. Answer (A) is incorrect. In order to determine the stability of a web woven by a male versus a female spider, one would need information not given herein. Answer (B) is incorrect. There is no evidence for this conclusion. Answer (C) is incorrect. No evidence is given upon which to base this conclusion.

4. The correct answer is (D). Using the information given, one may form a mental picture of the wheel because of the mention of the spoke, the center, and the parallel bands; a lacy tablecloth because of the "delicacy and symmetry" mentioned; a geometric figure because of the emphasis upon the symmetry of the design. Therefore, all answers are correct.

5. The correct answer is (D). The author uses the word disturbed in connection with the description of the pattern. Answer (A) is incorrect. While the statement is true, it is NOT the best answer for the use of the word disturbed. Answer (B) is incorrect. Erratic behavior has no base in the word in question. Answer (C) is incorrect. The spider did react and did spin.

6. The correct answer is (A). Titles require the mention of the important words or topics with which the article deals. This one is about "spiders" and "drugs"; therefore, this would be the best title. Answer (B) is incorrect. "Insects" are not mentioned in the article. Answer (C) is incorrect. The beauty of the web is described to make the point of difference; however, the focus is not the web. Answer (D) is incorrect. The word disturbed is in the article as is the word spiders; however, the cause of the "disturbance" is the focus, not the disturbance itself.

At this point, you should have a fairly clear understanding of what will be required of you on the Verbal Reasoning section of the MCAT. As you go through the practice tests in this book, take the time to refer back to this chapter if you have any questions or difficulty with any of the material in this section of the test.

Unit 2

One of the most important tools available to man, regardless of occupation or profession, is the ability to communicate—verbally and nonverbally. Certainly the art of written communication is vital. The physician must be able to articulate in writing records and/or medical histories with clarity and precision as well as communicate directly with patients, colleagues, and other professionals when the need arises. Perhaps the greatest need for clarity and precision in written communication comes when the physician must collaborate with others to formulate policy, present proposals, and persuasively direct decisions concerning health care. The myth about the physician and his or her poor handwriting on prescriptions will not be dismissed in the foreseeable future, but today's physician can make great inroads toward dismissing the myth that health-care professionals are a part of the technical profession that limits itself to the bare essentials of communication. In a world that is increasingly technology-driven, patients in the care of physicians require communication that is expressive, articulate, and filled with the compassion that drives one into the practice of medicine.

Increasingly, medical school admissions indicate, and faculty members underscore, the vitality of superior writing skills on the part of their students. In response to these requests, this section has been added to the MCAT in order to more properly evaluate the communication skills of aspiring physicians with the goal of demonstrating clarity, cohesion, organization, analysis, and presentation. These results will be used in the medical school admissions procedure to evaluate candidates based upon their communication skills, in addition to the factual responses required on the remainder of the MCAT.

The Writing Sample of the MCAT consists of two 30-minute essays that have been designed to measure skills in:

1. brainstorming a topic to develop a thesis or main idea;

2. organizing information and ideas in a clear and logical manner;

3. analyzing and synthesizing ideas into concepts and explaining, persuading, and informing;

4. presenting ideas into a logical, cohesive whole; and

5. writing with clarity while following the accepted practices of English grammar, syntax, punctuation, diction, and vocabulary expected in a first draft within a given time limit.

DEFINITION

An essay, by definition, is a structured, creative, written composition dealing with a specific and limited subject from a more or less personal point of view. For the physician, the essay format provides the opportunity to analyze situations, people, and circumstances in order to preserve them for further use and for sharing. The permanence of the written essay allows the physician not only to preserve the ideas of the moment, but to preserve self and professional integrity and discovery. The writer benefits from the written essay as much as the reader, for in presentation the author learns more about the subject, self, and the profession of medicine itself, while sharpening thinking and organizational skills that are beneficial in all parts of life. Since the essay is a reflection of the author, it provides the thrill and satisfaction by preserving ideas, insight, emotion, attitude, knowledge, and application possessed by the author alone. The finished product is both personally and professionally rewarding.

SUGGESTIONS FOR WRITING THE MCAT ESSAY

The structure of the MCAT essay varies somewhat from the traditional essay consisting of a prompt (statement) that is designed to evoke from the writer an expository (explanatory) response that may express an opinion, discuss a philosophy, or describe a policy in a clear and concise but original manner. The structure is simple: The first section will make the statement of opinion, philosophy, or policy; the second section will explain or interpret the statement in a thorough and insightful manner; the third section explores the statement through the use of illustrations—either real or hypothetical—providing examples that present oppositions and/or contradictions; the fourth step is to discuss ways in which the contradictions of the third step and the statement in the second step may be reconciled while applying the writer's knowledge and understanding of the topic to the conflicts raised while reinforcing the initial statement; the fifth and last step is to draw the entire presentation into a cohesive conclusion that will leave the reader with an understanding of the author's position on the principle raised by the writing.

TIPS ON WRITING THE MCAT ESSAY

THINKING

Before beginning any writing, carefully think through the writing prompt: consider the issues involved and as many of the possible responses as possible while you focus on the task at hand:

1. Will your response require persuading, explaining, informing, or comparing?

2. Will you need to supply specific details, and if so, do you have those details readily available within your immediate knowledge?

3. Are you prepared to present conflict or contradictions that you can easily analyze and apply?

A clear understanding of the question will help you to determine the scope or extent of your essay and determine how you must limit it within the time parameters provided.

PLANNING

With the task firmly established in your mind, your next step is to plan your approach. Develop a thesis statement—a one-sentence overview of all you want to say, in which you clearly state the controlling ideas you will present. *Note:* This is of paramount importance to your presentation and conclusion because it not only identifies your main idea but provides a channel for stating your position. As well, this statement provides and dictates the basic content and development of your essay. You may discover that you can rewrite this statement as your essay develops, but you will not want to change its focus, which would be counterproductive to the time limit under which you are laboring. With an effectively developed central statement or thesis, you should briefly and roughly outline the body of your essay based upon the steps presented above; jot down ideas for details, examples, or illustrations that will help you to prove the validity of your position when faced with contradictions. *Note:* A sample listing, roughly done, will be adequate since this section of the exam is timed and will not permit or count extensive outlines. Rather, your outline should be a skeleton upon which you will build the points, details, and illustrations of your essay. During this stage, you also determine your pattern of organization, which should be dictated by the five steps already outlined.

COMPOSING

This is the actual writing of the essay. Using the thesis (central) statement and the rough outline as a guide, you should expand your ideas until they grow and your essay takes shape. Do not allow the outline to become overly restrictive. New ideas may emerge as you write. Feel free to include them *if* they support your thesis and improve the essay; however, do not be guilty of overkill. Once you have made your point, move on.

In terms of structure, there are three necessary elements—an introduction, body, and conclusion. The introduction provides an overview and a narrowing of the writing sample or prompt; the body is the actual presentation of your opinion, philosophy, or information followed by the possible conflicts explained and illustrated and the explanation of the resolution of the contradictions to reinforce your premise; the conclusion is wrapping up the presentation so that the reader not only understands the premise, but is convinced of your approach to it.

POLISHING

Aware of the time restrictions, read over your essay carefully. You may add, delete, rearrange, substitute, and make other improvements to your presentation. Be careful not to change the focus or to present conflicting ideas. The primary emphasis on polishing is to proofread for errors in punctuation, spelling, usage, and facts. No matter how effectively you have developed your content, errors in grammar and mechanics will detract; but the presentation of false or contradictory details will destroy its validity.

ESSAY SCORING/EVALUATION

The essays you write will be scored holistically, which means that each essay is judged as a whole rather than upon its separate sections. A single score is given to the writing itself. These essays are read by a group of trained readers who are experienced teachers and professionals. The performance of these readers is closely monitored throughout the scoring process to assure validity, clarity, and consistency among the group of readers. The scores are monitored to ensure fairness and accuracy.

A total of four readers will read your work; two separate readers will read the first essay and two other readers will read your second essay. No reader sees the score of another reader while scoring on a six-point scale, explained below. Each Writing Sample score is a function of the scores assigned by two readers. If the two scores are more than one point apart, a supervisory reader determines the final score.

The final scores given to each of the two essays are added together and converted to an alphabetic score for reporting. The range is low to high. The Writing Sample score is transmitted to medical schools containing percentile data and score distribution.

Responses that are blank, written in a language than English, or illegible are not scored. Obvious attempts to avoid the purpose of the writing prompt or to present a personal platform or agenda will be considered not scorable. The exclusion of either of the essays will render a score of "X" for the writing sample.

The following is an explanation of the score requirements:

- A paper earning the score of 6 (highest) will demonstrate clarity, depth, evidence of higher-level thinking in a focused and coherent manner with developed main ideas, and a mature use of the English language;
- The score of 5 will demonstrate clarity of thought with some depth, a focused and coherent treatment of the statement, with major ideas that are well-developed, and a strong control of the English language;
- The score of 4 will demonstrate clarity of thought and may demonstrate depth with a coherent and focused approach to the subject, adequate development and control of the English language;
- The score of 3 will demonstrate clarity but lack depth, while being coherent but lacking focus; major ideas will be developed somewhat; control of the English language will be evident with some mechanical errors;
- The score of 2 will demonstrate problems with clarity and depth as well as cohesion and focus; major ideas will lack development; there will be numerous errors in mechanics and usage;
- The score of 1 will demonstrate a lack of understanding of the writing assignment with serious problems of organization and development; numerous errors in mechanics and usage will render the ideas difficult to follow.

SAMPLE IDEAS AND RESPONSES

Following are four sample writing prompts for the MCAT writing sample.

SAMPLE ITEM 1

One of the greatest benefits to Americans is their freedom of speech.

Write a unified essay in which you perform the following tasks: explain what you think the statement means; describe specific situations in which Americans may benefit from freedom of speech; discuss ways that freedom might be contradicted or misused; provide evidence of how the misuse can be interpreted as beneficial; conclude with a justification for the statement.

SAMPLE ITEM 2

Today's society proves that "what goes around comes around."

Write a unified essay in which you perform the following tasks: explain what you think the statement means; describe specific situations in which the statement is true; discuss ways that the statement may not be proven; provide evidence of what this means to today's society; conclude with a justification of the positive or negative implications.

SAMPLE ITEM 3

A major concern in America on the part of many politicians is that each young person is entitled to a free college education.

Write a unified essay in which you perform the following tasks: explain what you think the statement means; describe specific situations in which there are indications that America's youth deserve a free education; discuss ways that such a practice might not be advantageous to the youth and to the nation; provide evidence of what this means to today's society; conclude with a justification of the positive or negative implications.

SAMPLE ITEM 4

The choice of a life's work and/or profession must be based upon realistic expectations rather than hopes and dreams.

Write a unified essay in which you perform the following tasks: explain what you think the statement means; describe specific situations in which knowing what is real in the choice of a career should motivate a choice; discuss ways that one's dreams and hopes should also be a factor in determining a life's work; provide evidence of what this means to today's society; conclude with a justification of the positive or negative implications.

Unit 3

Clearly, a good knowledge of basic mathematical skills is essential in order to be able to solve the many quantitative problems that appear on the MCAT. This section contains a review of the fundamental numerical skills that you will need to know for the test. Its purpose is not to give you a total review of all mathematics, but to refresh you on topic areas with which you should be familiar. Should you have difficulty with any of the topics covered in this review, it is suggested that you go back to a textbook for a more detailed explanation.

PROPERTIES OF NUMBERS

SYSTEMS OF NUMBERS

Within the real number system, numbers of various kinds can be identified. The numbers that are used for counting

$$1, 2, 3, 4, 5, \ldots$$

are called the natural numbers or positive integers. The positive integers, together with 0, are called the set of whole numbers. The positive integers, together with 0 and the negative integers

$$-1, -2, -3, -4, -5, \ldots$$

make up the set of integers.

A real number is said to be a rational number if it can be written as the ratio of two integers, where the denominator is not 0. Thus, for example, numbers such as

$$-16, \tfrac{2}{3}, -\tfrac{5}{6}, 0, 25, 12\tfrac{5}{8}$$

are rational numbers.

Any real number that cannot be expressed as the ratio of two integers is called an irrational number. Numbers such as $\sqrt{3}$, $-\sqrt{5}$, and π are irrational. Finally, the set of rational numbers, together with the set of irrational numbers, is called the set of real numbers.

ROUNDING OF NUMBERS

From time to time, an MCAT question will ask you to round an answer to a particular decimal place. The rules for rounding a number are very simple. In the case of whole numbers, begin by locating the digit to which the number is being rounded. Then, if the digit just to the right is 0, 1, 2, 3, or 4, leave the located digit alone. Otherwise, increase the located digit by 1. In either case, replace all digits to the right of the one located with 0s.

When rounding decimal numbers, the rules are similar. Again, begin by locating the digit to which the number is being rounded. As before, if the digit just to the right is 0, 1, 2, 3, or 4, leave the located digit alone. Otherwise, increase the located digit by 1. Finally, drop all the digits to the right of the one located.

Examples

Round the following as indicated.

1. 6,342 to the nearest 10

     Begin by locating the ten's digit, which is a 4. The number to the right of the 4 is a 2. Thus, drop the 2 and replace it with a 0, yielding 6,340.

2. 392.461 to the nearest tenth

     The tenth's digit is 4. The digit just to the right of it is 6, so increase the tenth's digit by 1, making it a 5. Drop the two digits to the right of this. The answer is 392.5

3. .0472 to the nearest thousandth

     Following the rules above, we obtain .047

PRECISION IN MEASUREMENT AND COMPUTATIONS WITH APPROXIMATE NUMBERS

Any measurement made in a scientific experiment is never exact; it is always approximate. *Precision* is a measure of how close we are to the true measurement. It is determined by the smallest unit of measure used to make the measurement.

For example, consider a measurement of 16,235 kilometers. Since the unit of measure used in this example is the kilometer, we say that the measurement is precise to the nearest kilometer. The maximum possible error is always one half of the unit that was used to make the measurement. This means that the true measure in this problem is somewhere between 16,235 ± 0.5 kilometers.

As another example, consider a measurement of 16,550 kilometers. If the unit of measurement in this example is tens of kilometers, we say that the measurement is precise to the nearest 10 kilometers. Thus, the true measurement is somewhere between 16,550 ± 5 kilometers.

Finally, consider a length measurement of $1\frac{5}{16}''$. If the unit of measurement is sixteenths of an inch, the measurement is precise to the nearest sixteenth of an inch, and the true measurement is somewhere between $1\frac{9}{32}''$ and $1\frac{11}{32}''$.

Since measurement is approximate, we often need to perform computations with approximate numbers. The result of a computation with approximate numbers can never be more accurate than the least accurate number involved in the computation.

To add or subtract approximate numbers, thus, perform the operations in the way you normally would, then round the result to the unit of the least precise number involved. Similarly, to multiply or divide approximate numbers, perform the operations as you usually would, and then round the answer to the number of decimal places in the least precise number involved.

Examples

1. 1.8 + 2.586 + 4.34 = 8.726. Since 1.8 is the least precise number, we present the answer as 8.7.

2. 5.67 × 2.6 = 14.742. The answer would be presented as 14.7.

SYSTEMS OF MEASUREMENTS

THE ENGLISH SYSTEM

When taking the MCAT, you will need to be able to compute using both the English system of measurement and the metric system. It may also be necessary for you to convert measurements from one system to the other, but in such cases, you will be given the appropriate conversion factors.

Make sure that you have the following relationships within the English system memorized:

Conversion Factors for Length
36 inches = 3 feet = 1 yard
12 inches = 1 foot
5,280 feet = 1,760 yards = 1 mile

Conversion Factors for Volume
2 pints = 1 quart
16 fluid ounces = 1 pint
8 pints = 4 quarts = 1 gallon

Conversion Factors for Weight
16 ounces = 1 pound
2,000 pounds = 1 ton

These conversion factors enable you to change units within the English system.

Examples

1. How many feet are in 5 miles?

$$5 \text{ miles} \times \frac{5{,}280 \text{ feet}}{1 \text{ mile}} = 26{,}400 \text{ feet}$$

Notice how the unit of "miles" cancels out of the numerator and denominator.

2. How many ounces are in 2 tons?

$$2 \text{ tons} \times \frac{2{,}000 \text{ pounds}}{1 \text{ ton}}$$
$$\times \frac{16 \text{ ounces}}{1 \text{ pound}} = 64{,}000 \text{ ounces}$$

Notice how the units of "tons" and "pounds" cancel out of the numerator and denominator.

THE METRIC SYSTEM

In the metric system, distance or length is measured in meters. Similarly, volume is measured in liters, and mass is measured in grams. The prefixes below are appended to the beginning of these basic units to indicate other units of measure with sizes equal to each basic unit multiplied or divided by powers of 10.

$$\text{giga} = 10^9$$
$$\text{mega} = 10^6$$
$$\text{kilo} = 10^3$$
$$\text{hecto} = 10^2$$
$$\text{deka} = 10^1$$
$$\text{deci} = 10^{-1}$$
$$\text{centi} = 10^{-2}$$
$$\text{milli} = 10^{-3}$$
$$\text{micro} = 10^{-6}$$
$$\text{nano} = 10^{-9}$$
$$\text{pico} = 10^{-12}$$

From the table above, we can see, for example, that a kilometer is 1,000 times as long as a meter, 100,000 times as long as a centimeter, and 1,000,000 times as a long as a millimeter. Similarly, a centigram is $\frac{1}{100}$ the size of a gram.

Conversions among metric units can be made quickly by moving decimal points.

Examples

a. Convert 9.43 kilometers to meters.

Since meters are smaller than kilometers, our answer will be larger than 9.43. There are 1,000 meters in a kilometer, so we move the decimal point three places over to the right. 9.43 kilometers is equal to 9,430 meters.

b. Convert 512 grams to kilograms.

Since kilograms are more massive than grams, our answer must less than 512. There are 10^{-3} kilograms in a gram, so we move the decimal point three places to the left. 512 grams are equal to .512 kilograms.

Conversions Between the English and the Metric Systems

Conversions between the English and metric systems are accomplished in the same way as conversions within the English system. Recall that any problem that requires you to make such a conversion will include the necessary conversion factors.

Examples

1. If 1 meter is equivalent to 1.09 yards, how many yards are in 10 meters?

$$10 \text{ meters} \times \frac{1.09 \text{ yards}}{1 \text{ meter}} = 10.9 \text{ yards.}$$

2. If 1 yard is equivalent to .914 meters, how many meters are there in 24 yards?

$$24 \text{ yards} \times \frac{.914 \text{ meters}}{1 \text{ yard}} = 21.94 \text{ meters.}$$

PERCENT PROBLEMS

When doing percent problems, it is usually easier to change the percent to a decimal or a fraction before computing. When we take a percent of a certain number, that number is called the base, the percent we take is called the rate, and the result is called the percentage or part. If we let B represent the base, R the rate, and P the part, the relationship between these quantities is expressed by the following formula:

$$P = R \times B$$

All percent problems can be done with the help of this formula.

Example 1

In a class of 24 students, 25% received an A. How many students received an A? The number of students (24) is the base, and 25% is the rate. Change the rate to a fraction for ease of handling and apply the formula.

$$25\% = \frac{25}{100} = \frac{1}{4}$$

$$P = R \times B$$

$$= \frac{1}{4} \times \frac{24}{1}$$

$$= 6 \text{ students}$$

To choose between changing the percent (rate) to a decimal or a fraction, simply decide which would be easier to work with. In Example 1, the fraction was easier to work with because cancellation was possible. In Example 2, the situation is the same except for a different rate. This time the decimal form is easier.

Example 2

In a class of 24 students, 29.17% received an A. How many students received an A?

$$29.17\% = .2917$$

$$P = R \times B$$

$$= .2917 \times 24$$

$$= 7 \text{ students}$$

$$\begin{array}{r} .2917 \\ \times\ 24 \\ \hline 1.1668 \\ 5.834 \\ \hline 7.0008 \end{array}$$

PERCENT OF INCREASE OR DECREASE

This kind of problem is not really new but follows immediately from the previous problems. First calculate the amount of increase or decrease. This amount is the P (percentage or part) from the formula $P = R \times B$. The base, B, is the original amount, regardless of whether there was a loss or gain.

Example

By what percent does Mary's salary increase if her present salary is $20,000 and she accepts a new job at a salary of $28,000?

Amount of increase is:

$$\$28,000 - \$20,000 = \$8000$$

$$P = R \times B$$

$$\$8000 = R \times \$20,000$$

Divide each side of the equation by $20,000. Then:

$$\frac{\overset{40}{\cancel{8000}}}{\underset{100}{\cancel{20,000}}} = \frac{40}{100} = R = 40\% \text{ increase}$$

POWERS AND ROOTS

EXPONENTS

The product $10 \times 10 \times 10$ can be written 10^3. We say 10 is raised to the *third power*. In general, $a \times a \times a \ldots a$ n times is written a^n. The *base a* is raised to the nth power, and n is called the exponent.

Examples

$3^2 = 3 \cdot 3$ read "3 squared"
$2^3 = 2 \cdot 2 \cdot 2$ read "2 cubed"
$5^4 = 5 \cdot 5 \cdot 5 \cdot 5$ read "5 to the fourth power"

If the exponent is 1, it is usually understood and not written; thus, $a^1 = a$.

Negative exponents are given meaning by the definition $a^{-n} = \dfrac{1}{a^n}$. Thus, for example, $5^{-2} = \dfrac{1}{5^2}$.

By definition, we say that $a^0 = 1$. We have thus given meaning to all integral exponents.

There are five rules for computing with exponents. In general, if k and m are integers, and a and b are any numbers:

Rule 1: $a^k \times a^m = a^{k+m}$

Rule 2: $\dfrac{a^k}{a^m} = a^{k-m}$

Rule 3: $(a^k)^m = a^{km}$

Rule 4: $(ab)^m = a^m \times b^m$

Rule 5: $\left(\dfrac{a}{b}\right)^m = \dfrac{a^m}{b^m}$

Examples

Rule 1: $2^2 \cdot 2^3 = 4 \times 8 = 32$

and $2^2 \cdot 2^3 = 2^5 = 32$

Rule 2: $\dfrac{3^5}{3^7} = \dfrac{243}{2187} = \dfrac{1}{9} = \dfrac{1}{3^2} = 3^{-2}$

and $\dfrac{3^5}{3^7} = 3^{(5-7)} = 3^{-2}$

Rule 3: $(3^2)^3 = 9^3 = 729$

and $(3^2)^3 = 3^6 = 729$

Rule 4: $(3 \times 4)^2 = 12^2 = 144$

and $(3 \times 4)^2 = 3^2 \times 4^2$

$= 9 \times 16 = 144$

Rule 5: $\left(\dfrac{6}{2}\right)^4 = 3^4 = 81,$

and $\left(\dfrac{6}{2}\right)^4 = \dfrac{6^4}{2^4}$

$= \dfrac{1,296}{16} = 81$

SCIENTIFIC NOTATION

Any number can be written as the product of a number between 1 and 10 and some power of 10. A number written this way is said to be written in scientific notation.

To express a number in scientific notation, begin by repositioning the decimal point, so that the number becomes a number between 1 and 10. (That is, place the decimal point so that there is one digit to its left.) Then, the appropriate power of 10 can be determined by counting the number of places that the decimal point has been moved. The following examples will clarify this concept.

Examples

Write the following numbers in scientific notation:

a. 640,000

In writing this number as 6.4, the decimal point is moved 5 places to the left. Thus, $640,000 = 6.4 \times 10^5$.

b. 2,730,000

To change this number to 2.730, the decimal point needs to be moved 6 places to the left. Thus, $2,730,000 = 2.73 \times 10^6$.

c. .00085

To change this number to 8.5, the decimal point must be moved 4 places to the right. Thus, $.00085 = 8.5 \times 10^{-4}$.

d. .000000562

To change this number to 5.62, the decimal point needs to be moved 7 places to the right. Thus, $.000000562 = 5.62 \times 10^{-7}$.

Examples

Write the following numbers without scientific notation:

a. 3.69×10^3

Since $10^3 = 1,000$, we see that $3.69 \times 10^3 = 3.69 \times 1,000 = 3,690$.

b. 6.7×10^{-4}

Since $10^{-4} = .0001$, $6.7 \times 10^{-4} = 6.7 \times .0001 = .00067$

ROOTS

The definition of roots is based on exponents. If $a^n = c$, where a is the base and n the exponent, a is called the nth root of c. This is written $a = \sqrt[n]{c}$. The symbol $\sqrt{\ }$ is called a *radical sign*. Since $5^4 = 625$, $\sqrt[4]{625} = 5$, and 5 is the fourth root of 625. The most frequently used roots are the second (called the square) root and the third (called the cube) root. The square root is written $\sqrt{\ }$ and the cube root is written $\sqrt[3]{\ }$.

SQUARE ROOTS

If c is a positive number, there are two values, one negative and one positive, which when multiplied together will produce c.

Example

$+4 \times (+4) = 16$ and $-4 \times (-4) = 16$
The positive square root of a positive number c is called the *principal* square root of c (briefly, the square root of c) and is denoted by $\sqrt{c}$:

$$\sqrt{144} = 12$$

If $c = 0$, there is only one square root, 0. If c is a negative number, there is no real number that is the square root of c:

$$\sqrt{-4} \text{ is not a real number}$$

CUBE ROOTS

Both positive and negative numbers have real cube roots. The cube root of 0 is 0. The cube root of a positive number is positive; that of a negative number is negative.

Examples

$2 \times 2 \times 2 = 8$;

therefore, $\sqrt[3]{8} = 2$

$-3 \times (-3) \times (-3) = -27$;

therefore, $\sqrt[3]{-27} = -3$

Each number has only one real cube root.

FRACTIONAL EXPONENTS

The definitions of exponents can be extended to include fractional exponents. In particular, roots of numbers can be indicated by fractions with a numerator of 1. For example, $\sqrt{2}$ can be written as $2^{1/2}$. Similarly, $\sqrt{7} = 7^{1/3}$. Using rules 1–5 above, we can also make sense of any negative fractional exponents.

Examples

a. $8^{-1/2} = \dfrac{1}{\sqrt{8}}$

b. $7^{-5/2} = (7^{-5})^{1/2} = \left(\dfrac{1}{16,807}\right)^{1/2}$

$= \dfrac{1}{\sqrt{16,807}} \approx .0077$

Note that from Rule 4 we can determine that $(a \times b)^{1/k} = a^{1/k} \times b^{1/k}$. Written in radical notation, this expression becomes $\sqrt{a \times b} = \sqrt{a} \times \sqrt{b}$. This statement justifies the technique we use for the simplification of square roots, which is discussed next.

SIMPLIFYING SQUARE ROOTS

Example 1

Simplify $\sqrt{98}$

$$\sqrt{98} = \sqrt{2 \times 49}$$

$$= \sqrt{2} \times \sqrt{49} \quad \text{where 49 is a square number}$$

$$= \sqrt{2} \times 7$$

Therefore, $\sqrt{98} = 7\sqrt{2}$, and the process terminates because there is no whole number whose square is 2. $7\sqrt{2}$ is called a radical expression or simply a *radical*.

Example 2

Which is larger, $2\sqrt{75}$ or $6\sqrt{12}$?

These numbers can be compared if the same number appears under the radical sign. Then the greater number is the one with the larger number in front of the radical sign.

$$\sqrt{75} = \sqrt{25 \times 3} = \sqrt{25} \times \sqrt{3} = 5\sqrt{3}$$

Therefore:

$$2\sqrt{75} = 2(5\sqrt{3}) = 10\sqrt{3}$$

$$\sqrt{12} = \sqrt{4 \times 3} = \sqrt{4} \times \sqrt{3} = 2\sqrt{3}$$

Therefore:

$$6\sqrt{12} = 6(2\sqrt{3}) = 12\sqrt{3}$$

since $12\sqrt{3} > 10\sqrt{3}$,

$$6\sqrt{12} > 2\sqrt{75}$$

Radicals can be added and subtracted only if they have the same number under the radical sign. Otherwise, they must be reduced to expressions having the same number under the radical sign.

Example

Add $2\sqrt{18} + 4\sqrt{8} - \sqrt{2}$.

$$\sqrt{18} = \sqrt{9 \times 2} = \sqrt{9} \times \sqrt{2} = 3\sqrt{2}$$

Therefore: $2\sqrt{18} = 2(3\sqrt{2}) = 6\sqrt{2}$

and $\sqrt{8} = \sqrt{4 \times 2} = \sqrt{4} \times \sqrt{2} = 2\sqrt{2}$

Therefore: $4\sqrt{8} = 4(2\sqrt{2}) = 8\sqrt{2}$

giving $2\sqrt{18} + 4\sqrt{8} - \sqrt{2}$

$$= 6\sqrt{2} + 8\sqrt{2} - \sqrt{2} = 13\sqrt{2}$$

Radicals are multiplied using the rule that

$$\sqrt[k]{a \times b} = \sqrt[k]{a} \times \sqrt[k]{b}$$

Example

$$\sqrt{2}(\sqrt{2} - 5\sqrt{3}) = \sqrt{4} - 5\sqrt{6}$$
$$= 2 - 5\sqrt{6}$$

A quotient rule for radicals similar to the product rule is:

$$\sqrt[k]{\frac{a}{b}} = \frac{\sqrt[k]{a}}{\sqrt[k]{b}}$$

Example

$$\sqrt{\frac{9}{4}} = \frac{\sqrt{9}}{\sqrt{4}} = \frac{3}{2}$$

ALGEBRA

ALGEBRAIC EXPRESSIONS

If we are given an expression and numerical values to be assigned to each letter, the expression can be evaluated.

Example

The formula for temperature conversion is:

$$F = \frac{9}{5}C + 32$$

where C stands for the temperature in degrees Celsius and F for degrees Fahrenheit. Find the Fahrenheit temperature that is equivalent to 20°C.

$$F = \frac{9}{5}(20°C) + 32 = 36 + 32 = 68°F$$

To solve verbal problems, it is necessary to be able to translate verbal expressions to algebraic ones:

Verbal	Algebraic
Thirteen more than x	$x + 13$
Six less than twice x	$2x - 6$
The square of the sum of x and 5	$(x + 5)^2$
The sum of the square of x and the square of 5	$x^2 + 5^2$
The distance traveled by a car going 50 miles an hour for x hours	$50x$
The average of 70, 80, 85, and x	$\dfrac{70+80+85+x}{4}$

MULTIPLICATION

Multiplication of expressions is accomplished by using the *distributive property*. If the multiplier has only one term, then

$$a(b + c) = ab + ac$$

Example

$$9x(5m + 9q) = (9x)\,(5m) + (9x)\,(9q)$$
$$= 45mx + 81qx$$

When the multiplier contains more than one term and you are multiplying two expressions, multiply each term of the first expression by each term of the second and then add like terms. Follow the rules for signed numbers and exponents at all times.

Example

$$(3x+8)(4x^2+2x+1)$$
$$= 3x(4x^2+2x+1)$$
$$+ 8(4x^2+2x+1)$$
$$= 12x^3+6x^2+3x+32x^2+16x+8$$
$$= 12x^3+38x^2+19x+8$$

Algebraic expressions can be multiplied by themselves (squared) or raised to any power.

Example 1

$$(a+b)^2 = (a+b)(a+b) = a(a+b)+b(a+b)$$
$$= a^2+ab+ba+b^2$$
$$= a^2+2ab+b^2$$

Example 2

$$(a+b)(a-b) = a(a-b)+b(a-b)$$
$$= a^2-ab+ba-b^2$$
$$= a^2-b^2$$

FACTORING

When two or more algebraic expressions are multiplied, each is called a factor and the result is the *product*. The reverse process of finding the factors given the product is called *factoring*. A product can often be factored in more than one way. Factoring is useful in multiplication, division, and solving equations.

One way to factor an expression is to remove any single-term factor that is common to each of the terms and write it outside the parentheses. It is the distributive law that permits this.

Example

$3x^3 + 6x^2 + 9x = 3x(x^2 + 2x + 3)$

The result can be checked by multiplication.

Expressions containing squares can sometimes be factored into expressions containing letters raised to the first power only, called *linear fractions*. We have seen that

$(a + b)(a - b) = a^2 - b^2$

Therefore, if we have an expression in the form of a difference of two squares, it can be factored as:

$a^2 - b^2 = (a + b)(a - b)$

Example

Factor $4x^2 - 9$.

$4x^2 - 9 = (2x)^2 - (3)^2 = (2x + 3)(2x - 3)$

Again, the result can be checked by multiplication.

A third type of expression that can be factored is one containing three terms, such as $x^2 + 5x + 6$. Since

$$(x + a)(x + b) = x(x + b) + a(x + b)$$
$$= x^2 + xb + ax + ab$$
$$= x^2 + (a + b)x + ab$$

an expression in the form $x^2 + (a + b)x + ab$ can be factored into two factors of the form $(x + a)$ and $(x + b)$. We must find two numbers whose product is the constant in the given expression and whose sum is the coefficient of the term containing x.

Example I

Find factors of $x^2 + 5x + 6$

First find two numbers that, when multiplied, have +6 as a product. Possibilities are 2 and 3, −2 and −3, 1 and 6, −1 and −6. From these select the one pair whose sum is 5. The pair 2 and 3 is the only possible selection, and so:

$x^2 + 5x + 6 = (x + 2)(x + 3)$ written in either order

Example 2

Factor $x^2 - 5x - 6$.

Possible factors of −6 are −1 and 6, 1 and −6, 2 and −3, and −2 and 3. We must select the pair whose sum is −5. The only pair whose sum is −5 is 1 and −6, and so:

$x^2 - 5x - 6 = (x + 1)(x - 6)$

In factoring expressions of this type, notice that if the last sign is plus, both a and b have the same sign and it is the same as the sign of the middle term. If the last sign is minus, the numbers have opposite signs.

Many expressions cannot be factored.

DIVISION

Write the division example as a fraction. If numerator and denominator each contain one term, divide the numbers using laws of signed numbers, and use the laws of exponents to simplify the letter part of the problem.

Example

Method 1: Law of Exponents

$$\frac{36mx^2}{9m^2x} = 4m^1x^2m^{-2}x^{-1}$$

$$= 4m^{-1}x^1 = \frac{4x}{m}$$

Method 2: Cancellation

$$\frac{36mx^2}{9m^2x} = \frac{\overset{4}{\cancel{36mxx}}}{\underset{1}{\cancel{9mmx}}} = \frac{4x}{m}$$

If the divisor contains only one term and the dividend is a sum, divide each term in the dividend by the divisor and simplify as you did in Method 2.

Example 2

$$\frac{9x^3+3x^2+6x}{3x} = \frac{\overset{3x^2}{\cancel{9x^3}}}{\cancel{3x}} + \frac{\overset{x}{\cancel{3x^2}}}{\cancel{3x}} + \frac{\overset{2}{\cancel{6x}}}{\cancel{3x}}$$

$$= 3x^2 + x + 2$$

This method cannot be followed if there are two terms or more in the denominator since

$$\frac{a}{b+c} \neq \frac{a}{b} + \frac{a}{c}$$

In this case, write the example as a fraction. Factor the numerator and denominator if possible. Then use laws of exponents or cancel.

Example 3

Divide $x^3 - 9x$ by $x^3 + 6x^2 + 9x$.

Write as: $\dfrac{x^3-9x}{x^3+6x^2+9x}$

Both numerator and denominator can be factored to give:

$$\frac{x(x^2-9)}{x(x^2+6x+9)} = \frac{\cancel{x}\cancel{(x+3)}(x-3)}{\cancel{x}\cancel{(x+3)}(x+3)} = \frac{x-3}{x+3}$$

EQUATIONS

Solving equations is one of the major objectives in algebra. If a variable x in an equation is replaced by a value or expression that makes the equation a true statement, the value or expression is called a *solution* of the equation. (Remember that an equation is a mathematical statement that one algebraic expression is equal to another.)

EQUATIONS WITH ONE VARIABLE

An equation may contain one or more variables. We begin with one variable. Certain rules apply to equations whether there are one or more variables. The following rules are applied to give equivalent equations that are simpler than the original:

Addition: If $s = t$, then $s + c = t + c$.
Subtraction: If $s + c = t + c$, then $s = t$.
Multiplication: If $s = t$, then $cs = ct$.
Division: If $cs = ct$ and $c \neq 0$, then $s = t$.

To solve for x in an equation in the form $ax = b$ with $a \neq 0$, divide each side of the equation by a:

$$\frac{ax}{a} = \frac{b}{a} \text{ yielding } x = \frac{b}{a}$$

Then, $\dfrac{b}{a}$ is the solution to the equation.

Example 1

Solve $4x = 8$.

Write $\dfrac{4x}{4} = \dfrac{8}{4}$

$\qquad x = 2$

Example 2

Solve $2x - (x - 4) = 5(x + 2)$ for x.

$$2x - (x - 4) = 5(x + 2)$$

Remove parentheses by distributive law

$$2x - x + 4 = 5x + 10$$

Combine like terms.

$$x + 4 = 5x + 10$$

Subtract 4 from each side.

$$x = 5x + 6$$

Subtract $5x$ from each side.

$$-4x = 6$$

Divide each side by -4.

$$x = \dfrac{6}{-4}$$

Reduce fraction to lowest terms.

$$= -\dfrac{3}{2}$$

Negative sign now applies to the entire fraction.

LITERAL EQUATIONS

An equation may have other letters in it besides the variable (or variables). Such an equation is called a *literal equation*. An illustration is $x + b = a$, with x the variable. The solution of such an equation will not be a specific number but will involve letter symbols. Literal equations are solved by exactly the same methods as those involving numbers, but we must know which of the letters in the equation is to be considered the variable. Then the other letters are treated as constants.

Example 1

Solve $ax - 2bc = d$ for x.

$$ax = d + 2bc$$

$$x = \dfrac{d + 2bc}{a} \text{ if } a \neq 0$$

Example 2

Solve $ay - by = a^2 - b^2$ for y.

Factor out common term.

$$y(a - b) = a^2 - b^2$$

Factor expression on right side.

$$y(a - b) = (a + b)(a - b)$$

Divide each side by $a - b$ if $a \neq b$.

$$y = a + b$$

Example 3

Solve for S in the equation

$$\dfrac{1}{R} = \dfrac{1}{S} + \dfrac{1}{T}$$

Multiply every term by RST, the *LCD*:

$$ST = RT + RS$$

$$ST - RS = RT$$

$$S(T - R) = RT$$

$$S = \dfrac{RT}{T - R} \qquad \text{if } T \neq R$$

QUADRATIC EQUATIONS

An equation containing the square of an unknown quantity is called a *quadratic* equation. One way of solving such an equation is by factoring. If the product of two expressions is zero, at least one of the expressions must be zero.

Example 1

Solve $y^2 + 2y = 0$.

Remove common factor y

$$y(y + 2) = 0$$

$$y = 0 \quad \text{or} \quad y + 2 = 0$$

Since the product is 0, at least one of the factors must be 0.

$$y = 0 \quad \text{or} \quad y = -2$$

Check by substituting both values in the original equation:

$$(0)^2 + 2(0) = 0$$
$$(-2)^2 + 2(-2) = 4 - 4 = 0$$

In this case there are two solutions.

Example 2

Solve $x^2 + 7x + 10 = 0$.

$$x^2 + 7x + 10 = (x + 5)(x + 2) = 0$$
$$x + 5 = 0 \quad \text{or} \quad x + 2 = 0$$
$$x = -5 \quad \text{or} \quad x = -2$$

Check:

$$(-5)^2 + 7(-5) + 10 = 25 - 35 + 10 = 0$$

$$(-2)^2 + 7(-2) + 10 = 4 - 14 + 10 = 0$$

Not all quadratic equations can be factored using only integers, but solutions can usually be found by means of a formula. A quadratic equation may have two solutions, one solution, or occasionally no real solutions. If the quadratic equation is in the form $Ax^2 + Bx + C = 0$, x can be found from the following formula:

$$x = \frac{-B \pm \sqrt{B^2 - 4AC}}{2A}$$

Example

Solve $2y^2 + 5y + 2 = 0$ by formula. Assume $A = 2$, $B = 5$, and $C = 2$.

$$x = \frac{-5 \pm \sqrt{5^2 - 4(2)(2)}}{2(2)}$$

$$= \frac{-5 \pm \sqrt{25 - 16}}{4}$$

$$= \frac{-5 \pm \sqrt{9}}{4}$$

$$= \frac{-5 \pm 3}{4}$$

This yields two solutions:

$$x = \frac{-5 + 3}{4} = \frac{-2}{4} = \frac{-1}{2}$$

and

$$x = \frac{-5 - 3}{4} = \frac{-8}{4} = -2$$

So far, each quadratic we have solved has had two distinct answers, but an equation may have a single answer (repeated), as in

$$x^2 + 4x + 4 = 0$$
$$(x + 2)(x + 2) = 0$$
$$x + 2 = 0 \text{ and } x + 2 = 0$$
$$x = -2 \text{ and } x = -2$$

The only solution is -2.

It is also possible for a quadratic equation to have no real solution at all.

Example

If we attempt to solve $x^2 + x + 1 = 0$, by formula, we get:

$$x = \frac{-1 \pm \sqrt{1 - 4(1)(1)}}{2} = \frac{-1 \pm \sqrt{-3}}{2}$$

Since $\sqrt{-3}$ is not defined, this quadratic equation has no real answer.

LINEAR INEQUALITIES

For each of the sets of numbers we have considered, we have established an ordering of the members of the set by defining what it means to say that one number is greater than the other. Every number we have considered can be represented by a point on a number line.

An *algebraic inequality* is a statement that one algebraic expression is greater than (or less than) another algebraic expression. If all the variables in the inequality are raised to the first power, the inequality is said to be a *linear inequality*. We solve the inequality by reducing it to a simpler inequality whose solution is apparent. The answer is not unique, as it is in an equation, since a great number of values may satisfy the inequality.

There are three rules for producing equivalent inequalities:

1. The same quantity can be added or subtracted from each side of an inequality.

2. Each side of an inequality can be multiplied or divided by the same *positive* quantity.

3. If each side of an inequality is multiplied or divided by the same *negative* quantity, the sign of the inequality must be reversed so that the new inequality is equivalent to the first.

Example 1

Solve $5x - 5 > -9 + 3x$.

Add 5 to each side.

$5x > -4 + 3x$

Subtract $3x$ from each side.

$2x > -4$

Divide by $+2$.

$x > -2$

Any number greater than -2 is a solution to this inequality.

Example 2

Solve: $2x - 12 < 5x - 3$.

Add 12 to each side.

$2x < 5x + 9$

Subtract $5x$ from each side.

$-3x < 9$

Divide each side by -3, changing the sign of the inequality.

$x > -3$

Any number greater than -3—for example, $-2. -1, -\frac{1}{2}, 0, 1,$ or 4—is a solution to this inequality.

LINEAR EQUATIONS IN TWO UNKNOWNS

Graphing Equations

The number line is useful in picturing the values of one variable. When two variables are involved, a coordinate system is effective. The Cartesian coordinate system is constructed by placing a vertical number line and a horizontal number line on a plane so that the lines intersect at their zero points. This meeting place is called the *origin*. The horizontal number line is called the x axis, and the vertical number line (with positive numbers above the x axis) is called the y axis. Points in the plane correspond to ordered pairs of real numbers.

Example

The points in this example are:

x	y
0	0
1	1
3	−1
−2	−2
−2	1

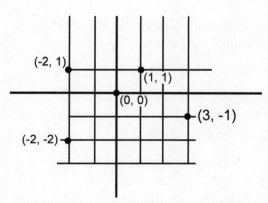

A first-degree equation in two variables is an equation that can be written in the form $ax + by = c$, where a, b, and c are constants. *First-degree* means that x and y appear to the first power. *Linear* refers to the graph of the solutions (x, y) of the equation, which is a straight line. We have already discussed linear equations of one variable.

Example

Graph the line $y = 2x - 4$.

First make a table and select small integral values of x. Find the value of each corresponding y and write it in the table:

x	y
0	−4
1	−2
2	0
3	2

If $x = 1$, for example, $y = 2(1) - 4 = -2$. Then plot the four points on a coordinate system. It is not necessary to have four points; two would do since two points determine a line, but plotting three or more points reduces the possibility of error.

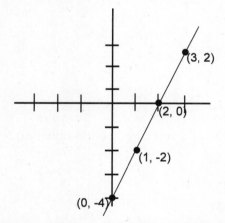

After the points have been plotted (placed on the graph), draw a line through the points and extend it in both directions. This line represents the equation $y = 2x - 4$.

Solving Simultaneous Linear Equations

Two linear equations can be solved together (simultaneously) to yield an answer (x, y) if it exists. On the coordinate system, this amounts to drawing the graphs of two lines and finding their point of intersection. If the lines are parallel and therefore never meet, no solution exists.

Simultaneous linear equations can be solved in the following manner without drawing graphs. From the first equation find the value of one variable in terms of the other; substitute this value in the second equation. The second equation is now a linear equation in one variable and can be solved. After the numerical value of the one variable has been found, substitute that value into the first equation to find the value of the second variable. Check the results by putting both values into the second equation.

Example 1

Solve the system

$2x + y = 3$
$4x - y = 0$

From the first equation, $y = 3 - 2x$. Substitute this value of y into the second equation to get

$$4x - (3 - 2x) = 0$$
$$4x - 3 + 2x = 0$$
$$6x = 3$$
$$x = \frac{1}{2}$$

Substitute $x = \frac{1}{2}$ in the first of the original equations:

$$2\left(\frac{1}{2}\right) + y = 3$$
$$1 + y = 3$$
$$y = 2$$

Check by substituting both x and y values into the second equation:

$$4\left(\frac{1}{2}\right) - 2 = 0$$
$$2 - 2 = 0$$

Example 2

A change-making machine contains \$30 in dimes and quarters. There are 150 coins in the machine. Find the number of each type of coin.

Let x = number of dimes and y = number of quarters. Then:

$x + y = 150$

Since $.25y$ is the product of a quarter of a dollar and the number of quarters, and $.10x$ is the amount of money in dimes,

$.10x + .25y = 30$

Multiply the last equation by 100 to eliminate the decimal points:

$10x + 25y = 3000$

From the first equation, $y = 150 - x$. Substitute this value in the equivalent form of the second equation.

$$10x + 25(150 - x) = 3000$$
$$-15x = -750$$
$$x = 50$$

This is the number of dimes. Substitute this value in $x + y = 150$ to find that the number of quarters, $y = 100$.

Check:

$.10(50) + .25(100) = 30$

$\$5 + \$25 = \$30$

EXPONENTIAL EQUATIONS

An exponential equation is an equation whose variable appears in a exponent. Such equations can be solved by algebraic means if it is possible to express both sides of the equation as powers of the same base.

Example 1

Solve $5^{2x-1} = 25$

Rewrite the equation as $5^{2x-1} = 5^2$. Then it must be true that $2x - 1 = 2$. This means that $x = \dfrac{3}{2}$.

Example 2

Solve $9^{x+3} = 27^{2x}$.

Rewrite the left side of the equation as $(3^2)^{x+3} = 3^{2x+6}$. Rewrite the right side of the equation as $(3^3)^{2x} = 3^{6x}$. Then, it must be true that $2x + 6 = 6x$. This means that $x = \dfrac{3}{2}$.

Exponential equations in which the bases cannot both be changed to the same number can be solved by using logarithms.

RATIO AND PROPORTION

Many problems in arithmetic and algebra can be solved using the concept of *ratio* to compare numbers. The ratio of a to b is the fraction $\dfrac{a}{b}$. If the two ratios $\dfrac{a}{b}$ and $\dfrac{c}{d}$ represent the same comparison, we write:

$$\frac{a}{b} = \frac{c}{d}$$

This equation (statement of equality) is called a *proportion*. A proportion states the equivalence of two different expressions for the same ratio.

Example 1

In a class of 39 students, 17 are men. Find the ratio of men to women.

39 students − 17 men = 22 women

Ratio of men to women is $\dfrac{17}{22}$, also written 17:22.

Example 2

A fertilizer contains 3 parts nitrogen, 2 parts potash, and 2 parts phosphate by weight. How many pounds of fertilizer will contain 60 pounds of nitrogen?

The ratio of pounds of nitrogen to pounds of fertilizer is 3 to $3 + 2 + 2 = \frac{3}{7}$. Let x be the number of pounds of mixture. Then:

$$\frac{3}{7} = \frac{60}{x}$$

Multiply both sides of the equation by $7x$ to get:

$3x = 420$

$x = 140$ pounds

Variation

The terminology of variation is useful for describing a number of situations that arise in science. If x and y are variables, then *y is said to vary directly as x* if there is a non-zero constant *km* such that $y = kx$.

Similarly, we say that *y varies inversely as x* if $y = \frac{k}{x}$ for some non-zero constant k. To say that *y varies inversely as the square of x* means that $y = \frac{k}{x^2}$ for some non-zero constant k. Finally, to say *y varies jointly as s and t* means that $y = kst$ for some non-zero constant k.

Example

Boyle's law says that, for an enclosed gas at a constant temperature, the pressure p varies inversely as the volume v. If $v = 10$ cubic inches when $p = 8$ pounds per square inch, find v when $p = 12$ pounds per square inch.

Since p varies inversely as v, we have $p = \frac{k}{v}$, for some value of k. We know that when $p = 8$, $v = 10$, so $8 = \frac{k}{10}$. This tells us that the value of k is 80, and we have $p = \frac{80}{v}$. For $p = 12$, we have $12 = \frac{80}{v}$, or $v = \frac{80}{12} = 6.67$ cubic inches.

LOGARITHMS

The Meaning of Logarithms

The logarithm of a number is the power to which a given base must be raised to produce the number. For example, the logarithm of 25 to the base 5 is 2, since 5 must be raised to the second power to produce the number 25. The statement "the logarithm of 25 to the base 5 is 2" is written as $\log_5 25 = 2$.

Note that every time we write a statement about exponents, we can write an equivalent statement about logarithms. For example, $\log_3 27 = 3$ since $3^3 = 27$, and $\log_8 4 = \frac{2}{3}$, since $8^{2/3} = 4$.

An important by-product of the definition of logarithms is that we cannot determine values for $\log_a x$ if x is either zero or a negative number. For example, if $\log_2 0 = b$, then $2^b = 0$, but there is no exponent satisfying this property. Similarly, if $\log_2(-8) = b$, then $2^b = -8$, and there is no exponent satisfying this property.

While logarithms can be written to any base, logarithms to the base 10 are used so frequently that they are called common logarithms, and the symbol "log" is used to stand for "$\log_{10}$".

Examples

1. Write logarithmic equivalents to the follow statements about exponents:

   a. $2^5 = 32$

   The statement $2^5 = 32$ is equivalent to $\log_2 32 = 5$.

   b. $12^0 = 1$

   The statement $12^0 = 1$ is equivalent to $\log_{12} 1 = 0$.

2. Use the definition of logarithm to evaluate the following:

a. $\log_6 36$

$\log_6 36 = 2$, since $6^2 = 36$

b. $\log_4\left(\dfrac{1}{16}\right)$

$= -2$ since $4^{-2} = \dfrac{1}{16}$.

PROPERTIES OF LOGARITHMS

Since logarithms are exponents, they follow the rules of exponents previously discussed. For example, when exponents to the same base are multiplied, their exponents are added; thus we have the rule: $\log_a xy = \log_a x + \log_a y$. The three most frequently used rules of logarithms are:

Rule 1: $\log_a xy = \log_a x + \log_a y$

Rule 2: $\log_a\left(\dfrac{x}{y}\right) = \log_a x - \log_a y$

Rule 3: $\log_a x^b = b\log_a x$

Examples

Rule 1: $\log_3 14 = \log_3(7\cdot2) = \log_3 7 + \log_3 2$

Rule 2: $\log\left(\dfrac{13}{4}\right) = \log 13 - \log 4$

Rule 3: $\log_7 \sqrt{5} = \log_7(5^{1/2}) = \left(\dfrac{1}{2}\right)\log_7 5$

By combining these rules, we can see, for example, that $\log\left(\dfrac{5b}{7}\right) = \log 5 + \log b - \log 7$.

SOLVING EXPONENTIAL EQUATIONS BY USING LOGARITHMS

Exponential equations for which both sides cannot be written as exponents to the same power can be solved by using logarithms.

Example

Solve $3^{2x} = 4^{x-1}$

Begin by taking the logarithm of both sides. We could take the logarithm with respect to any base; in this example, to keep things simple, we will take the logarithm to the base 10.

$\log 3^{2x} = \log 4^{x-1}$

$2x\log 3 = (x - 1)\log 4$

$2x\log 3 = x\log 4 - \log 4$

$2x\log 3 - x\log 4 = -\log 4$

$x(2\log 3 - \log 4) = -\log 4$

$x = \dfrac{-\log 4}{(2\log 3 - \log 4)}$

We now need to obtain values for log 3 and log 4. These can be obtained from either a table of logarithms or a scientific calculator. We obtain log 3 = 0.4771, and log 4 = 0.6021. Thus,

$x = \dfrac{-(0.6021)}{[2(0.4771) - 0.6021]} = \dfrac{-0.6021}{0.3521} = -1.7100$

TRIANGLES AND THE PYTHAGOREAN THEOREM

TRIANGLES

A triangle is a polygon of three sides. Triangles are classified by measuring their sides and angles. The sum of the angles of a plane triangle is always 180°. The symbol for a triangle is Δ. The sum of any two sides of a triangle is always greater than the third side.

Equilateral

Equilateral triangles have equal sides and equal angles. Each angle measures 60° because $\frac{1}{3}(180°) = 60°$.

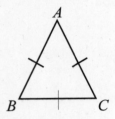

$AB = AC = BC$.
$\angle A = \angle B = \angle C = 60°$.

Isosceles

Isosceles triangles have two sides equal. The angles opposite the equal sides are equal. The two equal angles are sometimes called the *base* angles and the third angle is called the *vertex* angle. Note that an equilateral triangle is isosceles.

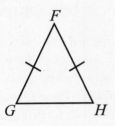

$FG = FH$.
FG ≠ GH.
$\angle G = \angle H$.
$\angle F$ is vertex angle.
$\angle G$ and $\angle H$ are base angles.

Scalene

Scalene triangles have all three sides of different length and all angles of different measure. In scalene triangles, the shortest side is opposite the angle of smallest measure, and the longest side is opposite the angle of greatest measure.

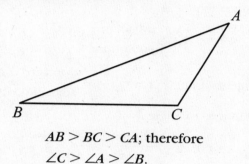

$AB > BC > CA$; therefore
$\angle C > \angle A > \angle B$.

Right

Right triangles contain one right angle. Since the right angle is 90°, the other two angles are complementary. They may or may not be equal to each other. The side of a right triangle opposite the right angle is called the *hypotenuse*. The other two sides are called *legs*. The *Pythagorean theorem* states that the square of the length of the hypotenuse is equal to the sum of the squares of the lengths of the legs.

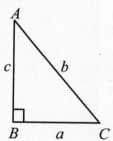

AC is the hypotenuse.
AB and BC are legs.
$\angle B = 90°$.
$\angle A + \angle C = 90°$.
$a^2 + c^2 = b^2$.

Examples

If ABC is a right triangle with right angle at B, and if $AB = 6$ and $BC = 8$, what is the length of AC?

$$AB^2 + BC^2 = AC^2$$
$$6^2 + 8^2 = 36 + 64 = 100 = AC^2$$
$$AC = 10$$

If the measure of angle A is 30°, what is the measure of angle C?

Since angles A and C are complementary:

$$30° + C = 90°$$
$$C = 60°$$

If the lengths of the three sides of a triangle a, b, and c and the relation $a^2 + b^2 = c^2$ holds, the triangle is a right triangle and side c is the hypotenuse.

Example

Show that a triangle of sides 5, 12, and 13 is a right triangle.

The triangle will be a right triangle if $a^2 + b^2 = c^2$.

$$5^2 + 12^2 = 13^2$$
$$25 + 144 = 169$$

Therefore, the triangle is a right triangle and 13 is the length of the hypotenuse.

TRIGONOMETRY

Trigonometry enables you to solve problems that involve finding measures of unknown lengths and angles.

THE TRIGONOMETRIC RATIOS

Every right triangle contains two acute angles. With respect to each of these angles, it is possible to define six ratios, called the trigonometric ratios, each involving the lengths of two of the sides of the triangle. For example, consider the following triangle *ABC*.

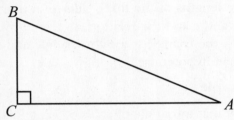

In this triangle, side *AC* is called the side adjacent to angle *A*, and side *BC* is called the side opposite angle *A*. Similarly, side *AC* is called the side opposite angle *B*, and side *BC* is called the side adjacent to angle *B*. Of course, side *AB* is referred to as the hypotenuse with respect to both angles *A* and *B*.

The six trigonometric ratios with respect to angle A, along with their standard abbreviations, are given below:

Sine of angle $A = \sin A = \dfrac{\text{opposite}}{\text{hypotenuse}} = \dfrac{BC}{AB}$

Cosine of angle *A*

$= \cos A = \dfrac{\text{adjacent}}{\text{hypotenuse}} = \dfrac{AC}{AB}$

Tangent of angle $A = \tan A = \dfrac{\text{opposite}}{\text{adjacent}} = \dfrac{BC}{AC}$

Cotangent of angle *A*

$= \cot A = \dfrac{\text{adjacent}}{\text{opposite}} = \dfrac{AC}{AB}$

Secant of angle *A*

$= \sec A = \dfrac{\text{hypotenuse}}{\text{adjacent}} = \dfrac{AB}{AC}$

Cosecant of angle *A*

$= \csc A = \dfrac{\text{hypotenuse}}{\text{opposite}} = \dfrac{AB}{BC}$

The last three ratios are actually the reciprocals of the first three, in particular:

$$\cot A = \frac{1}{\tan A}$$

$$\sec A = \frac{1}{\cos A}$$

$$\csc A = \frac{1}{\sin A}$$

Also note that:

$$\frac{\sin A}{\cos A} = \tan A, \text{ and } \frac{\cos A}{\sin A} = \cot A.$$

In order to remember which of the trigonometric ratios is which, you can memorize the well-known acronym: **SOH–CAH–TOA**. This stands for: **S**ine is **O**pposite over **H**ypotenuse, **C**osine is **A**djacent over **H**ypotenuse, **T**angent is **O**pposite over **A**djacent.

Example

Consider right triangle *DEF* below, whose sides have the lengths indicated. Find sin *D*, cos *D*, tan *D*, sin *E*, cos *E*, and tan *E*.

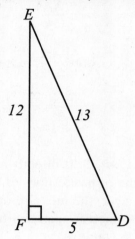

$$\sin D = \frac{EF}{ED} = \frac{12}{13} \qquad \sin E = \frac{DF}{ED} = \frac{5}{13}$$

$$\cos D = \frac{DF}{ED} = \frac{5}{13} \qquad \cos E = \frac{EF}{ED} = \frac{12}{13}$$

$$\tan D = \frac{EF}{DF} = \frac{12}{5} \qquad \tan E = \frac{DF}{EF} = \frac{5}{12}$$

Note that the sine of *D* is equal to the cosine of *E*, and the cosine of *D* is equal to the sine of *E*.

Example

In right triangle *ABC*, $\sin A = \frac{4}{5}$. Find the values of the other 5 trigonometric ratios.

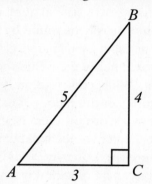

Since the sine of *A* = opposite over hypotenuse = $\frac{4}{5}$, we know that *BC* = 4, and *AB* = 5. We can use the Pythagorean theorem to determine that *AC* = 3. Then:

$$\cos A = \frac{3}{5}, \tan A = \frac{4}{3}, \cot A = \frac{3}{4},$$

$$\sec A = \frac{5}{3}, \csc A = \frac{5}{4}.$$

TRIGONOMETRIC RATIOS FOR SPECIAL ANGLES

The actual values for the trigonometric ratios for most angles are irrational numbers, whose values can most easily be found by looking in a trig table or using a calculator. On the MCAT, you will not need to find the values for such trig functions; you can simply leave the answer in terms of the ratio. For example, if the answer to a word problem is 35 tan 37°, the correct answer choice will be, in fact, 35 tan 37°. There are, however, a few angles whose ratios can be obtained exactly. The ratios for 30°, 45°, and 60° can be determined from the properties of the 30–60–90 right triangle and the 45–45–90 right triangle. First of all, note that the Pythagorean theorem can be used to determine the following side and angle relationships in 30–60–90 and 45–45–90 triangles:

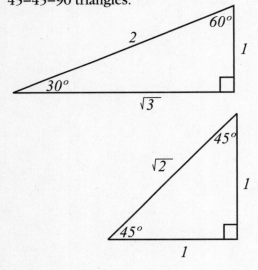

From these diagrams, it is easy to see that:

$$\sin 30° = \frac{1}{2}, \cos 30° = \frac{\sqrt{3}}{2},$$

$$\tan 30° = \frac{1}{\sqrt{3}} = \frac{\sqrt{3}}{3}$$

$$\sin 60° = \frac{\sqrt{3}}{2}, \cos 60° = \frac{1}{2}, \tan 60° = \sqrt{3}$$

$$\sin 45° = \cos 45° = \frac{1}{\sqrt{2}} = \frac{\sqrt{2}}{2}, \tan 45° = 1$$

Example

From point A, which is directly across from point B on the opposite sides of the banks of a straight river, the measure of angle CAB to point C, 35 meters upstream from B, is 30. How wide is the river?

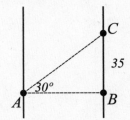

To solve this problem, note that

$$\tan A = \frac{\text{opposite}}{\text{adjacent}} = \frac{BC}{AB} = \frac{35}{AB}.$$

Since the measure of angle A is 30°, we have

$$\tan 30° = \frac{35}{AB}. \text{ Then:}$$

$$AB = \frac{35}{\tan 30°} = \frac{35}{\sqrt{3}/3} = \frac{105}{\sqrt{3}}.$$

Therefore, the width of the river is $\frac{105}{\sqrt{3}}$ meters, or approximately 60 meters wide.

THE PYTHAGOREAN IDENTITIES

There are three fundamental relationships involving the trigonometric ratios that are true for all angles and are helpful when solving problems. They are:

$$\sin^2 A + \cos^2 A = 1$$
$$\tan^2 A + 1 = \sec^2 A$$
$$\cot^2 A + 1 = \csc^2 A$$

These three identifies are called the Pythagorean identities since they can be derived from the Pythagorean theorem. For example, in triangle ABC below:

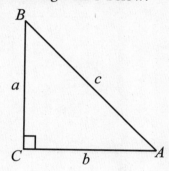

$$a^2 + b^2 = c^2$$

Dividing by c^2, we obtain,

$$\frac{a^2}{c^2} + \frac{b^2}{c^2} = 1, \text{ or}$$

$$\left(\frac{a}{c}\right)^2 + \left(\frac{b}{c}\right)^2 = 1.$$

Now, note that $\frac{a}{c} = \sin A$ and $\frac{b}{c} = \cos A$. Substituting these values in, we obtain $\sin^2 A + \cos^2 A = 1$. The other two identities are similarly obtained.

Example

If, in triangle ABC, $\sin A = \frac{7}{9}$, what are the values of $\cos A$ and $\tan A$?

Using the first of the trigonometric identities, we obtain:

$$\left(\frac{7}{9}\right)^2 + \cos^2 A = 1$$

$$= \frac{49}{81} + \cos^2 A = 1$$

$$\cos^2 A = 1 - \frac{49}{81}$$

$$\cos A = \sqrt{\frac{32}{81}}$$

$$= \frac{4\sqrt{2}}{9}$$

Then, since $\tan A = \frac{\sin A}{\cos A}$, we have

$$\tan A = \frac{\left(\frac{7}{9}\right)}{\left(\frac{4\sqrt{2}}{9}\right)} = \frac{7}{4\sqrt{2}} = \frac{7\sqrt{2}}{8}.$$

TRIGONOMETRY WORD PROBLEMS

1. The road to a bridge above a highway is 500 feet long. The road makes an angle of 30° with the horizontal. Find the height of the bridge.

2. At a point 15 feet from the base of a tree, the angle of elevation to its top is 60°. Find the height of the tree.

3. A ladder leans against a building, touching it at a point 18 feet above the ground. If the ladder makes an angle of 45° with the ground, how long is the ladder?

Solutions

1.

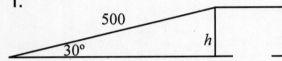

$$\sin 30° = \frac{h}{500}$$

Thus, $h = 500 \sin 30° = 500 \left(\frac{1}{2}\right) = 250$

The bridge is 250 feet high.

2.

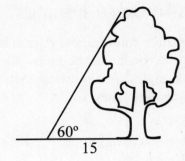

$$\tan 60° = \frac{h}{15}$$

Thus, $15 \tan 60° = h$ and $h = 15 (\sqrt{3})$.

The height of the tree is $15 \sqrt{3}$ feet.

3.

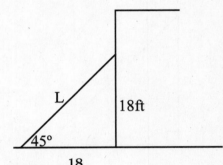

$$\sin 45° = \frac{18}{L}$$

Thus, $L = \dfrac{18}{\sin 45°} = \dfrac{18}{\dfrac{\sqrt{2}}{2}} = \dfrac{36}{\sqrt{2}}$

$$= \frac{36\sqrt{2}}{2} = 18\sqrt{2}$$

The ladder is $18\sqrt{2}$ feet long.

COORDINATE GEOMETRY

Coordinate geometry gives us an effective way to picture the relationships between two variables.

Recall that the general equation of a line has the following form:

$$Ax + By + C = 0,$$

where A and B are constants and are not both 0. This means that if you were to find all of the points (x, y) that satisfy the above equation, they would all lie on the same line as graphed on a coordinate axis.

If the value of B is not 0, a little algebra can be used to rewrite the equation in the form

$$y = mx + b,$$

where m and b are two constants. Since the two numbers m and b determine this line, let's see what their geometric meaning is. First of all, note that the point $(0, b)$ satisfies the above equation. This means that the point $(0, b)$ is one of the points on the line; in other words, the line crosses the y-axis at the point b. For this reason, the number b is called the **y-intercept** of the line.

To interpret the meaning of m, choose any two points on the line. Let us call these points (x_1, y_1) and (x_2, y_2). Both of these points must satisfy the equation of the line above, and so:

$$y_1 = mx_1 + b \text{ and } y_2 = mx_2 + b.$$

If we subtract the first equation from the second we obtain

$$y_2 - y_1 = m(x_2 - x_1),$$

and solving for m, we find

$$m = \frac{(y_2 - y_1)}{(x_2 - x_1)}$$

The above equation tells us that the number m in the equation $y = mx + b$ is the ratio of the difference of the y-coordinates to the difference of the x-coordinates. This number is called the **slope** of the line. Therefore, the ratio $m = \dfrac{(y_2 - y_1)}{(x_2 - x_1)}$ is a measure of the number of units the line rises (or falls) in the y direction for each unit moved in the x direction. Another way to say this is that the slope of a line is a measure of the rate at which the line rises (or falls). Intuitively, a line with a positive slope rises from left to right; one with a negative slope falls from left to right.

Because the equation $y = mx + b$ contains both the slope and the y-intercept, it is called the **slope-intercept** form of the equation of the line. This, however, is not the only form in which the equation of the line can be written.

If the line contains the point (x_1, y_1), its equation can also be written as:

$$y - y_1 = m(x - x_1).$$

This form of the equation of a line is called the **point-slope** form of the equation of a line, since it contains the slope and the coordinates of one of the points on the line.

Two lines are parallel if and only if they have the same slope. Two lines are perpendicular if and only if their slopes are negative inverses of each other. This means that if a line has a slope m, any line perpendicular to this line must have a slope of $-1/m$. Also note that a horizontal line has a slope of 0. For such a line, the slope-intercept form of the equation reduces to $y = b$.

131

Finally, note that if $B = 0$ in the equation $Ax + By + C = 0$, the equation simplifies to

$Ax + C = 0$,

and represents a vertical line (a line parallel to the y-axis) that crosses the x-axis at $^{-C}/_A$. Such a line is said to have no slope.

Example 1

Find the slope and the y-intercept of the following lines.

a. $y = 5x - 7$

b. $3x + 4y = 5$

a. $y = 5x - 7$ is already in slope-intercept form. The slope is 5, and the y-intercept is −7.

b. Write $3x + 4y = 5$ in slope-intercept form:

$4y = -3x + 5$

$$y = \left(\frac{-3}{4}\right)x + \left(\frac{5}{4}\right)$$

The slope is $^{-3}/_4$, and the y-intercept is $^5/_4$. This means that the line crosses the y-axis and the point $^5/_4$, and for every 3 units moved in the x-direction, the line falls 4 units in the y-direction.

Example 2

Find the equations of the following lines:

a. the line containing the points (4, 5) and (7,11)

b. the line containing the point (6, 3) and having slope 2

c. the line containing the point (5,2) and parallel to $y = 4x + 7$

d. the line containing the point (−2, 8) and perpendicular to $y = -2x + 9$

a. First, we need to determine the slope of the line.

$$m = \frac{11-5}{7-4} = \frac{6}{3} = 2.$$

Now, using the point-slope form: $y - 5 = 2(x - 4)$. If desired, you can change this to the slope-intercept form: $y = 2x - 3$.

b. Since we know the slope and a point on the line, we can simply plug into the point-slope form: $y - 3 = m(x - 6)$ to obtain $y - 3 = (x - 6)$.

c. The line $y = 4x + 7$ has a slope of 4. Thus, the desired line can be written as $y - 2 = 4(x - 5)$.

d. The line $y = -2x + 9$ has a slope of −2. The line perpendicular to this one has a slope of ½. The desired line can be written as $y - 8 = \left(\frac{1}{2}\right)(x + 2)$.

PROBABILITY

Probability is the branch of mathematics that gives you techniques for dealing with uncertainties. Intuitively, probability can be thought of as a numerical measure of the likelihood, or the chance, that an event will occur.

A probability value is always a number between 0 and 1. The nearer a probability value is to 0, the more unlikely the event is to occur; a probability value near 1 indicates that the event is almost certain to occur. Other probability values between 0 and 1 represent varying degrees of likelihood that an event will occur.

In the study of probability, an *experiment* is any process that yields one of a number of well-defined outcomes. By this we mean that on any single performance of an experiment, one and only one of a number of possible outcomes will occur. Thus, tossing a coin is an experiment with two possible outcomes: heads or tails. Rolling a die is an experiment with 6 possible outcomes; playing a game of hockey is an experiment with three possible outcomes (win, lose, tie).

In some experiments, all possible outcomes are equally likely. In such an experiment, with, say, n possible outcomes, we assign a probability of $\frac{1}{n}$ to each outcome. Thus, for example, in the experiment of tossing a coin, for which there are two equally likely outcomes, we would say that the probability of each outcome is ½. In the experiment of tossing a die, for which there are 6 equally likely outcomes, we would say that the probability of each outcome is ⅙.

How would you determine the probability of obtaining an even number when tossing a die? Clearly, there are three distinct ways

that an even number can be obtained: tossing a 2, a 4, or a 6. The probability of each one of these three outcomes is ⅙. The probability of obtaining an even number is simply the sum of the probabilities of these three favorable outcomes, that is to say, the probability of tossing an even number is equal to the probability of tossing a 2, plus the probability of tossing a 4, plus the probability of tossing a 6, which is

$$\frac{1}{6} + \frac{1}{6} + \frac{1}{6} = \frac{3}{6} = \frac{1}{2}.$$

This result leads us to the fundamental formula for computing probabilities for events with equally likely outcomes:

The probability of an event occurring =

$$\frac{\text{(The number of favorable outcomes)}}{\text{(The total number of possible outcomes)}}$$

In the case of tossing a die and obtaining an even number, as we saw, there are 6 possible outcomes, three of which are favorable, leading to a probability of $\frac{3}{6} = \frac{1}{2}$.

Example 1

What is the probability of drawing one card from a standard deck of 52 cards and having it be a king? When you select a card from a deck, there are 52 possible outcomes, 4 of which are favorable. Thus, the probability of drawing a king is $\frac{4}{52} = \frac{1}{13}$.

Example 2

Human eye color is controlled by a single pair of genes, one of which comes from the mother and one of which comes from the father, called a genotype. Brown eye color, B, is dominant over blue eye color ℓ. Therefore, in the genotype Bℓ, which consists of one brown gene B and one blue gene ℓ, the brown gene dominates. A person with Bℓ genotypes will have brown eyes.

If both parents have genotype Bℓ, what is the probability that their child will have blue eyes? To answer the question, we need to consider every possible eye color genotype for the child. They are given in the table below:

mother \ father	B	ℓ
B	BB	Bℓ
ℓ	ℓB	$\ell\ell$

The four possible genotypes for the child are equally likely, so we can use the formula above to compute the probability. Of the four possible outcomes, blue eyes can occur only with the $\ell\ell$ genotype, so only one of the four possible outcomes is favorable to blue eyes. Thus, the probability that the child has blue eyes is ¼.

Two events are said to be independent if the occurrence of one does not affect the probability of the occurrence of the other. For example, if a coin is tossed and a die is thrown, obtaining heads on the coin and obtaining a 5 on the die are independent events. On the other hand, if a coin is tossed three times, the probability of obtaining heads on the first toss and the probability of obtaining tails on all three tosses are not independent. In particular, if heads is obtained on the first toss, the probability of obtaining three tails becomes 0.

When two events are independent, the probability that they both happen is the product of their individual probabilities. For example, the probability of obtaining heads when a coin is tossed is ½, and the probability of obtaining 5 when a die is thrown is ⅙; thus, the probability of both of these events happening is $\left(\dfrac{1}{2}\right)\left(\dfrac{1}{6}\right) = \dfrac{1}{12}$.

In a situation where two events occur one after the other, be sure to correctly determine the number of favorable outcomes and the total number of possible outcomes.

Example 3

Consider a standard deck of 52 cards. What is the probability of drawing two kings in a row, if the first card drawn is replaced in the deck before the second card is drawn? What is the probability of drawing two kings in a row if the first card drawn is not replaced in the deck?

In the first case, the probability of drawing a king from the deck on the first attempt is ⁴⁄₅₂. If the selected card is replaced in the deck, the probability of drawing a king on the second draw is also ⁴⁄₅₂, and, thus, the probability of drawing two consecutive kings would be

$$\left(\frac{\overset{1}{\cancel{4}}}{52}\right)\left(\frac{\overset{1}{\cancel{4}}}{52}\right) = \frac{1}{2,074}.$$

On the other hand, if the first card drawn is a king and is not replaced, there now only three kings in a deck of 51 cards, and the probability of drawing the second king becomes ³⁄₅₁. The overall probability, thus, would be

$$\left(\frac{\overset{1}{\cancel{4}}}{52}\right)\left(\frac{3}{51}\right) = \frac{3}{2,652}.$$

STATISTICS

Statistics is the study of collecting, organizing, and analyzing data. There are several important numerical measures for data that you should be familiar with prior to taking the MCAT.

MEASURES OF LOCATION

Measures of location describe the "centering" of a set of data; that is, they are used to represent the central value of the data. There are three common measures of central location. The one that is typically the most useful (and certainly the most common) is the *arithmetic mean*, which is computed by adding up all of the individual data values and dividing by the number of values.

Example 1

A researcher wishes to determine the average (arithmetic mean) amount of time a particular prescription drug remains in the bloodstream of users. She examines five people who have taken the drug and determines the amount of time the drug has remained in each of their bloodstreams. In hours, these times are: 24.3, 24.6, 23.8, 24.0, and 24.3. What is the mean number of hours that the drug remains in the bloodstream of these experimental participants?

To find the mean, we begin by adding up all of the measured values. In this case, $24.3 + 24.6 + 23.8 + 24.0 + 24.3 = 121$. We then divide by the number of participants (5), and obtain $\frac{121}{5} = 24.2$ as the mean.

Example 2

Suppose the participant with the 23.8-hour measurement had actually been measured incorrectly, and a measurement of 11.8 hours obtained instead. What would the mean number of hours have been?

In this case, the sum of the data values is only 109, and the mean becomes 21.8.

This example exhibits the fact that the mean can be greatly "thrown off" by one incorrect measurement. Similarly, one measurement that is unusually large or unusually small can have great impact upon the mean. A measure of location that is not impacted as much by extreme values is called the median. The median of a group of numbers is simply the value in the middle when the data values are arranged in numerical order. This numerical measure is sometimes used in the place of the mean when we wish to minimize the impact of extreme values.

Example 3

What is the median value of the data from example 1? What is the median value of the modified data from example 2?

Note that in both cases, the median is 24.3. Clearly, the median was not impacted by the one unusually small observation in example 2.

In the event that there are an even number of data values, we find the median by computing the number halfway between the two values in the middle (that is, we find the mean of the two middle values).

Another measure of location is called the mode. The mode is simply the most frequently occurring value in a series of data. In the examples above, the mode is 24.3. The mode is determined in an experiment when we wish to know which outcome has happened the most often.

MEASURES OF VARIABILITY

Measures of location provide only information about the "middle" value. They tell us nothing, however, about the spread, or the variability, of the data. Yet sometimes knowing the variability of a set of data is very important. To see why, examine the example below.

Consider an individual who has the choice of getting to work using either public transportation or his/her own car. Obviously, one consideration of interest would be the amount of travel time associated with these two different ways of getting to work. Suppose that over the period of several months, the individual uses both modes of transportation the same number of times and computes the mean for both. It turns out that both methods of transportation average 30 minutes. At first glance, it might appear, therefore, that both alternatives offer the same service. However, let's take a look at the actual data, in minutes:

Travel time using a car: 28, 28, 29, 29, 30, 30, 31, 31, 32, 32

Travel time using public transportation: 24, 25, 26, 27, 28, 29, 30, 33, 36, 42

Even though the average travel time is the same (30 minutes), do the alternatives possess the same degree of reliability? For most people, the variability exhibited for public transportation would be of concern. To protect against arriving late, one would have to allow for 42 minutes of travel time using public transportation, but with a car one would only have to allow a maximum of 32 minutes. Also of concern are the wide extremes that must be expected when using public transportation.

Thus, we can see that when we look at a set of data, we may wish to not only consider the average value of the data, but also the variability of the data.

The easiest way to measure the variability of the data is to determine the difference between the largest and the smallest values. This is called the range.

Example 4

Determine the range of the data from example 1 and example 2 above.

The range of the data from example 1 is $24.6 - 23.8 = 0.8$. The range of the data in example 2 is $24.6 - 11.8 = 12.8$. Note how the one faulty measurement in example 2 has totally changed the range. For this reason, it is usually desirable to use another, more reliable, measure of variability, called the standard deviation.

The standard deviation is an extremely important measure of variability; however, it is rather complicated to compute. On the MCAT, you will never be asked to compute a standard deviation; you simply must know how to interpret one when you see it.

To understand the meaning of the standard deviation, suppose that you have a set of data which has a mean of 120 and a standard deviation of 10. As long as this data is "normally distributed" (most reasonable sets of data are), we can conclude that approximately 68 percent of the data values lie within one standard deviation of the mean. This means, in this case, that 68 percent of the data values lie between $120 - 10 = 110$ and $120 + 10 = 130$. Similarly, about 95 percent of the data values will lie within 2 standard deviations from the mean; that is, in this case, between 100 and 140. Finally, about 99.7 percent (which is to say, virtually all) of the data will lie within three standard deviations from the mean. In this case, this means that almost all of the data values will fall between 90 and 150.

CORRELATION

Very often, researchers need to determine whether any relationship exists between two variables that they are measuring. For example, they may wish to determine whether an increase in one variable implies that a second variable is likely to have increased as well, or whether an increase in one variable implies that another variable is likely to have decreased.

The *correlation coefficient* is a single number that can be used to measure the degree of the relationship between two variables. Again, on the MCAT, you will not be expected to compute the value of a correlation coefficient; however, you must be able to interpret them.

The value of a correlation coefficient can range between −1 and +1. A correlation of +1 indicates a perfect positive correlation; the two variables under consideration increase and decrease together. A correlation of −1 is a perfect negative correlation; when one variable increases, the other decreases, and vice versa. If the correlation is 0, there is no relationship between the behavior of the variables.

Consider a correlation coefficient that is a positive fraction. Such a correlation represents a positive relationship; as one variable increases, the other will tend to increase. The closer that correlation coefficient is to 1, the stronger the relationship will be. Now, consider a correlation coefficient which is a negative fraction. Such a correlation represents a negative relationship; as one variable increases, the other will tend to decrease. The closer the correlation coefficient is to −1, the stronger this inverse relationship will be.

As an example, consider the relationship between height and weight in human beings. Since weight tends to increase as height increases, you might expect that the correlation coefficient for the variables of height and weight would be near +1. On the other hand, consider the relationship between maximum pulse rate and age. In general, maximum pulse rate decreases with age, so you might expect that the correlation coefficient for these two variables would be near −1.

One common mistake in the interpretation of correlation coefficients that you should avoid making is the assumption that a high coefficient indicates a cause and effect relationship. This is not always the case. An example that is frequently given in statistics classes is the fact that there is a high correlation between gum chewing and crime in the United States. That is to say, as the number of gum chewers went up, there was a similar increase in the number of crimes committed. Obviously, this does not mean that there is any cause and effect between chewing gum and committing a crime. The fact is, simply, that as the population of the United States increased, both gum chewing and crime increased.

The following graphs are three "scatterplots" depicting the relationships between two variables. In the first, the plotted points almost lie on a straight line going up to the right. This is indicative of a strong positive correlation (a correlation near +1). The second scatterplot depicts a strong negative correlation, and the final scatterplot depicts two variables that are unrelated and probably have a correlation that is close to 0.

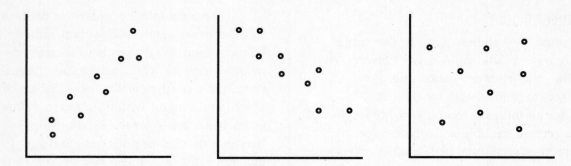

SCALARS AND VECTORS

There are two kinds of physical quantities that are dealt with extensively in science and mathematics. One quantity has magnitude only, and the other has magnitude and direction. A quantity that has magnitude only is called a *scalar* quantity. The length of an object expressed in a particular unit of length, mass, time, and density are all examples of scalars. A quantity that has both magnitude and direction is called a *vector*. Forces, velocities, and accelerations are examples of vectors.

It is customary to represent a vector by an arrow. The length of the arrow represents the magnitude of the vector, and the direction in which the arrow is pointing represents the direction. Thus, a force, for example, could be represented graphically by an arrow pointing in the direction in which the force acts and having a length (in some convenient unit of measure) equal to the magnitude of the force. The vector below, for example, represents a force of magnitude three units, acting in a direction 45° above the horizontal.

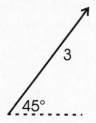

Two vectors are said to be equal if they are parallel, have the same magnitude (length), and point in the same direction. Thus, the two vectors **V** and **U** in the diagram below are equal. If a vector has the same magnitude as **U** but points in the opposite direction, it is denoted as −**U**.

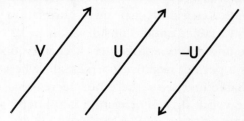

OPERATIONS ON VECTORS

To find the sum of two vectors **A** and **B**, we draw from the head of vector **A** a vector equal to **B**. The sum of **A** and **B** is then defined as the vector drawn from the foot of **A** to the head of **B**.

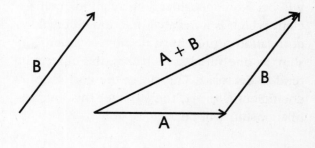

This technique of vector addition can enable us to compute the net effect of two different forces applied simultaneously to the same body.

Example

Two forces, one of magnitude $3\sqrt{3}$ pointing to the east and one of magnitude 3 pointing to the north, act on a body at the same time. Determine the direction in which the body will move and the magnitude of the force with which it will move.

Begin by drawing vectors **OA** and **OB** representing the two forces. Redraw vector **OB** on the tip of **OA**. Then, draw in the vector **OC**, which represents the sum of the two vectors. The body will move in the direction in which this vector is pointing, with a force equal to the magnitude of the vector.

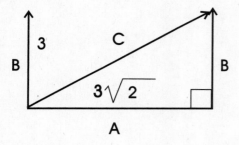

Since **OA** and **OB** operate at right angles to each other, we can use the Pythagorean theorem to determine the magnitude of the *resultant* vector.

$$(3\sqrt{2})^2 + 3^2 = C^2$$
$$27 + 9 = C^2$$
$$36 = C^2$$
$$6 = C$$

Further, by recalling the properties of the 30-60-90 triangle, we can see that the resultant force is 30° to the horizontal. Thus, the body will move with a force of 6 units at an angle of 30° to the horizontal.

To subtract the vector **U** from the vector **V**, we first draw the vectors from a common origin. Then, the vector extending from the tip of **U** to the tip of **V** and pointing to the tip of **V** is defined as the difference **V − U**.

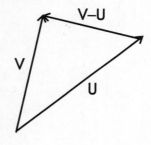

Unit 4

CHEMISTRY

1 H 1.0																	2 He 4.0
3 Li 6.9	4 Be 9.0											5 B 10.8	6 C 12.0	7 N 14.0	8 O 16.0	9 F 19.0	10 Ne 20.2
11 Na 23.0	12 Mg 24.3											13 Al 27.0	14 Si 28.1	15 P 31.0	16 S 32.1	17 Cl 35.5	18 Ar 39.9
19 K 39.1	20 Ca 40.1	21 Sc 45.0	22 Ti 47.9	23 V 50.9	24 Cr 52.0	25 Mn 54.9	26 Fe 55.8	27 Co 58.9	28 Ni 58.7	29 Cu 63.5	30 Zn 65.4	31 Ga 69.7	32 Ge 72.6	33 As 74.9	34 Se 79.0	35 Br 79.9	36 Kr 83.8
37 Rb 85.5	38 Sr 87.6	39 Y 88.9	40 Zr 91.2	41 Nb 92.9	42 Mo 95.9	43 Tc (98)	44 Ru 101.1	45 Rh 102.9	46 Pd 106.4	47 Ag 107.9	48 Cd 112.4	49 In 114.8	50 Sn 118.7	51 Sb 121.8	52 Te 127.6	53 I 126.9	54 Xe 131.3
55 Cs 132.9	56 Ba 137.3	57 La* 138.9	72 Hf 178.5	73 Ta 180.9	74 W 183.9	75 Re 186.2	76 Os 190.2	77 Ir 192.2	78 Pt 195.1	79 Au 197.0	80 Hg 200.6	81 Tl 204.4	82 Pb 207.2	83 Bi 209.0	84 Po (209)	85 At (210)	86 Rn (222)
87 Fr (223)	88 Ra 226.0	89 Act† 227.0	104 Unq (261)	105 Unp (262)	106 Unh (263)	107 Uns (262)	108 Uno (265)	109 Une (267)									

*	58 Ce 140.1	59 Pr 140.9	60 Nd 144.2	61 Pm (145)	62 Sm 150.4	63 Eu 152.0	64 Gd 157.3	65 Tb 158.9	66 Dy 162.5	67 Ho 164.9	68 Er 167.3	69 Tm 168.9	70 Yb 173.0	71 Lu 175.0
†	90 Th 232.0	91 Pa (231)	92 U 238.0	93 Np (237)	94 Pu (244)	95 Am (243)	96 Cm (247)	97 Bk (247)	98 Cf (251)	99 Es (252)	100 Fm (257)	101 Md (258)	102 No (259)	103 Lr (260)

1. Isotopes of an element all contain the same:

   A. gram formula mass
   B. gram atomic mass
   C. number of neutrons
   D. number of protons

The correct answer is (D). An element is defined by its number of protons. An isotope is defined as a form of an element that varies in the number of neutrons. Therefore, isotopes vary in mass and number of neutrons, but the number of protons is the same. **Topic:** The Atom

2. If we exclude Helium, all of the inert gases have:

   A. different numbers of electrons in their outer orbits
   B. eight electrons in their outer orbits
   C. eighteen electrons in their outer orbits
   D. filled outer orbits

The correct answer is (B). The inert gases, excluding helium, all have eight electrons in their outermost orbit, thus rendering them unreactive. Filling orbits 3, 4, 5, and beyond with the maximum of 18, 32, 50, etc., respectively, does not appear to be necessary in order for these elements to be inert. **Topic:** The Atom

3. Electron configuration is usually written in terms of additional electrons from group _____ elements.

   A. 8
   B. 18
   C. 2
   D. 4

The correct answer is (B). Scientists refer back to the inert gas, or group 18 element, on the row previous to the element in question and indicate any additional orbital information with the appropriate s, p, d, f information, e.g., manganese would be [Ar]$4s^2 3d^5$ **Topic:** The Atom

4. Potassium-40 has more _____ than Potassium-39.

   A. electrons
   B. protons
   C. neutrons
   D. ions

The correct answer is (C). These two substances are isotopes of the same element; therefore, they have the same number of protons and electrons. It is the varying number of neutrons that define an isotope and cause the mass to be different. **Topic:** Components of the Atom

5. Under ordinary conditions, if an element becomes a positive ion it:

   A. has converted a neutron into a proton
   B. has lost electrons
   C. has gained protons
   D. is a nonmetal

The correct answer is (B). **Topic:** Components of the Atom

6. The diagram ↑↓ indicates:

   A. the charge on an atom
   B. the proton placement
   C. the direction of two neutron charges
   D. the spin of two electrons

The correct answer is (D). Arrows are used to indicate the spin of electrons. **Topic:** Placement of Electrons—Energy Levels

7. The maximum number of electrons that can fit in energy level #5 is:

   A. 18
   B. 50
   C. 64
   D. 32

The correct answer is (B). Using the formula $2n^2$ to calculate the number of electrons that fill an energy level, where n = the number of the energy level, we get a maximum of 50 electrons for the 5th level. **Topic:** Placement of Electrons—Energy Levels

8. Using the periodic table, the atomic number for antimony is:

A. 15
B. 51
C. 121.76
D. 122

The correct answer is (B). The atomic number is the smaller of the two numbers indicated and always a whole number. Answer (D) is a whole number, but it was rounded off from the decimal number that is the natural abundance atomic mass. **Topic:** Periodic Table

9. Of the four elements given, which would have properties most similar to potassium?

A. Argon
B. Magnesium
C. Nitrogen
D. Iodine

The correct answer is (B). Magnesium, like potassium, is a metal. **Topic:** Periodic Table

10. A bromide ion contains _____ electrons.

A. 34
B. 35
C. 36
D. 80

The correct answer is (C). Since a bromine atom is in the Group 17 elements, it has a tendency to gain one electron to become a bromide ion. The atomic number of 35 indicates that it has 35 protons and 35 electrons in the neutral state with the outermost orbit needing one more electron in order to be filled. When this occurs, the bromide ion acquires a negative charge and now holds 36 electrons. **Topic:** Periodic Table

11. $[Kr]4d^{10}5s^25p^2$ is the electron configuration for:

A. Krypton
B. Scandium
C. Silicon
D. Tin

The correct answer is (D). The electron configuration indicated includes Krypton, element number 36, plus 14 more electrons, giving the electron total found in Tin, element #50. **Topic:** Periodic Table

12. All gases:

A. have high densities
B. have no definite shape or volume
C. are lighter than air
D. exhibit similar chemical behavior

The correct answer is (B). **Topic:** Gases

13. Ideal gas molecules:

A. move very slowly
B. have strong attractive forces
C. move in curved paths
D. have zero volume

The correct answer is (D). **Topic:** Gases

14. Which solids conduct electricity?

A. Ionic
B. Metallic
C. Molecular
D. All of these

The correct answer is (B). Metals are surrounded by a large number of highly mobile valence electrons. **Topic:** Liquids and Solids

15. Viscosity:

    A. decreases as temperature increases
    B. increases as temperature increases
    C. does not depend on temperature
    D. stays constant from liquid to liquid

The correct answer is (A). Viscosity is dependent on intermolecular forces. As the temperature increases, these attractive forces begin to break down with the increase in motion that comes with an increase in temperature. **Topic:** Liquids and Solids

16. When the vapor pressure of a liquid equals atmospheric pressure, the liquid will:

    A. boil
    B. freeze
    C. sublime
    D. ignite

The correct answer is (A). Raising the vapor pressure of a liquid to atmospheric pressure causes the liquid to freely and rapidly pass into the atmosphere. This is called boiling. **Topic:** Phase Changes

17. Evaporation:

    A. occurs at the same rate for all liquids
    B. increases as temperature increases
    C. is in equilibrium with condensation
    D. is the same thing as boiling

The correct answer is (B). As temperature increases, kinetic theory states that the motion of particles also increases. In a liquid, this would cause more and more particles to escape. This would cause evaporation to increase. **Topic:** Phase Changes

18. Which type of formula best shows how atoms combine in a molecule?

    A. Molecular
    B. Empirical
    C. Structural
    D. Chemical

The correct answer is (C). By definition, the structural formula of a molecule best shows the placement of atoms and the bonds that keep them together. **Topic:** Chemical Compounds

19. Ionic compounds are always:

    A. electrically neutral
    B. made up of atoms that share electrons
    C. polyatomic cations
    D. the same as molecules

The correct answer is (A). They are the result of positive ions and negative ions combining in exact ratios to neutralize any excess charge. **Topic:** Chemical Compounds

20. A group of atoms united by covalent bonds is a(n):

    A. cation
    B. molecule
    C. ionic compound
    D. octet

The correct answer is (B). **Topic:** Chemical Compounds

21. A chemical reaction has not occurred if the products have:

    A. the same mass as the reactants
    B. less total bond energy than the reactants
    C. more total bond energy than the reactants
    D. the same chemical properties as the reactants

The correct answer is (D). Definition of a chemical reaction. **Topic:** Balanced Chemical Equations

22. When balancing a chemical equation, use coefficients to:

    A. make atoms of all elements equal to the same number
    B. change the valence number of the atom
    C. use the correct chemical formula
    D. satisfy the law of conservation of mass

The correct answer is (D). The formulas of both the reactants and the products cannot be changed to account for more or less material. Only by changing the coefficients of the materials involved can you balance a chemical equation. **Topic:** Balanced Chemical Equations

23. Of the following chemical equations, the only one that is both combustion and decomposition is:

    A. $C(s) + O_2(g) \rightarrow CO_2(g)$
    B. $2C_4H_{10}(l) + 13O_2(g) \rightarrow 8CO_2(g) + 10H_2O(g)$
    C. $2H_2O_2(l) \rightarrow 2H_2O(l) + O_2(g)$
    D. $4Fe(s) + 3O_2(s) \rightarrow 2Fe_2O_3(s)$

The correct answer is (B). This is the only choice in which something is decomposed using oxygen and yielding carbon dioxide. **Topic:** Balanced Chemical Equations

24. Which of the following would be the most concentrated solution?

    A. 220 g of $C_{12}H_{22}O_{11}$ in 1 kg of water
    B. 150,000 ppm of $C_{12}H_{22}O_{11}$ in water
    C. 10% solution of in $C_{12}H_{22}O_{11}$ water
    D. 1 mole of $C_{12}H_{22}O_{11}$ in 1 L of water

The correct answer is (D). A mole is the largest number of particles of all four. **Topic:** Solutions

25. The compound that will most likely dissolve in water:

    A. is not a dipole
    B. has effective poles in different position
    C. has effective poles in the same position
    D. contains hydrogen sulfide

The correct answer is (B). This is the best situation in which the bipolar nature of water will have the most effect. **Topic:** Solutions

26. Molecules that have both polar and nonpolar regions:

    A. are likely to be flammable
    B. could act as emulsifying agents
    C. will not dissolve in any solvent
    D. are unstable

The correct answer is (B). Emulsifying agents serve to disperse nonpolar substances in polar substances. **Topic:** Solutions

27. A solution of a weak base dissolved in water will:

    A. conduct an electric current as well as a strong acid
    B. taste sour
    C. feel slippery
    D. react with metal to produce H_2 gas

The correct answer is (C). The base will retain its slippery quality but not have any of the others listed. **Topic:** Bases

28. By the Arrhenius definitions, a base:

    A. produces an H^+ ion in water
    B. reacts with a metal to produce H_2
    C. feels slippery on the skin
    D. produces an OH^- ion in water

The correct answer is (D). Simple definition of an Arrhenius base. **Topic:** Bases

29. A substance that can act as an acid or a base is:

   A. a conjugate acid
   B. a conjugate base
   C. amphoteric
   D. methane

The correct answer is (C). Simple definition of amphoteric. **Topic:** Acids

30. The addition of an excess of a strong acid to a weak base in water produces:

   A. an acidic salt solution
   B. a basic salt solution
   C. a neutral salt solution
   D. pure water

The correct answer is (A). There is more than enough acid to combine with all the base to produce the salt with some acid left over to lower the pH somewhat. **Topic:** Acids

31. Pure water has a neutral pH because:

   A. it completely dissociates
   B. $[H_3O^+]$ and $[OH^-]$ are equal
   C. all amphoteric compounds are neutral
   D. it does not dissociate

The correct answer is (B). Water (H_2O) dissociates into equal numbers of H^+ ions, which combine with the available H_2O molecules to produce H_3O^+ ions, and OH^- ions. Water does not completely dissociate. There would be no water left. **Topic:** pH

32. A pH indicator changes color due to:

   A. the heat of acidification
   B. an increase in either K_a or K_b
   C. an equilibrium shift resulting from an increase in $[H_3O^+]$ or $[OH^-]$
   D. hydrogen ion donors reaching an equilibrium with hydrogen ion acceptors

The correct answer is (C). This shift brings about the color change in substances we use as indicators. **Topic:** pH

33. The compound BaO is a(n):

   A. acidic anhydride
   B. basic anhydride
   C. salt
   D. buffer

The correct answer is (B). When mixed in water, BaO reacts to form $Ba(OH)_2$. **Topic:** Buffers

34. A good buffer could be a mixture of:

   A. ammonia and NaOH
   B. acetic acid and HCl
   C. acetic acid and sodium acetate
   D. a strong acid and a strong base

The correct answer is (C). Acetate ions readily accept H^+ ions leaving few H_3O^+ ions in solution so the pH changes only slightly. **Topic:** Buffers

35. In a chemical cell composed of two half-cells, ions are allowed to flow from one half-cell to the other by means of:

   A. electrodes
   B. a wire
   C. a voltmeter
   D. a salt bridge

The correct answer is (D). The classic setup for a chemical cell. **Topic:** Electrochemistry

36. In a voltaic cell, reduction occurs at the:

A. anode
B. electrolyte
C. salt bridge
D. cathode

The correct answer is (D). Reduction is the acceptance of electrons, which are available at the negative half-cell or the cathode. **Topic:** Electrochemistry

37. When the enthalpy of the products is greater than the enthalpy of the reactants, the reaction:

A. releases heat
B. absorbs heat
C. is spontaneous
D. can do work

The correct answer is (B). The products absorb the heat in what is known as an endothermic reaction. **Topic:** Thermodynamics

38. In all spontaneous processes:

A. enthalpy decreases
B. free energy increases
C. useful work can be performed
D. $S_{universe}$ decreases

The correct answer is (C). A spontaneous process is one that can proceed on its own without any outside intervention. **Topic:** Thermodynamics

39. The activation energy is the amount of energy necessary to form the:

A. products
B. catalyst
C. reaction mechanism
D. activated complex

The correct answer is (D). Once this level is reached, the reaction proceeds on its own. **Topic:** Rates of Reaction

40. The rate of a particular reaction doubles for each 10°C increase in temperature. If the reaction takes 200 seconds to be completed at 30°C, at 70°C it will require:

A. 12.5 seconds
B. 1,000 seconds
C. 100 seconds
D. 160 seconds

The correct answer is (A). Collision theory states that the faster the particles move, the more likely they are to collide. Temperature raises the kinetic energy [motion] of particles. **Topic:** Rates of Reaction

41. Which of the following is not a pure substance?

A. Milk
B. Hydrogen
C. Water
D. Oxygen

The correct answer is (A). Milk is a mixture of a variety of substances. It is not composed of one thing only. **Topic:** Characteristics of Mixtures and Compounds

42. A homogenous mixture can be separated by all of the following methods except:

A. distillation
B. chromatography
C. crystallization
D. filtration

The correct answer is (D). Choices A through C involve methods that are able to distinguish between molecules. The spaces between fibers are too large in filter paper to use this to separate molecules in most homogenous mixtures. **Topic:** Characteristics of Mixtures and Compounds

43. When the equation $Al + Br_2 \rightarrow AlBr_3$ is balanced, the coefficient for Al is:

A. 1
B. 2
C. 3
D. 4

The correct answer is (B). $2AL + Br^2 \rightarrow 2AlBr_3$ **Topic:** Reactions

44. Two or more substances combine to form one substance in a:

A. direct combination reaction
B. single-replacement reaction
C. decomposition reaction
D. double-replacement reaction

The correct answer is (B). The definition of an S-R type of a reaction. **Topic:** Reactions

45. An equation is balanced by:

A. changing subscripts
B. erasing elements as necessary
C. adding coefficients
D. adding elements as necessary

The correct answer is (C). In order to balance an equation we manipulate the coefficients. Once the formula for a substance is know, it cannot be changed. **Topic:** Reactions

46. Enzymes are a type of:

A. nucleic acid
B. protein
C. lipid
D. carbohydrate

The correct answer is (B). **Topic:** Enzymes

47. DNA is a type of:

A. protein
B. enzyme
C. base
D. nucleic acid

The correct answer is (D). **Topic:** Enzymes

48. The model that describes enzyme activity as being based on a change in shape of the molecule is called the:

A. Pauli principle
B. induced fit model
C. lock and key model
D. tertiary folding model

The correct answer is (B). The enzyme changes shape or conformation as it interacts with its substrate. **Topic:** Enzymes

49. On the Kelvin scale, 37°C equals:

A. 236°K
B. 273°K
C. 310°K
D. 337°K

The correct answer is (C). Kelvin temperatures are °C + 273°. **Topic:** Temperature Conversions

50. On the Celsius scale, 1016°K is equal to:

A. 743°C
B. 1289°C
C. 273°C
D. −273°C

The correct answer is (A). Celsius temperatures are °K − 273°. **Topic:** Temperature Conversions

51. Who first developed the atomic theory of matter?

A. Benjamin Franklin
B. Democritus
C. John Dalton
D. François Joule

The correct answer is (C). Dalton was one of the first to explain the behavior of matter in terms of atoms. **Topic:** Formulas and Laws

52. "An orbital can hold a maximum of 2 electrons" is a consequence of:

A. the Pauli exclusion principle
B. Hund's Rule
C. the Bohr atom
D. the Aufbau principle

The correct answer is (A). This is Pauli's fundamental observation concerning the placement of the electrons. **Topic:** Formulas and Laws

53. Where "n" is a quantum level, the maximum number of electrons in that level is given by the formula:

A. $n + 2$
B. $2n^2$
C. $2n$
D. $n^2 - 2n$

The correct answer is (B). The basic formula for calculating the maximum number of electrons in each orbit. **Topic:** Formulas and Laws

54. "If a change in conditions is imposed on a system at equilibrium, the equilibrium position will change in the direction that tends to reduce that change," is a statement of:

A. Hund's Rule
B. LeChatelier's Principle
C. Gibb's free energy condition
D. Hess's Rule

The correct answer is (B). This is LeChatelier's statement regarding equilibrium. **Topic:** Formulas and Laws

55. Carbon is unique in that it can:

A. form covalent bonds
B. become a metal
C. bond with other nonmetals
D. form long chains of atoms

The correct answer is (D). Forming covalent bonds is not as unique as the long chain polymers that carbon forms. **Topic:** Organic: General Considerations

56. Which of the following is not an organic compound?

A. CO_2
B. C_5H_{12}
C. $C_{12}H_{22}O_{11}$
D. C_2H_3O

The correct answer is (A). The end product of combustion and respiration, CO_2, is generally not considered an organic molecule. **Topic:** Organic: General Considerations

57. Which of the following does not represent an allotrope of carbon?

A. Graphite
B. Fullerene
C. Lead
D. Diamond

The correct answer is (C). Lead is an entirely different element and not a form of carbon. **Topic:** Organic: General Considerations

58. Polymers are formed by joining individual units called:

A. plastics
B. carbon
C. minimers
D. monomers

The correct answer is (D). Polymers are defined as large molecules formed by joining monomers together. **Topic:** Organic: General Considerations

59. Proteins are made by:

  A. monomerization
  B. polymerization
  C. cellular respiration
  D. double replacement

The correct answer is (B). Since proteins are polymers of amino acids (monomers), the process of making a protein is called polymerization. **Topic:** Organic: General Considerations

60. In water, most hydrocarbons are:

  A. insoluble
  B. soluble
  C. reactive
  D. more dense

The correct answer is (A). Most nonpolar hydrocarbons do not dissolve in water. **Topic:** Organic: General Considerations

61. C_6H_{12} could be a(n):

  A. alkane
  B. alkyne
  C. alkene
  D. benzene

The correct answer is (C). The presence of one unsaturated bond in C_6H_{12} gives the formula indicated. **Topic:** Hydrocarbons

62. Which of the following formulas represents a noncyclic alkane?

  A. C_3H_6
  B. C_8H_{14}
  C. C_5H_{10}
  D. C_6H_{14}

The correct answer is (D). Having no unsaturated bonds, noncyclic alkanes are given by the formula C_nH_{n+2}. **Topic:** Hydrocarbons

63. A six-carbon hydrocarbon that has two major resonance structures is:

  A. hexane
  B. hexene
  C. cyclane
  D. benzene

The correct answer is (D). The double bonds in benzene have two dominant, resonant arrangements. **Topic:** Hydrocarbons

64. A saturated hydrocarbon always has:

  A. only single bonds
  B. at least one double or triple bond
  C. a ring
  D. more carbon atoms than hydrogen atoms

The correct answer is (A). The definition of a saturated bond is a single bond (sharing of one pair of electrons) so a hydrocarbon with only single bonds is called a saturated hydrocarbon. **Topic:** Alkanes

65. The general formula for a noncyclic alkane is:

  A. C_nH_{2n}
  B. C_nH_n
  C. C_nH_{2n+2}
  D. C_nH_{2n-2}

The correct answer is (C). **Topic:** Alkanes

66. Cyclic hydrocarbons with only single bonds are called:

  A. cycloalkenes
  B. cycloalkanes
  C. cyclobenzenes
  D. cycloalkynes

The correct answer is (B). Alkanes have no double, triple, or aromatic (unsaturated) bonds. **Topic:** Cycloalkanes

67. Which of the following could be a cycloalkane?

    A. C_5H_{12}
    B. C_5H_{10}
    C. C_8H_{20}
    D. $C_{10}H_{22}$

The correct answer is (B). Unlike the noncyclic alkanes, the cycloalkanes are given by the formula C_nH_{2n}. **Topic:** Cycloalkanes

68. The general formula for a noncyclic monoalkene is:

    A. C_nH_{2n}
    B. C_nH_n
    C. C_nH_{2n+2}
    D. C_nH_{2n-2}

The correct answer is (A). **Topic:** Alkenes

69. Which of the following is an example of a noncyclic monoalkene?

    A. C_3H_6
    B. C_8H_{14}
    C. C_5H_{12}
    D. C_6H_{14}

The correct answer is (A). Such alkenes are given by the formula C_nH_{2n}. **Topic:** Alkenes

70. Alkynes differ from other hydrocarbons in that they contain:

    A. all single bonds
    B. some double bonds
    C. at least one triple bond
    D. oxygen

The correct answer is (C). **Topic:** Alkynes

71. Which of the following could be an alkyne?

    A. C_2H_6
    B. C_2H_2
    C. C_2H_4
    D. None of these

The correct answer is (B). This is ethyne (acetylene). **Topic:** Alkynes

72. Aromatics typically contain a(n):

    A. benzene ring
    B. alkane
    C. cycloalkane
    D. isomer of pentane

The correct answer is (A). The characteristic aroma of many compounds comes from the addition of a benzene ring to a larger molecule. **Topic:** Aromatics

73. Nearly all alkyl and aryl halides form Grignard reagents when reacting with:

    A. Lithium
    B. Manganese
    C. Magnesium
    D. Mercury

The correct answer is (C). The definition of a Grignard reagent. **Topic:** Grignard Reagents

74. Which of the following is not an example of an industrial/commercial product made using Grignard reagents?

    A. Vitamins
    B. Motor fuel additives
    C. Inorganic additives
    D. Synthetic perfumes

The correct answer is (C). Grignard reagents are used in the organic field. **Topic:** Grignard Reagents

75. Alcohols contain a:

    A. hydroxyl group
    B. carbonyl group
    C. carboxyl group
    D. benzene ring

The correct answer is (A). **Topic:** Alcohols

76. The general formula for an alcohol is:

    A. RX
    B. ROR′
    C. RCOOH
    D. ROH

The correct answer is (D). The distinguishing characteristic of alcohols is the −OH group. **Topic:** Alcohols

77. Two classes of organic compounds that contain nitrogen are:

    A. alcohols and ethers
    B. esters and carboxylic acids
    C. amines and amides
    D. aldehydes and ketones

The correct answer is (C). **Topic:** Amines

78. The general formula for an amine is:

    A. $R\text{-}NH_4$
    B. $R\text{-}NH_3$
    C. $R\text{-}NH_2$
    D. none of these

The correct answer is (C). **Topic:** Amines

79. The general formula for an amide is:

    A. $R\text{-}CONH_2$
    B. $R\text{-}COOH$
    C. $R\text{-}CH_3OH$
    D. $R\text{-}NH_3$

The correct answer is (A). **Topic:** Amides

80. Amide bonds link together the monomers in a:

    A. protein
    B. carbohydrate
    C. lipid
    D. nucleic acid

The correct answer is (A). Amide bonds are also known as peptide bonds, the basic linkage in the formation of proteins. **Topic:** Amides

81. The reduction of a primary alcohol will produce a(n):

    A. aldehyde
    B. amide
    C. alkane
    D. benzene ring

The correct answer is (C). Primary alcohols can be formed when a hydroxyl group replaces a hydrogen in an alkane. Reduction of the alcohol replaces the OH with the hydrogen in a reversal of the formation of the alcohol. **Topic:** Alcohols

82. The difference between the structures of aldehydes and ketones is:

    A. type of functional group
    B. kind of atoms in the molecules
    C. placement of the functional group in the molecule
    D. ability to form hydrogen bonds

The correct answer is (C). An aldehyde has a carbonyl group at the end of a hydrocarbon chain whereas the ketones have their carbonyl groups in the interior of hydrocarbon chains. **Topic:** Aldehydes and Ketones

83. The condensed structural formula CH_3CH_2CHO signifies a(n):

    A. alcohol
    B. aldehyde
    C. ketone
    D. carboxylic acid

The correct answer is (B). This places the carbonyl group at the end, making this an aldehyde using the designation R-CHO. **Topic:** Aldehydes and Ketones

84. The general formula for carboxylic acids is:

    A. R-CHO
    B. R-COOH
    C. R-COR′
    D. R-NH$_2$

The correct answer is (B). **Topic:** Carboxylic Acids

85. The most polar organic acids are:

    A. amides
    B. ethers
    C. alcohols
    D. carboxylic acids

The correct answer is (D). The carboxylic end of the molecule is an electron-rich area because both oxygens have unshared electron pairs. **Topic:** Carboxylic Acids

86. The general formula for an ester is:

    A. R-COOH
    B. R-CHO
    C. R-COOR′
    D. R-O-R′

The correct answer is (C). **Topic:** Esters

87. The IUPAC name for ethyl butyl ether is:

    A. ethoxybutane
    B. ethylbutyrate
    C. butylethoxate
    D. butryic ethoxide

The correct answer is (A). **Topic:** Ethers

88. The biomass evident in a particular biome on the Earth consists of:

    A. almost all the water and minerals
    B. all the organic substances
    C. abiotic factors
    D. none of the above

The correct answer is (B). All of the organic material in the environment makes up what we call the biomass. **Topic:** Final remarks

89. Biochemistry is the study of:

    A. photosynthesis
    B. cellular respiration
    C. the chemicals of life
    D. hydrocarbons

The correct answer is (C). **Topic:** Areas of Biochemistry

90. The pH of the blood:

    A. stays in the narrow range of 7.35–7.45
    B. is usually below 7
    C. must be above 8
    D. can vary by as much as one or two points on the pH scale.

The correct answer is (A). The pH of the blood must stay within a very narrow range and is helped to do that by certain buffers in the blood. **Topic:** pH

91. Buffers in the blood are mainly there to control the constant production, by most physiological activities, of:

   A. acids
   B. bases
   C. lipids
   D. hydrocarbons

The correct answer is (A). Most physiological activities in the body produce acids which are controlled by the presence of buffers. **Topic:** Buffers—Biochemistry

92. Amino acids always contain C, H, O, and

   A. S
   B. N
   C. Cl
   D. P

The correct answer is (B). The amino group is so named because it contains nitrogen. **Topic:** Amino acids

93. Biochemists call the amide bond between amino acids a(n):

   A. amino bond
   B. peptide bond
   C. protein bond
   D. hydrated bond

The correct answer is (B). **Topic:** Peptides

94. Proteins are polymers made up of hundreds of monomers called:

   A. lipids
   B. saccharides
   C. nucleotides
   D. amino acids

The correct answer is (D). **Topic:** Proteins

95. The most specialized type of proteins are called:

   A. vitamins
   B. enzymes
   C. glycerols
   D. hormones

The correct answer is (B). **Topic:** Enzymes

96. Glucose and other biomolecules like it that serve to store energy that can be released when needed by cells, belong to a group called:

   A. nucleic acids
   B. carbohydrates
   C. amines
   D. proteins

The correct answer is (B). **Topic:** Carbohydrates

97. Which of the following does not belong in the lipid group?

   A. Fats
   B. Disaccharides
   C. Oils
   D. Waxes

The correct answer is (B). These are members of the carbohydrate group. **Topic:** Lipids

98. DNA is a polymer that includes:

   A. lipids
   B. carbohydrates
   C. nucleic acids
   D. B and C

The correct answer is (D). **Topic:** Nucleic Acids

99. DNA monomers contain one less oxygen than the corresponding monomers of:

A. alpha proteins

B. RNA

C. BNA

D. phospholipids

The correct answer is (B). The structure of DNA and RNA are alike with the exception of one less oxygen in the S-carbon sugar of DNA, hence the name Deoxyribonucleic Acid. **Topic:** Nucleic Acids

100. DNA molecules are made up of long chains of monomers called:

A. nucleic acids

B. nucleotides

C. bases

D. 5-carbon sugars

The correct answer is (B). **Topic:** Nucleic Acids

PHYSICS

1. An object is dropped from a plane that is 2 kilometers above the ground. One tenth of a second after it is dropped the object would have an acceleration of:

A. 9.8 m/s^2

B. more than 9.8 m/s^2

C. 4.9 m/s^2

D. less than 9.8 m/s^2

The correct answer is (D). The acceleration of gravity decreases as you move above sea level. **Topic:** Accelerated Motion

2. A ball tied to a rope and swung in a circle will have:

A. uniform acceleration and uniform velocity

B. a changing acceleration and uniform velocity

C. uniform acceleration and a changing velocity

D. a changing acceleration and a changing velocity

The correct answer is (D). If the object is traveling in a circle, the speed would remain constant but the direction would be changing, so the velocity would be changing. If the velocity is changing, the acceleration must also change. **Topic:** Accelerated Motion

3. When analyzing a distance-time graph, a car's motion would not be considered to be uniform if:

A. the graph was a horizontal line

B. the graph was a vertical line

C. the graph was a curving line

D. all of the above

The correct answer is (C). The slope of a curved line is not constant so the speed of the car must not be constant. **Topic:** Accelerated Motion

4. A foul ball is hit straight up in the air with a speed of 85 miles/hr. How high does the ball go?

A. 74.5 meters

B. 76.9 meters

C. 65.7 meters

D. 83.2 meters

The correct answer is (A). The ball is hit at 38 m/s and will continue moving upwards for 3.9 s before it begins to fall. The distance the ball travels upward is dependent only on the time it takes to reach its highest point. **Topic:** Accelerated Motion

155

5. A ball with mass of 6 kilograms and a ball with a mass of 2 kilograms are dropped off the World Trade Center. Both balls have a circumference of 1 meter. Which statement is true?

   A. Air resistance is greater on the 6 kilogram ball.

   B. Gravity acts with 3 times the force on the 6 kilogram ball.

   C. The 6 kilogram ball will strike the pavement first.

   D. The 2 kilogram ball will strike the pavement first.

The correct answer is (B). The heavier an object is the greater the force that is acting on it, but there is also more mass for that force to accelerate. **Topic:** Accelerated Motion

6. A force causes a 200-pound person to slide across a frictionless surface with an acceleration of 3.2 m/s². What is the magnitude of the force?

   A. 290.9 kg m/s²

   B. 128,000 kg m/s²

   C. 290 N

   D. 305 N

The correct answer is (C). Use the formula F = ma and 1 kg = 2.2 lbs. **Topic:** Forces and Motion

7. If a bowling ball with a weight of 19.6 Newtons is taken to the Moon and allowed to fall from a height of 10 meters, what will its acceleration be?

   A. 1.6 m/s²

   B. 4.9 m/s²

   C. 3.2 m/s²

   D. 3.24 m/s²

The correct answer is (A). The Moon has an acceleration due to gravity ⅙ that of the Earth. Note that the weight of the bowling ball is irrelevant to the problem. **Topic:** Forces and Motion

8. Which of the following statements is correct?

   A. The weight of an object is independent of its mass.

   B. An object will weigh more in an airplane than it will on the ground.

   C. Moving an object vertically will change its weight.

   D. Moving an object horizontally will change its weight.

The correct answer is (C). The higher above sea level an object is the less gravity will affect it. **Topic:** Forces and Motion

9. Jim gets in a car and drives 40 m/s east to Judy's house and stops to pick her up. He then drives at 35 m/s back to his house. Judy lives 5 km from Jim, and the trip takes a total of 30 minutes. The net acceleration of Jim's car will be:

   A. 9 m/s²

   B. 135 m/s²

   C. 1.8 m/s²

   D. 0

The correct answer is (D). The resultant velocity is zero because the car started and ended in the same place. Therefore, the net acceleration must also be zero. **Topic:** Forces and Motion

10. An ultralight flying at 20 miles per hour touches down in a cow pasture. If it is decelerating at a rate of 4.5 m/s, how long does the pasture have to be for the plane to come to a complete stop?

   A. 8.8 meters
   B. 8.8 kilometers
   C. 8.8 hectometers
   D. 33 feet

The correct answer is (A). Convert mph to m/s and then use the formula: original velocity^2 = 2as. **Topic:** Forces and Motion

11. Concurrent forces of 50 N east and 70 N at 30° north of east act on a ball. What is the resultant force?

   A. 104 N 26° north of east
   B. 104 N 26° east of north
   C. 10.4 N 26° north of east
   D. 104 N 60° east of north

The correct answer is (A). Use the law of cosines to determine the magnitude of the resultant and then use the law of sines to determine the direction. Do not forget that the resultant vector is drawn from the tail of the first vector to the head of the second vector. **Topic:** Forces and Motion

12. A lawn mower is pushed across a field. Person A kicks it with a force of 5 N and a direction of 270°. Person B kicks it with a force of 4 N and a direction of 135°. Person C kicks it with a force of 3 N and a direction of 45°. What direction will it go?

   A. Northeast
   B. Nowhere
   C. Southeast
   D. Northwest

The correct answer is (B). These vectors have a resultant vector of zero. **Topic:** Forces and Motion

13. A person throws an orange horizontally at 10 m/s from the top of a ladder 6 meters high. How far from the base of the ladder will the orange fall?

   A. 4 meters
   B. 3 meters
   C. 2 meters
   D. 1 meter

The correct answer is (C). You must determine how long the orange will remain in the air, and then use this time to determine the horizontal distance. **Topic:** Projectile Motion

14. A plane drops a turkey. If the loadmaster wants the turkey to land by his friend having a picnic, how far away must he release the turkey? The plane is flying at a height of 1.96 km and at a speed of .09 km/s.

   A. 1.8 km
   B. 2.3 km
   C. 180 meters
   D. 230 decameters

The correct answer is (A). **Topic:** Projectile Motion

15. A 150 g mass rests on a rough surface, which exerts a constant frictional force of 5 N. A 45 N force is applied to the mass, resulting in an acceleration of the mass. Determine the acceleration of the mass.

A. 267.0 m/s^2
B. 166 m/s^2
C. 0.13 m/s^2
D. 20.0 m/s^2

The correct answer is (A). You must convert g to kg and find the net force before using the equation: acceleration = force/mass
Topic: Friction

16. Sally picks up a box, weighing 15 N, that is resting on a table 1 meter high. She carries the box waist high (1.5 m) down a hallway that is 50 meters long. She then places the box on another table 1 meter high. How much work did she do on the box?

A. 57.5 J
B. 0 J
C. 25 J
D. 24.5 J

The correct answer is (B). The box did not gain any potential energy because it did not have a net change in height, so work was not done on the box. Work was done on Sally's muscles. **Topic:** Work and Power

17. Bob is pulling his bass boat onto his trailer. He is exerting a force of 13 N on the cable that is held at an angle of 60° from the horizontal. How much work is done when he pulls the boat 50 meters?

A. 321 Newton-meters
B. 32.5 J
C. 325 J
D. 321 J

The correct answer is (C). You have to find the horizontal component of the force, and then use this force and the distance to find the work. **Topic:** Work and Power

18. Bob is pulling his bass boat onto his trailer. He is exerting a force of 13 N on the cable that is held at an angle of 60° from the horizontal. He pulls the boat 50 meters in 5 minutes. Determine the power.

A. 64.2 watts
B. 6.5 watts
C. 1.1 kW
D. 1.1 W

The correct answer is (D). You have to convert minutes to seconds and recall P = W/t. **Topic:** Work and Power

19. A 200 g brick is lifted 5 m in the air. Determine the potential energy of the brick.

A. 9.8 J
B. 9,800 kg meter^2/s^2
C. 9,800 J
D. 49 J

The correct answer is (A). Convert the mass to kilograms, then use the equation: potential energy = (mass)(gravity)(height). **Topic:** Energy

20. A 200 g brick is slid along a frictionless surface with a speed of 5 m/s. Determine the kinetic energy of the brick.

    A. 2.5 J
    B. 2.5 kJ
    C. 1,000 J
    D. 500 J

The correct answer is (A). Convert g to kg. Kinetic energy = $\frac{1}{2}$(mass) (velocity^2) divided by 2. **Topic:** Energy

21. An electron is shot through a vacuum with a speed of 2.5×10^5 km/s. If the mass of the electron is 9.0×10^{-31} kg, determine the kinetic energy of the electron.

    A. 2.8×10^{-7} J
    B. 2.8×10^{-14} J
    C. 2.8×10^{17} J
    D. 2.8×10^{11} J

The correct answer is (B). Convert the speed to m/s then use the formula: Kinetic energy = $\frac{1}{2}$(mass)(velocity^2). **Topic:** Energy

22. A force of 15 N is applied to a concrete block with a mass of 1.5 kg. The force is applied for a total of 5 seconds. Determine the change in momentum.

    A. 65 Newton-seconds
    B. 65 J
    C. 75 Newton-seconds
    D. 75 J

The correct answer is (C). Impulse = change of momentum. Change of momentum = (mass)(change in velocity), and change in velocity = (force)(time)/(mass). **Topic:** Momentum

23. A 500 kg stock car is traveling a dirt track with a radius of 100 m. It takes 1.5 minutes to make one lap of the track. Determine the acceleration of the car.

    A. 15.5 m/s
    B. 30 m/s
    C. 10 m/s
    D. 10.5 m/s

The correct answer is (A). You have to determine the centripetal force and then determine the centripetal acceleration. Centripetal force = (mass)(4)(pi)(radius^2) divided by the period^2. Centripetal acceleration = velocity^2 divided by the radius. **Topic:** Uniform Circular Motion–Centripetal Acceleration.

24. In circular motion the centripetal force must be _____ to the object's instantaneous velocity.

    A. parallel
    B. at 45°
    C. at 60°
    D. perpendicular

The correct answer is (D). The force has to act perpendicular to the circular motion for the circular motion to continue. **Topic:** Uniform Circular Motion

25. Jake swings a bucket of water with a mass of 1.5 kg, in a circle that remains parallel to the ground. The bucket is 1 meter from his shoulder. If the bucket is swung at a rate of 2 rev/sec, determine the centripetal force.

A. 47 N
B. 4.7 N
C. 14.8 N
D. 1.48 N

The correct answer is (B).

Centripetal force $= \dfrac{(mass)(4)(pi)(radius^2)}{period^2}$.

Topic: Uniform Circular Motion

26. A car with a mass of 550 kg is traveling around a curve. It takes 25 seconds to get around the curve. If the centripetal force is 5.0 N, determine the centrifugal force.

A. 5.0 N
B. 50 N
C. 3.5 N
D. You need more information.

The correct answer is (A). Centripetal force must equal centrifugal force in magnitude if the car is going to stay on the road and go around the curve. The two forces act in opposite directions. **Topic:** Uniform Circular Motion

27. Fifty-one cubic meters of oxygen, under a pressure of 100 kPa, is compressed until its volume is 37 cubic meters. Determine the final pressure acting on the oxygen.

A. 73 kPa
B. 73 Pa
C. 140 kPa
D. 140 Pa

The correct answer is (C). Pressure(1) × Volume(1) = Pressure(2) × Volume(2). **Topic:** Fluids at Rest

28. A metal ball with a mass of 54 g is lowered into a vat of liquid. The ball displaces 35 ml of the liquid. What is the density?

A. .0015 g/ml
B. 1.5 g/ml
C. .01 g/ml
D. 3.2 kg/l

The correct answer is (B). Density = mass/volume. **Topic:** Fluids at Rest

29. One gallon of water has a mass of 3.6 kg. Find the specific gravity of an unknown liquid if one gallon of it has a mass of 4.2 kg.

A. 1.2
B. .86
C. 2.1
D. 8.6

The correct answer is (A). Specific gravity = mass of given volume divided by the mass of an equal volume of water. **Topic:** Fluids at Rest

30. In order for an object to float, which of the following statements must be true?

A. The gravitational force and the buoyant force must be equal.
B. The gravitational force must be greater than the buoyant force.
C. The mass of the object must be lighter than the mass of the fluid it is in.
D. The buoyant force must be greater than the gravitational force.

The correct answer is (D). **Topic:** Fluids at Rest

31. Two balls each with a mass of 5.3 kg are placed next to each other. What gravitational force do they exert on each other if their centers are 249 mm apart?

    A. 1.42×10^{-9} N
    B. 1.42×10^{-8} N
    C. 3.0×10^{-8} N
    D. 7.5×10^{-12} N

The correct answer is (C). Convert mm to m and then use the formula:

$$\text{Force} = \frac{(\text{Gravitational constant})(\text{mass1})(\text{mass2})}{\text{radius}^2}$$

where $G = \dfrac{6.67 \times 10^{-11} \text{ Newton-meters}^2}{\text{kg}^2}$.

Topic: Gravity

32. Convert 32° Celsius to Fahrenheit.

    A. 83.6° F
    B. 89.6° F
    C. 85.2° F
    D. 88.3° F

The correct answer is (B). Fahrenheit $= \dfrac{9}{5}$ Celsius + 32. **Topic:** Temperature Calculations and Measurement

33. Convert 23° Celsius to Kelvin.

    A. 296 K
    B. −250 K
    C. 250 K
    D. 123 K

The correct answer is (A). Kelvin = Celsius + 273 **Topic:** Temperature Calculations and Measurement

34. The specific heat of a substance is the amount of heat needed to raise the temperature of a unit mass of that substance through one degree. The correct metric units for specific heat are:

    A. joules per gram Celsius degree
    B. joules per kilogram Celsius degree
    C. joules per gram Kelvin
    D. kilojoules per gram Celsius degree

The correct answer is (A). **Topic:** Heat

35. A 30 g block of metal absorbs 5.016 kJ of heat when its temperature changes from 30° Celsius to 50° Celsius. Determine the specific heat of the metal.

    A. .008 J/g-Celsius degree
    B. .8 J/g-Celsius degree
    C. 8.4 kJ/g-Celsius degree
    D. 8.4 J/g-Celsius degree

The correct answer is (D).

$$\text{Specific Heat} = \frac{(\text{Change in thermal energy/mass})}{\text{Change in temperature}}.$$

Topic: Heat

36. The _____ states that when mechanical energy, electric energy, or any other kind of energy is converted to heat, all energy is conserved.

    A. first law of thermodynamics
    B. second law of thermodynamics
    C. third law of thermodynamics
    D. first law of heat

The correct answer is (A). **Topic:** Heat

37. The same amount of heat necessary to raise the temperature of 30 grams of water from 20° Celsius to 100° Celsius is added to 50 g of zinc. How much heat was added to the zinc?

A. 100 J
B. 10 J
C. 100°
D. 100.8 J

The correct answer is (B). Thermal energy = (mass)(specific heat)(change in temperature). The specific heat of water is $\dfrac{4.21 \text{ J}}{g - °C}$.

Topic: Heat

38. Which of the following statements is true?

A. The latent heat of vaporization for water is greater than that for ethyl alcohol, but less than that for sulfuric acid.
B. The latent heat of vaporization for sulfuric acid is greater than that for both water and ethyl alcohol.
C. The latent heat of vaporization for water is greater than that for both ethyl alcohol and sulfuric acid.
D. The latent heat of vaporization for ethyl alcohol is greater than that for both water and sulfuric acid.

The correct answer is (C). **Topic:** Heat

39. Heat is added to 50 grams of water in the liquid state at 0° Celsius until the temperature of the new gaseous water reaches 110° Celsius. How much heat is absorbed?

A. 113.000 J
B. 1010 J
C. 135 kJ
D. 113 kJ

The correct answer is (C). First you have to determine the heat necessary to move the water from 0 degree Celsius to 100° Celsius (remaining in the liquid state). Second, you have to determine the heat necessary to move the water at 100° Celsius in the liquid state to 100° Celsius in the gaseous state. Third, you have to determine the heat necessary to move the steam from 100° Celsius to 110° Celsius. **Topic:** Heat

40. 35 kJ of work is put into a frictionless roller coaster to raise it 50 meters to the top of the first hill. At the end of the ride the roller coaster still contains 3 kJ of potential energy. How much heat was generated by the roller coaster?

A. 3500 J
B. 35 kJ
C. 300 kJ
D. 32 kJ

The correct answer is (D). The initial work is converted to heat and potential energy. **Topic:** Thermodynamics

41. Thermodynamics dictates that the charge on a solid sphere will be spread:

    A. proportionally throughout, depending on distance from the center
    B. over its outer surface
    C. equally throughout
    D. none of the above

The correct answer is (B). This arrangement puts the electrons the farthest from each other, which causes a state of equilibrium to exist over the surface. **Topic:** Electrostatics

42. A force of 0.4 N is acting on a positive test charge of 3.5×10^{-4}C, which is in an electric field. Determine the size of the electric field intensity at the point where the positive charge is located.

    A. 1.143 N/C
    B. 114 N/C
    C. 1143 N/C
    D. Not enough information is given.

The correct answer is (C). Field intensity = Electric force/unit charge **Topic:** Electrostatics

43. Two parallel plates, 0.3 m apart, have a field intensity between the plates of 2256 N/C. What is the difference in potential between the two plates?

    A. 677 V
    B. 6768 V
    C. 3384 V
    D. 2256 V

The correct answer is (A). Potential difference = (Field intensity)(Distance) **Topic:** Electrostatics

44. A German scientist discovered that the ratio of the potential difference between the ends of a wire and the current flowing through the wire is:

    A. greater the further you get from the ends
    B. a value that fluctuates
    C. a constantly changing value
    D. a constant

The correct answer is (D). **Topic:** Electricity

45. A portable CD player uses two AAA batteries, arranged in series. It has an internal resistance of 0.5 ohms, and a current of 6 amperes. Determine the net voltage of the two batteries.

    A. 1.5 V
    B. 12 V
    C. 6 V
    D. 3 V

The correct answer is (D). Voltage = (Resistance)(Current). **Topic:** Electric Circuits

46. A series circuit has a toaster drawing 12 ohm, a light bulb drawing 88.8 ohm, and a light switch that has an internal resistance of .3 ohms (in the on position). The copper wire exhibits a resistance equal to .15 ohms. If a potential difference of 110 volts is applied to the circuit, with everything working, what would be the resistance of the circuit?

    A. 101.8 ohms
    B. 101 ohms
    C. 10.1 ohms
    D. 10.09 ohms

The correct answer is (B). Resistance in series = R1 + R2 +R3 + etc. Note that the voltage is irrelevant. **Topic:** Electric Circuits

47. A circuit has resistors with values of 36 ohms, 120 ohms, 96 ohms, and 1540 ohms connected in parallel with each other. If a potential difference of 110 volts is applied to the circuit, what will the total resistance be..

A. .005 ohms
B. .0006 ohms
C. 21 ohms
D. 500 ohms

The correct answer is (C). The total resistance of a parallel circuit is the inverse of the sum of the inverses of each resistance. **Topic:** Electric Circuits

48. If a flashlight has 5 dry cell batteries in series, each with a voltage of 1.5 volts, what is the potential difference in the circuit when the switch is in the on position?

A. 1.5 volts
B. 7.5 volts
C. It would depend on the total resistance.
D. It would depend on the current in the circuit.

The correct answer is (B). Batteries placed in series are added together to find the total voltage or potential difference. **Topic:** Electric Circuits

49. You are building a cabin in the mountains and it is too expensive to run an electric line to the cabin, so you are going to use photovoltaic panels to provide the necessary electricity. You will use a battery system to store the energy until it is needed. You purchase twelve 2-volt storage batteries from the telephone company. How would you arrange the batteries to provide a 12-volt D.C. source for your cabin?

A. Hook 6 of them up in series and keep the rest for spares.
B. Hook all of them up in series and use a voltage limiter.
C. Hook all of them up in parallel.
D. Hook six up in series and then connect these in parallel with the other six that are hooked in series.

The correct answer is (D). This arrangement will give you two sources of 12-volt D.C. energy. With the correct switch, when one bank is depleted the other bank can be used, so you will have a constant source of energy. **Topic:** Electric Circuit

50. James Prescott Joule (1818-1889) was know for his work involving

_____.

A. conservation of energy
B. movement of electrical current
C. acceleration of a falling object
D. quantum mechanics

The correct answer is (A). **Topic:** Electric Energy

51. What is the power of an electric motor when it is in a circuit with a potential difference of 110 V and a current of 12 amperes is flowing through the circuit?

A. 9.2 kW
B. 1091 W
C. 1.3 kW
D. 109 W

The correct answer is (C). Power = Potential difference × Current. **Topic:** Electric Energy

52. An AC generator develops a maximum voltage of 240 V in a circuit with a total resistance of 16 ohms. What is the effective voltage of the generator?

A. 240 V
B. 120 V
C. 169.7 V
D. 220 V

The correct answer is (C). The effective voltage = 0.707 (maximum voltage). **Topic:** Alternating Current

53. An AC generator develops a maximum voltage of 240 V in a circuit with a maximum current of 15 amperes. What is the resistance of the circuit?

A. 18.0 ohms
B. 16.0 ohms
C. 3600 ohms
D. .0625 ohms

The correct answer is (B). Resistance in an AC circuit = Effective voltage/effective current (or max voltage/max current). **Topic:** Alternating Current

54. A pulley is used to lift a huge stone weighing 250 N. A force of 75 N is applied to the rope on the pulley. What is the actual mechanical advantage of the pulley?

A. 0.004
B. 3.3
C. 1.65
D. 4.2

The correct answer is (B). Actual mechanical advantage = Force out/force In. **Topic:** Machines and Mechanical Advantage

55. A pulley is used to lift a 100 N concrete block 1 meter. A force of 50 N is applied to the pulley, which moves 2 meters. What is the actual mechanical advantage of the pulley?

A. 2
B. .5
C. 3
D. 2.5

The correct answer is (A). Actual mechanical advantage = Force out/force In. **Topic:** Machines and Mechanical Advantage

56. A machine uses 67 N-M of work to produce 45 N-M of work. What is the efficiency of the machine?

A. 1.49%
B. 74%
C. 53%
D. 67%

The correct answer is (D). Efficiency = (Work out/work in)(100%) **Topic:** Machines and Mechanical Advantage

57. What is the period of a pendulum 5.0 meters long that is set up in Houston, Texas?

   A. 4.5 seconds
   B. 3.2 seconds
   C. 2.2 seconds
   D. 1.2 seconds

The correct answer is (A). Period of a pendulum = (2)(pi)[the square root of (length/gravity)]. **Topic:** Simple Harmonic Motion

58. A(n) _____ wave is one in which the particles of a medium vibrate perpendicularly to the direction of the wave's path.

   A. standing
   B. electromagnetic
   C. transverse
   D. longitudinal

The correct answer is (C). **Topic:** Waves

59. What is the wavelength of a wave with a velocity of 32.0 m/s and a frequency of 15 Hz?

   A. 240 m
   B. 2.1 m
   C. .469 m
   D. 4.69 mm

The correct answer is (B). Wavelength = $\frac{velocity}{frequency}$. **Topic:** Waves

60. When two or more waves meet in the same medium, their displacements will add together. This process is called:

   A. amplification
   B. nodation
   C. construction
   D. interference

The correct answer is (D). **Topic:** Waves

61. _____ occurs when an erect pulse meets an inverted pulse. The amplitude of the resulting pulse is less than the amplitudes of either of the pulses that met.

   A. Destructive interference
   B. Constructive interference
   C. Amplitude destruction
   D. Nodal interference

The correct answer is (A). **Topic:** Waves

62. A wave with a wavelength of 0.5 meters and a frequency of 5 m/s is moving at 90° and meets an identical wave in the same medium moving at 270°. Assuming matched amplitudes, a(n) _____ is the result of this meeting.

   A. standing wave
   B. electrical wave
   C. nodal wave
   D. none of these are correct

The correct answer is (A). **Topic:** Waves

63. In general, most people can hear sound waves with frequencies between _____ and _____.

   A. 50 Hz, 2000 Hz
   B. 1000 Hz, 5000Hz
   C. 2000 Hz, 10000 Hz
   D. 500 Hz, 2500 Hz

The correct answer is (A). **Topic:** Sound Waves

64. A sound with a frequency of 1000 Hz and a intensity level of _____ would probably cause pain in most people.

   A. 90 dB
   B. 95 dB
   C. 110 dB
   D. 120 dB

The correct answer is (D). **Topic:** Sound Waves

65. When a baritone and a flute produce a sound with a frequency of 1000 Hz, they sound differently. This difference in sound is called _____.

   A. beat
   B. node
   C. timbre
   D. none of these

The correct answer is (C). **Topic:** Sound Waves

66. A police car driving down the freeway with its siren on will create sound waves. The sound waves in front of the car will have a higher pitch than the sound waves behind the car. This is a result of:

   A. interference
   B. destruction of air molecules
   C. nodal effect
   D. the Doppler effect

The correct answer is (D). **Topic:** Sound Waves

67. If a light ray strikes a reflecting surface at an angle of 35°, what will the angle of reflection be?

   A. 65°
   B. 35°
   C. 55°
   D. None of these

The correct answer is (A). The angle of reflection = angle of incidence. The angle of incidence is the angle between the incident ray and the normal line, which is perpendicular to the reflecting surface. **Topic:** Light Rays

68. A light ray enters, at an angle, a medium in which its velocity increases. The ray is refracted _____ the normal line.

   A. toward
   B. away from
   C. 90° from
   D. 45° from

The correct answer is (B). **Topic:** Light Rays

69. The index of refraction for a diamond would be _____ the index of refraction for a piece of quartz.

   A. one-half
   B. one-fourth
   C. two-thirds
   D. greater than

The correct answer is (D). The index of refraction for a diamond is 2.42, while that of a piece of quartz is 1.46. This makes the diamond much more desirable for a ring than the piece of quartz. **Topic:** Light Rays

70. A ray of light from the sun strikes a fish tank with an angle of incidence of 60°. What will the angle of refraction be as the ray leaves the tank?

   A. 30°
   B. 45°
   C. 60°
   D. 75°

The correct answer is (C). **Topic:** Light Rays

71. Total internal reflection will only occur if the angle of refraction is _____ the critical angle.

   A. 50% of
   B. greater than
   C. less than
   D. at least 90% of

The correct answer is (B). **Topic:** Light Rays

72. If the image is located the same distance from the mirror as the object, the same size as the object, and is erect but reversed right for left, then the light must be reflecting from a:

   A. concave mirror
   B. convex mirror
   C. spherical mirror
   D. plane mirror

The correct answer is (D). **Topic:** Mirrors

73. If you were interested in safety, you would use a _____ mirror to view the corner where two halls meet.

   A. concave
   B. convex
   C. spherical
   D. plane

The correct answer is (B). A convex mirror causes the light rays to spread out so that you would be able to see a larger area, even though it may be somewhat distorted. **Topic:** Mirrors

74. The focal point of a _____ is located halfway between the center of curvature and the center of the mirror's surface.

   A. concave mirror
   B. convex mirror
   C. spherical mirror
   D. plane mirror

The correct answer is (A). A concave mirror is a converging mirror. **Topic:** Mirrors

75. If the object is beyond the focal point, a _____ lens produces an image that is smaller than the original, virtual, and erect.

   A. concave
   B. convex
   C. spherical
   D. converging

The correct answer is (A). **Topic:** Lenses

76. If an object is placed beyond the focal point, a _____ lens produces an image that is smaller, inverted, and real.

   A. concave
   B. convex
   C. spherical
   D. diverging

The correct answer is (B). **Topic:** Lenses

77. A refracting telescope uses both an objective lens and an eyepiece lens. The eyepiece lens is _____ where the objective lens is convex.

   A. concave
   B. convex
   C. spherical
   D. diverging

The correct answer is (B). **Topic:** Lenses

78. It is thought that _____ with a mass about 300 times greater than the electron pass back and forth between neutrons and protons and are responsible for holding the nucleus together.

   A. leptons
   B. neutrinos
   C. mesons
   D. strings

The correct answer is (C). **Topic:** Composition of the Atom

79. When writing the symbol for isotopes the mass number is written to the _____ of the symbol for the element.

    A. lower right
    B. lower left
    B. upper right
    D. upper left

The correct answer is (D). **Topic:** Composition of the Atom

80. During a nuclear reaction, a gamma ray is emitted. The number of protons in the nucleus:

    A. remains the same
    B. increases by one
    C. decreases by one
    D. increases by two

The correct answer is (A). **Topic:** Composition of the Atom

81. The symbol for an alpha particle is the same as the symbol for a:

    A. hydrogen ion
    B. helium nucleus
    C. hydrogen atom
    D. neon atom

The correct answer is (B). **Topic:** Radioactivity

82. When writing the symbol for a beta particle the mass number is _____ and the atomic number is:

    A. 0, −1
    B. −1, 0
    C. 0, 0
    D. −1, −1

The correct answer is (A). **Topic:** Radioactivity

83. The half-life of I-131 is _____, and decay produces beta and gamma radiation.

    A. 5 seconds
    B. 138 days
    C. 8 days
    D. 10.6 hours

The correct answer is (C). **Topic:** Radioactivity

84. The binding energy of an isotope's nucleus typically takes units of:

    A. MV
    B. AMU
    C. kV
    D. MeV

The correct answer is (D). The mega electronvolt is the unit typically used to measure the binding energy of the nucleus. **Topic:** Nuclear Energy

85. _____ reactions, also called thermo-nuclear reactions, take place when temperatures reach the range of 2×10^7 K.

    A. Nuclear fission
    B. Nuclear fusion
    C. Hydrogenation
    D. None of these

The correct answer is (B). Unless cold fusion is perfected, the problem with commercial fusion reactions is the temperature at which they occur. **Topic:** Nuclear Energy

86. The principles of _____ explain the fact that light behaves both as particles and waves.

    A. photon theory
    B. quantum theory
    C. Planck's theory
    D. Keppler's theory

The correct answer is (B). **Topic:** Photons

87. The energy of a photon is:

    A. proportional to its wavelength

    B. inversely proportional to its wavelength

    C. proportional to its frequency

    D. both B and C

The correct answer is (D). **Topic:** Photons

88. The _____ supports the particle theory of light.

    A. photoelectric effect

    B. nuclear effect

    C. Planck's discharge effect

    D. polarization effect

The correct answer is (A). **Topic:** Photons

89. Visible light has wavelengths ranging from _____ m to _____ m.

    A. 3.80×10^{4}, 7.60×10^{2}

    B. 3.80×10^{-8}, 7.60×10^{-11}

    C. 3.80×10^{-2}, 7.60×10^{-6}

    D. 3.80×10^{-7}, 7.60×10^{-7}

The correct answer is (D). **Topic:** Atomic Energy Levels

90. When looking at the hydrogen spectrum, you would expect to see these colors.

    A. orange, yellow, violet

    B. red, green, blue

    C. yellow and green

    D. red and yellow

The correct answer is (B). **Topic:** Atomic Energy Levels

Unit 5

1. The size of a cell is important in all of the following **except:**

   A. Selecting the correct size needle for venipuncture.
   B. Recognizing cells using the microscope.
   C. Pinocytosis
   D. Phagocytosis

The correct answer is (C). Pinocytosis is the endocytosis (engulfing) of liquids, which would not be size dependent. **Topic:** Cells

2. Eukaryotic cell protoplasm includes:

   A. cytoplasm
   B. nucleoplasm
   C. protein
   D. all of the above

The correct answer is (D). The protoplasm can be divided into the cytoplasm and the nucleoplasm within the nuclear envelope. As would be expected, the protoplasm is composed mainly of protein, carbohydrate, lipid, water, and inorganic salts and oxygen. **Topic:** Cells

3. The properties of the typical animal cell vary with the function it has in the body. While alive, cells retain all these properties **except:**

   A. reproduction
   B. secretion
   C. respiration
   D. absorption

The correct answer is (A). Some cells, such as neurons, lose their ability to reproduce themselves when they are mature. **Topic:** Cells

4. Which group below names cells *each* with high numbers of mitochondria in the cell?

   A. liver cell, muscle cell
   B. fat cell, hair cell
   C. liver cell, fat cell
   D. fat cell, lung cell

The correct answer is (A). The components of a cell vary with the function of the cell. A cell that is involved in high energy production (oxidative respiration) contains a greater amount of mitochondria. **Topic:** Cells

5. Mitosis is associated with which group of responses?

   A. wound healing, cancer
   B. body maintenance, diplotene
   C. red blood cells, diversification
   D. cloning, haploid

The correct answer is (A). Mitosis is the duplication of a diploid cell. This maintains the organism or provides orderly growth. This ensures quality control (not diversification) but errors can occur and these errors are then reproduced resulting in uncontrolled growth (tumors, cancer). **Topic:** Cells

6. Choose the *incorrect* association regarding its histochemical use in cell microscopy:

   A. Mallory's stain : connective tissue
   B. Feulgen reaction : RNA
   C. Sudan IV : lipids
   D. Silver impregnation : nervous tissue

The correct answer is (B). The Feulgen reaction is a histochemical method used to stain and identify DNA but not RNA. The intensity of the stain is an indication of the amount of DNA present in the sample. **Topic:** Cells

7. Which response is *not* associated with the prokaryotic cell?

   A. Smaller than the eukaryotic cell
   B. Spirochetes
   C. Gram positive
   D. Organelles

The correct answer is (D). A *prokaryotic* cell, such as a bacteria, lacks an organized nucleus and cytoplasmic organelles. **Topic:** Cells

8. A *correct* taxonomy classification would be which one of the following?

   A. Fungi : Monera
   B. Sponges : Animalia
   C. Algae : Planta
   D. Virus : Monera

The correct answer is (B). Sponges are the only organisms on the list that are correctly placed in their taxonomic kingdom. **Topic:** Classification of Living Organisms

9. The *incorrect* human organ system association is:

   A. Muscular system : cardiac : striated : intercalated disk
   B. Nervous system : axon : myelin sheath : node of Ranvier
   C. Repiratory system : blood : hemo-globin : Bohr effect
   D. Renal system : nephron : loop of Henle : medulla

The correct answer is (B). The nervous system axon has no myelin sheath at the node of Ranvier. This is a very important concept for understanding the speed of impulse conduction in the myelinated fiber. **Topic:** Organization of the Human Body

10. The *incorrect* association with connective tissue is:

   A. blood matrix : plasma
   B. collagen : protein
   C. mast cell : histamine
   D. fibrocytes : ectoderm

The correct answer is (D). Fibrocytes are not associated with actoderm tissue. **Topic:** Organization of the Human Body

11. The *incorrect* axial skeleton association is:

   A. vertebral column : coccyx
   B. skull : mandible
   C. thorax : scapula
   D. All of the above associations are correct.

The correct answer is (C). The scapula is part of the appendicular skeleton. **Topic:** Skeletal System

12. The *incorrect* appendicular skeleton association is:

A. Pectoral girdle : scapula : clavical : glenoid
B. Pelvic girdle : ilium : ischium : sacrum
C. Upper appendage : humerus : carpal : phalange
D. All of the above associations are true.

The correct answer is (B). The pelvic girdle (an ilium, an ischium, and a pubis on each side that are fused to each to form a partial ring that is completed as each side) is attached to the lateral aspect of the sacrum, which is part of the axial skeleton. **Topic:** Skeletal System

13. An *incorrect* statement about the Haversian system in bone is:

A. Longitudinal central canals contain blood vessels and nerves.
B. The lacunae contain blood vessels to nourish the bone.
C. The Haversian system is the major component of most compact bone.
D. All of the above statements are true.

The correct answer is (B). As seen under the microscope, the Haversian unit consists of a *central canal*, which contains blood vessels and nerves running up and down the bone. Each central canal is surrounded by concentric rings (lamellae) of calcified bone. The osteocyte lies within these rings in a space termed a *lacuna*. **Topic:** Skeletal System

14. The *correct* pairing of synovial joints is:

A. ball and socket joint: ankle
B. hinge joint: elbow
C. plane joint: intervertebral
D. All of the above are correct.

The correct answer is (B). The ligaments holding the bones together form an enclosing capsule. An example is the *hinge*; flexion and extension in one plane: knee, elbow. **Topic:** Skeletal System

15. The correct association with vertebrate muscle is:

A. Smooth muscle: iris of eye: involuntary
B. Smooth muscle: multinucleate: involuntary
C. Cardiac muscle: unbranching: automaticity
D. All of the above are correct.

The correct answer is (A). *Smooth* muscle consists of nonstriated smooth sheets of long tapered cells. Smooth muscle is under the control of the ANS autonomic nervous system (involuntary). It is found in the intestinal tract (viscera), the walls of the blood vessels, the iris of the eye, and in the reproductive organs. **Topic:** Muscular System

16. The correct set of associations with skeletal muscle is:

  A. voluntary, striated, epithelium
  B. involuntary, striated, endothelium
  C. voluntary, striated, endomysium
  D. involuntary, striated, branching

The correct answer is (C). Skeletal muscle (also called voluntary muscle and striated muscle), consists of elongated unbranching multinucleated cells (or fibers), which appear striated under the light microscope. Endomysium envelopes the single muscle cell (fiber) and carries the capillaries. **Topic:** Muscular System

17. Generally held true associations of skeletal muscle attachment are:

  A. origin, proximal, sphincter
  B. origin, proximal, small range of motion
  C. insertion, proximal, small range of motion
  D. origin, distal, large range of motion

The correct answer is (B). The *origin* is the end of the muscle that does not move very much when contracted. The origin is usually closer to the midline of the body and is the more proximal attachment. **Topic:** Muscular System

18. "Twisting" the ankle so as to stretch the lateral ligaments of the ankle is:

  A. Extension
  B. Eversion
  C. Inversion
  D. Flexion

The correct answer is (C). *Inversion* is rotation of the sole of the foot inward. **Topic:** Muscular System

19. A muscle name that gives its origin and insertion is:

  A. flexor carpi radialis
  B. levator scapulae
  C. serratus posterior superior
  D. None of the above.

The correct answer is (D). Muscles are named by the their attachments, function, location, or shape. **Topic:** Muscular System

20. The myofibril band that shortens during contraction is:

  A. A band
  B. I band
  C. A and I bands
  D. None of the above.

The correct answer is (B). The myofibrils each contain thin actin filaments and thick myosin filaments arranged longitudinally. The filaments overlap each other creating a pattern of striations. The I band is greatly reduced during contraction. **Topic:** Muscular System

21. The composition of the myofilaments of the muscle fiber are most completely described by:

  A. thin actin, thick myosin
  B. thick actin, thin myosin, triads
  C. thin actin, tropomyosin, troponin
  D. None of the above.

The correct answer is (A). The active contractile elements of the muscle fiber are the longitudinal rod shaped myofibrils (or fibrils). These myofibrils form the striations seen on skeletal muscle. The myofibrils each contain thin actin myofilaments (filaments) and thick myosin myofilaments (filaments) arranged longitudinally. **Topic:** Muscular System

22. The triad of the muscle myofiber is best described by:

A. Three T tubules meeting at the Z line.
B. Two T tubules and one terminal cisternae.
C. One T tubule and two terminal cisternae.
D. None of the above.

The correct answer is (C). The triad consists of: 1 cisternae-1T tubule-1 cisternae. This sarcolemma tubule-sarcoplasmic reticulum system serves to conduct the action potential into the muscle cell, which causes release of calcium stored in the sarcoplasmic reticulum. The myofibril response is contraction. **Topic:** Muscular System

23. Which is the correct association with the excitation of the gastrocnemius muscle?

A. action potential, acetylcholine, nicotinic receptor
B. action potential, norepinephrine, nicotinic receptor
C. action potential, norepinephrine, muscarinic receptor
D. action potential, acetylcholine, muscarinic receptor

The correct answer is (A). The action potential, arriving at the end of the neuron, increases the permeability of the nerve ending to calcium, causing exocytosis of the acetycholine (Ach) vesicles into the synaptic cleft. Ach binds to these nicotinic receptors on the junctional folds of the motor end plate. **Topic:** Muscular System

24. Select the false statement regarding skeletal muscle contraction at the cellular level.

A. Each motor neuron innervates more than one nerve fiber.
B. A muscle of precision has a motor neuron, which innervates fewer muscle fibers.
C. The action potential triggers release of calcium from the terminal cisternae.
D. All of the statements are true.

The correct answer is (D). The motor unit consists of a single motor neuron and all the skeletal muscle cells (fibers) that it inervates. A muscle of precision, the hand or eye, has a motor neuron that innervates fewer muscle fibers. **Topic:** Muscular System

25. The best association with the muscle twitch is:

A. a series of contractions
B. one contraction, then relaxation
C. contraction phase
D. tetany

The correct answer is (B). A single action potential that causes a brief contraction followed by relaxation is called a muscle twitch. **Topic:** Muscular System

26. The false statement about tetanus of a skeletal muscle is:

A. Incomplete tetanus occurs when periods of incomplete relaxation occur between the summated stimuli.
B. Summation occurs because the contractile mechanism has no refractory period.
C. Summation of contractions is independent of twitch duration
D. Complete tetanus occurs if there is no muscle relaxation between stimuli.

The correct answer is (C). A muscle that is repeatedly stimulated without allowing relaxation to occur produces a response added to the previous response. This is known as *summation* of contractions. Summation occurs because the contractile mechanism has no refractory period. **Topic:** Muscular System

27. The incorrect statement of energy sources for contraction of skeletal muscle is:

A. Each myosin bridge contains ATP.
B. Bridge linking is inhibited by the troponin—tropomyosin complex blocking access to actin.
C. The limiting factors are available ATP and calcium.
D. All of the above are true.

The correct answer is (D). Energy release allows the ratcheted action of the myosin bridges attaching and releasing the actin heads, sliding the actin in toward the center over the myosin. The limiting factors are available ATP and calcium. The relaxation process occurs when the nerve impulse decreases and the sarcoplasmic reticulum no longer releases calcium ions but reabsorbs it. The calcium is no longer available to complex with troponin and blocking of the actin heads occurs. **Topic:** Muscular System

28. The types of muscle fibers include:

A. Type I, and red
B. Type I, and slow
C. Type I, and oxidative
D. All of the above are true.

The correct answer is (D). Skeletal muscle may look the same under the light microscope, but it is really a mix of different fiber types. **Topic:** Muscular System

29. The circulatory system does not participate in which of the following:

A. blood clotting
B. regulation of body temperature
C. erythropoiesis
D. All of the above are functions of the circulatory system.

The correct answer is (D). The function of the circulatory system includes regulation of waste from the tissues to the kidneys; of carbon dioxide to the lungs; of hormones and cell regulatory substances; of body temperature; of blood clotting; and of control and production of blood components. **Topic:** Circulatory Systems

30. The correct circulation system association is:

A. Vein, large lumen, thick wall, deoxygenated blood
B. Pulmonary artery, deoxygenated blood
C. Lymphatic, no smooth muscle, valves
D. All of the above are correct.

The correct answer is (B). The *pulmonary* circulation consists of the vessels of the lungs where the oxygen enters the blood and carbon dioxide leaves. Arteries carry blood away from the heart and veins toward the heart. The pulmonary artery is the only artery carrying deoxygenated blood. **Topic:** Circulatory Systems

31. During strenuous activity, the athletic heart cardiac output increases because:

A. The heart rate increases
B. The stroke volume increases
C. Both A and B
D. The cardiac output does not increase.

The correct answer is (C). The blood follows a closed path with the four chambered heart as the pump. The cardiac output is the amount pumped in a minute (80 ml × 72 = 5760 ml). With strenuous activity, the conditioned heart's cardiac output can increase to 30–35 liters per minute because both the heart rate and the stroke volume increase. **Topic:** Circulatory Systems

32. Correct associations with the heart are:

A. Passage into the right atria is guarded by a semilunar valve.
B. Passage into the right ventricle is guarded by a tricuspid valve.
C. Chordae tendineae anchor the semilunar valves.
D. All of the above are correct.

The correct answer is (B). Blood from the superior and inferior vena cavae enters the right atrium. The passage into the right ventricle is guarded by a tricuspid valve. The tricuspid valve prevents regurgitation (backflow) of blood into the atria during ventricular contraction (systole). **Topic:** Circulatory Systems

33. An incorrect statement about the blood is:

A. Lymphocytes are mainly formed in the lymph nodes.
B. Monocytes at the site of an infection become activated macrophages.
C. Basophils and eosinophils participate in the inflammatory response.
D. All of the above are true.

The correct answer is (D). *Lymphocytes* are mainly formed in the lymph nodes, thymus, and spleen from precursor cells from the bone marrow. They are the mainstay cell of the immune system. **Topic:** Circulatory Systems

34. Considering the anatomy of the respiratory tree, there are no cilia in:

   A. primary bronchi
   B. trachea
   C. bronchioles
   D. alveoli

The correct answer is (D). The trachea and primary bronchi have cartilage, a small amount of smooth muscle, and are lined with pseudostratified ciliated columnar epithelium with goblet cells. Continued branching within the lung structure brings significant changes. Bronchioles have ciliated columnar epithelium, which changes to non-ciliated cuboidal near the alveoli. **Topic:** Circulatory Systems

35. Which measure of pulmonary ventilation does change with activity?

   A. tidal volume
   B. vital capacity
   C. residual volume
   D. All of the above change with activity.

The correct answer is (A). The volume of air inspired with each breath, the *tidal volume*, is approximately 500 ml. This can be increased significantly by increasing the volume inspired and the rate of inspiration. **Topic:** Respiratory System

36. A true statement about inspiration and expiration is:

   A. Tidal volume is the volume of air moving in with each inspiration.
   B. Residual volume is the volume of air not available for gas exchange.
   C. Vital capacity is the volume of air moving in with each inspiration.
   D. All of the above are false.

The correct answer is (A). The tidal volume (TV) is the amount of air that moves into or out of the lungs with each inspiration or expiration. **Topic:** Respiratory System

37. A true statement regarding ventilation is:

   A. A gas diffuses from an area of high pressure to an area of low pressure.
   B. The rate of diffusion depends on the concentration gradient and the nature of the barrier separating the areas.
   C. The lungs are stretched when first inflated at birth and will collapse if the seal is lost.
   D. All of the above are true.

The correct answer is (D). A gas expands to fill the volume available to it. A gas diffuses from an area of high pressure to an area of low pressure, and the rate of diffusion depends on the concentration gradient and the nature of the barrier separating the areas. The lungs and the chest wall are elastic and separated from each other by a thin film of fluid, which provides surface tension. They thus resist separation. **Topic:** Respiratory System

38. The control of respiration is most closely associated with:

   A. pH, partial pressure of oxygen, respiratory control center

   B. pH in blood and CSF, partial pressure of carbon dioxide and oxygen, respiratory control center

   C. pH in blood and CSF, partial pressure of oxygen, respiratory control center

   D. carotid bodies, aortic bodies, 4th ventricle, respiratory control center

The correct answer is (B). The *respiratory control center* in the medulla receives increased impulses if any increase in acidity (lowering the pH) or carbon dioxide concentration or a drop in oxygen concentration is detected by the carotid and aortic bodies in the blood vessels, or by sensors in the CSF of the 4th ventricle. **Topic:** Respiratory System

39. A necessary factor involved in diffusion of a gas across the alveolus is:

   A. concentration gradient

   B. permeable membrane

   C. moisture

   D. All of the above are true.

The correct answer is (D). The exchange of gases requires: (1) a moist; (2) permeable surface area of sufficient size; and (3) separating a concentration gradient. **Topic:** Respiratory System

40. The *incorrect* association of oxygen transport is:

   A. Oxygen moves from the alveoli to the blood down its partial pressure gradient.

   B. Hemoglobin has 2 polypeptide chains, four heme groups and 4 iron atoms.

   C. One hemoglobin can bind 4 molecules of oxygen (O_2).

   D. Hemoglobin more easily gives up oxygen in high partial pressures of carbon dioxide.

The correct answer is (B). Hemoglobin has four polypeptide chains, four heme groups, and four iron atoms. **Topic:** Respiratory System

41. An incorrect association of carbon dioxide transport is:

   A. Carbon dioxide, blood plasma, carbonic anhydrase

   B. Carbon dioxide, carbonic anhydrase, hydrogen ions

   C. Carbon dioxide, carbonic anhydrase, bicarbonate ion

   D. Carbon dioxide, carbonic anhydrase, water

The correct answer is (A). With the help of the carbonic anhydrase enzyme found in the RBC but not in the plasma, the carbonic acid dissociates into hydrogen ions and bicarbonate ions. **Topic:** Respiratory System

42. Chemical regulation of respiration is associated with all of the following **except:**

A. Aortic bodies, type I cells
B. Carotid bodies, type I cells
C. acidosis, hypercapnia
D. All of the above are true associations.

The correct answer is (D). The respiratory system is always undergoing small adjustments to keep conditions optimum in the body. The chemical state of the blood controls the signals to the nervous control and includes all of the above. **Topic:** Respiratory System

43. An incorrect association with the kidney structure is:

A. Bowman's capsule, glomerulus, afferent capillary
B. cortex, medulla, renal pelvis
C. Bowman's capsule, proximal convoluted tubule, ureter
D. distal convoluted tubule, collecting duct, calyces

The correct answer is (C). **Topic:** Urinary System

44. All of the following are true associations of the ureter **except:**

A. smooth muscle, peristaltic contractions
B. renal pelvis
C. pudendal nerves
D. All of the above are true associations.

The correct answer is (C). The bladder, which holds 500 ml of urine, is lined with transitional epithelium, and there are three muscular layers to the detrusor muscle. The urethral opening is located in the most dependent part of the bladder. Further outside of the bladder, the sphincter of the membranous urethra (*external urethral sphincter*) encircles the urethra and is innervated by the pudendal nerves. **Topic:** Urinary System

45. Tubular filtrate is normally hypertonic in the lumen of:

A. proximal convoluted tubule
B. distal convoluted tubule
C. ascending loop of Henle
D. descending loop of Henle

The correct answer is (D). The thin descending loop, straight, with flat epithelial cells, is *permeable* to water. The fluid becomes hypertonic because water moves out of the tubule into the hypertonic interstitium created by the next part of the loop tubule. **Topic:** Urinary System

46. ADH secretion is associated with:

   A. the anterior pituitary
   B. conserving body water
   C. the proximal convoluted tubule
   D. all of the above

The correct answer is (B). If the blood passing through the capillaries of the *hypothalamus* is hypertonic, the hypothalamus secretes antidiuretic hormone (ADH) into the *posterior* pituitary, which releases ADH into the blood. The stimulation of the hypothalamus also causes the sensation of thirst, and if the water intake is increased, more water is added to the blood. **Topic:** Urinary System

47. True associations of the skin include all but:

   A. touch, pressure, temperature, and pain.
   B. epithelium
   C. epidermis, dermis,
   D. All of the above are true associations of the skin.

The correct answer is (D). *Epithelium* forms the surface lining of most surfaces in the body and epidermis is the outer epithelial surface of the skin. The skin is a sensory organ, sensing touch, pressure, temperature, and pain. Skin is composed of the epidermis and the dermis. **Topic:** Integumentary (Skin) System

48. Which of the following is not true of sweat glands?

   A. Eccrine glands are small sweat glands of the simple tubular type.
   B. Sweat glands are an epidermal invagination into the dermis.
   C. Sweat glands are very numerous except in thick skin, palms, and soles.
   D. Apocrine sweat glands develop at puberty.

The correct answer is (C). There are two types of sweat glands, *eccrine* and apocrine. The eccrine are small sweat glands of the simple tubular type and are very numerous in thick skin, palms, and soles. **Topic:** Integumentary (Skin) System

49. All of the following are true **except:**

   A. Epidermal invagination into the dermis differentiates into hair follicles.
   B. Hair growth is cyclic.
   C. Connective tissue, with its blood capillaries, indents the base of the germinal matrix.
   D. A bundle of skeletal muscle fibers attaches to the hair follicle.

The correct answer is (D). The hair follicle is surrounded by a connective tissue sheath. A bundle of *smooth* muscle fibers, the arrector pili muscle, attaches to this connective tissue sheath of the hair follicle and passes up to the papillary layer of the dermis. **Topic:** Integumentary (Skin) System

50. All of the following are true of a finger nail **except:**

   A. The nail plate rests on the avascular nail bed.

   B. The deeper cells of the nail groove proliferate to become the nail matrix.

   C. The nail plate is composed of cornified epithelial cells.

   D. The nail is formed by the invagination of the epithelium of the dorsal side of the phalange into the dermis.

The correct answer is (A). The cells of the nail matrix proliferate and the upper layer differentiates to form a layer of hard keratin, the *nail plate*. The matrix continues to proliferate and the hard nail is pushed out of the nail groove over the distal epidermis, the nail bed. The nail plate rests on this very vascular nail bed. The nail bed contains abundant blood vessels and sensory *nerve* endings. **Topic:** Integumentary (Skin) System

51. The essential fat soluble vitamins are:

   A. A, D, E, K, B12

   B. A, D, E, K, which function as coenzymes.

   C. A, D, E, K, which do not function as coenzymes.

   D. None of the above is correct.

The correct answer is (C). If the body can not make a needed substance from smaller building blocks, it is called essential and must be supplied in the diet. Some fat must be eaten to supply the essential fat soluble vitamins A, D, E, and K, and the essential fatty acids, linolenic, linoleic, and arachidonic acids. **Topic:** Digestive System and Nutrition

52. The digestive system muscle layers are arranged in the general pattern of:

   A. inner circular under the mucosa, middle longitudinal, and outer circular

   B. inner longitudinal, middle circular, and outer longitudinal

   C. inner longitudinal under the mucosa, middle circular, and no outer

   D. inner circular, middle circular, and outer longitudinal

The correct answer is (B). The walls of the GI tract follow the same general pattern of tissues: inner mucosal lining, 3 muscle layers, and serosa. The muscle layers are arranged: inner longitudinal under the mucosa, middle circular, and outer longitudinal. **Topic:** Digestive System and Nutrition

53. The role of the liver in digestion involves all but:

   A. formation of bile salts

   B. secretion of bile

   C. sphincter of Oddi

   D. enterohepatic circulation

The correct answer is (C). The bile is released into the *duodenum* of the small intestine at the duodenal papilla, where it is usually joined by the pancreatic duct and guarded by the sphincter of Oddi. **Topic:** Digestive System and Nutrition

54. All of the following are correct associations of the GI system **except:**

A. esophagus: no digestion, peristalsis
B. stomach: mainly enzymes, acid, no peristalsis
C. duodenum: adds the most enzymes
D. large intestine: mostly water reabsorption

The correct answer is (B). The digestive system softens, mixes, adds enzymes and emulsifiers, moves, and absorbs the food in a coordinated manner to sustain the organism. The stomach adds acid, enzymes, hormones, intrinsic factor, and churns the food, turning it into a partially digested chyme that enters the duodenum though the pyloric sphincter. The antrum, pylorus, and upper duodenum function as a unit and contraction of the antrum is followed in a peristaltic wave to the duodenum. **Topic:** Digestive System and Nutrition

55. Qualities or properties of intestinal motility are all of the following **except:**

A. Muscle layers are inner longitudinal, middle circular, outer longitudinal.
B. Peristaltic activity occurs with or without extrinsic innervation.
C. eristaltic activity can be increased or decreased by autonomic innervation.
D. All of the above are true.

The correct answer is (D). The walls of the GI tract follow the same general pattern of tissues of inner mucosal lining, 3 muscle layers, and external serosa. The muscle layers are arranged as inner longitudinal under the mucosa, middle circular, and outer longitudinal. There are two types of movement, segmental *contractions* and peristaltic waves, both requiring an intact myenteric nerve plexus but not an extrinsic nerve supply. Peristaltic activity can be increased or decreased by autonomic innervation but it occurs with or without extrinsic innervation. **Topic:** Digestive System and Nutrition

56. The following are true of the innervation of the intestine **except:**

A. Innervation of the intestinal tract is divided into intrinsic and extrinsic.
B. Intrinsic innervation is the myenteric plexus and Auerbach's plexus.
C. Intrinsic networks are interconnected and form the enteric nervous system.
D. Parasympathetic cholinergic generally increases GI stimulation.

The correct answer is (B). Innervation of the intestinal tract is divided into intrinsic and extrinsic. There are two nerve networks that are intrinsic to the gastrointestinal tract, the myenteric plexus or Auerbach's plexus and the submucous plexus or Meissner's plexus. **Topic:** Digestive System and Nutrition

57. The following are true of the digestive juices **except:**

    A. Saliva has alpha amylase and lingual lipase.

    B. Stomach juice has hydrochloric acid, pepsin, mucin, and intrinsic factor.

    C. Trypsin, chymotrypsin, and carboxypeptidase are inactive proteases.

    D. Amylase digests starch and glycogen.

The correct answer is (C). Trypsin, chymotrypsin, and carboxypeptidase are active proteases, which are secreted as an inactive form and activated in the duodenum. **Topic:** Digestive System and Nutrition

58. The following are true of the hormones of the intestine **except:**

    A. Gastrin stimulates gastric acid and pepsin, has trophic action on the mucosa.

    B. CCK contracts gallbladder, increases secretion of enzyme pancreatic juice.

    C. Secretin increases secretion an alkaline pancreatic juice.

    D. All of the above are true.

The correct answer is (D). *Gastrin* is secreted by the G cell of the mucosa of the stomach and has two main actions, stimulation of gastric acid and pepsin, and a trophic action on the mucosa of the stomach and small intestine. *CCK* or cholecystokinin-pancreozymin, is secreted by endocrine cells in the upper small intestine causing contraction of the *gallbladder* (bile) and the secretion of an enzyme rich pancreatic juice. Secretin is secreted by S cells in the mucosa of the upper SI. Secretin increases the bicarbonate secretion of the pancreas and biliary tract, producing an alkaline pancreatic juice. **Topic:** Digestive System and Nutrition

59. The following are true statements about digestion **except:**

A. Digestion is the breakdown of food into small units to be absorbed.
B. Lactose intolerance is the result of a missing disaccharide enzyme, lactase.
C. Missing enzymes can result in serious health problems.
D. All of the above are true.

The correct answer is (D). *Digestion* is the mechanical and chemical breakdown of food into units small enough to be absorbed and utilized by the body. When the glucose/galactose transporter is defective glucose and galactose malabsorption occurs, resulting in severe diarrhea. Lactose intolerance is the result of a missing disaccharide enzyme, lactase. **Topic:** Digestive System and Nutrition

60. All but one of the following are part of nervous tissue.

A. Glial, neuroglia, neurons, microglia, oligodendrogliocytes, astrocytes
B. Schwann, neurons, microglia, oligodendrogliocytes, astrocytes
C. Schwann, glial, neuroglia, neurons, microglia, astrocytes
D. All of the above are cells of nervous tissue

The correct answer is (D). **Topic:** Nervous System

61. The following are true about the axon **except:**

A. all myelinated
B. all efferent processes of the cell
C. are peripheral or central processes
D. All of the above are true about axons.

The correct answer is (A). The cell process that conducts depolarization away from the cell body, efferent process, is the axon. Usually there is only one axon, of variable length and thickness, and it can be myelinated or unmyelinated. **Topic:** Nervous System

62. All but one of the following are types of neurons.

A. sensory, interneuron, and motor
B. unipolar, bipolar, and multipolar
C. unipolar, bipolar, multipolar, and microglia
D. afferent, efferent, and interneuron

The correct answer is (C). Nervous tissue consists of neurons and support cells for the neurons. Glial cells or neuroglia are the supporting cells. There are many times more glial cells than neurons. Neurons can also be grouped by the number of cell *processes* extending from the cell body, unipolar, bipolar, and multipolar. **Topic:** Nervous System

63. Correct neuron terminology includes all of the following **except:**

A. neuron cell bodies, outside the CNS, ganglion (ganglia)
B. neuron cell bodies, layers, cortex
C. neuron cell bodies, inside the CNS, nucleus (nuclei)
D. All of the above are correct terminology for neuron cell bodies.

The correct answer is (D). Neuron cell *bodies* (soma) in a group because of similar function but located outside the central nervous system, are called a *ganglion* (ganglia). When neuron cell bodies group inside the CNS, usually with information from the same area or sense, they are called a nucleus. Cortex is a term for a collection of neuron cell bodies arranged in layers. **Topic:** Nervous System

64. The incorrectly matched cell with its function is which of the following:

A. microglia—trophic
B. oligodendrogliocytes—myelination
C. astrocytes—blood brain barrier
D. Schwann cells—myelination

The correct answer is (A). *Microglia* enter the nervous system from the blood and are the scavenger cells of the nervous system. **Topic:** Nervous System

65. The false statement about the central nervous system is which of the following?

A. Dura mater meningeal layer provides support.
B. Subdural space contains some CSF or cerebrospinal fluid.
C. Arachnoid meningeal covering is a weblike layer.
D. All of the above are true.

The correct answer is (B). The space between the arachnoid and the pia is the *subarachnoid space* and contains some CSF or *cerebrospinal fluid*. **Topic:** Nervous System

66. The following associations of the peripheral nervous system are true **except:**

A. peripheral nervous system has somatic and autonomic divisions
B. somatic system consists of cranial nerves and spinal nerves
C. parasympathetic system is from thoracic and lumbar spinal segments
D. autonomic system is internal activities, sympathetic and parasympathetic

The correct answer is (C). The *parasympathetic* system motor outflow is from the *cranial* nerves and the sacral spinal nerves. The *sympathetic* motor outflow is from the thoracic and lumbar spinal segments, functioning to prepare the body for flight or fight. **Topic:** Nervous System

67. True associations of the reflex arc are all of the following **except:**

A. efferent sensory neuron, synapse, afferent motor neuron, polysynaptic

B. knee jerk, a stretch reflex

C. afferent sensory neuron, synapse, efferent motor neuron, monosynaptic

D. All of the above are true of the reflex arc.

The correct answer is (A). The arc is stereotyped and specific both in stimulus and response. The arc consists of a sensory receptor, an afferent neuron, an efferent neuron, and an effector. **Topic:** Nervous System

68. True associations of the visual system are all of the following except:

A. Eyeball is protected superiorly by the frontal bone.

B. Six pairs of extrinsic muscles innervated by CN III, CN IV, CN VI.

C. Optic nerve is CN I.

D. All of the above are true associations of the visual system.

The correct answer is (C). The eye is a complex sensory receptor that detects electromagnetic energy in the range of visible light waves. It is only part of the visual system, which also includes the optic nerve, CN II, the visual pathways to the brain, the muscles of eye movement, CN III, CN IV, CN VI, the eyelids, and lacrimal glands and ducts. **Topic:** Organs of Special Sense

69. The hearing apparatus consists of all of the following **except:**

A. organ of Corti, cochlear duct, basilar membrane

B. the external ear, middle ear, the cochlea, cranial nerve VIII

C. tectorial membrane, saccule, stereocilia, hair cell, cranial nerve VIII

D. malleus, incus, stapes, oval window

The correct answer is (C). Summary of path of sound: air to bone to fluid to nerve: external ear, external auditory canal, tympanic membrane; middle ear: malleus, incus, stapes, oval window; inner ear: cochlear apparatus: cochlear duct (organ of Corti), basilar membrane, hair cell, afferent CN VIII, brainstem. The semicircular canals, utricle, and saccule are concerned with equilibrium. **Topic:** Organs of Special Sense

70. Decreased functioning of cranial nerve I may be due to all but one of the following:

A. cribriform plate fracture

B. anosmia, hyposmia

C. adaptation

D. frontal lobe tumor

The correct answer is (B). Damage to the nerves results in anosmia, the absence of the sense of smell, or hyposmia, the diminished sense of smell. Hyposmia occurs with age due to an increase in the threshold concentration for detection of an odor. **Topic:** Organs of Special Sense

71. All but one of the following are true about the sense of taste.

    A. The four basic tastes are sweet, salty, bitter, and sour.
    B. The vallate papilla is the largest but the fewest in number.
    C. Taste buds are found only on the tongue.
    D. The tongue contains three types of papillae.

The correct answer is (C). Taste buds can also be found in the mucosa of the palate, pharynx, and epiglottis not associated with papillae. **Topic:** Organs of Special Sense

72. All but one of the following statements is true about the anterior pituitary.

    A. Five of the hormones secreted are tropic hormones.
    B. Anterior and intermediate pituitary lobes develop from Rathke's pouch.
    C. Anterior lobe does not have a typical endocrine structure.
    D. Anterior lobe has a special portal vessel connection with the brain.

The correct answer is (C). The anterior lobe has a typical endocrine structure, cell cords with an interlacing fenestrated capillary network, cell granules full of stored hormone. **Topic:** Endocrine System

73. The following are true associations of the thyroid gland **except:**

    A. Thyroid path of migration fails to obliterate, the thyroglossal duct remains.
    B. Hypothalamus secretes thyroid releasing factor, TSH-RF.
    C. Posterior pituitary secretes thyroid stimulating hormone, TSH.
    D. Endocrine gland producing thyroxin, triiodothyronine, and calcitonin.

The correct answer is (C). The anterior pituitary detects the increased level of TSH-RF and secretes a thyroid stimulating hormone, TSH. **Topic:** Endocrine System

74. The following are true statements about the parathyroid gland **except:**

    A. Parathyroid PTH increases blood calcium.
    B. Calcitonin decreases the absorption of calcium.
    C. Parathyroid releases calcitonin at detected high levels of blood calcium.
    D. Low blood calcium levels can cause muscle tetany.

The correct answer is (C). The parathyroid increases the concentration of available calcium by releasing PTH when it detects low level of blood calcium. This PTH acts on the intestines to act with a vitamin D metabolite to increase the absorption of calcium from the available food, acts on the bones to remove calcium and on the kidneys to decrease the excretion of calcium. **Topic:** Endocrine System

75. The endocrine activity of the pancreas includes all but one of the following:

A. "D" cells of the islets secrete somatostatin
B. "A" (alpha) cells secrete glucagon
C. "B" cells (beta) secrete insulin
D. "F" cells produce pancreatic enzymes

The correct answer is (D). *"F" cells* produce *pancreatic polypeptide,* which slows the absorption of food. Its secretion increases with the presence of protein, fasting, exercise, and acute hypoglycemia and decreases by somatostatin and IV glucose. **Topic:** Endocrine System

76. Correct statements about the adrenal cortex are all but one of the following:

A. Adrenal cortex develops from mesoderm.
B. CRH stimulates the anterior pituitary to secrete ACTH.
C. Mineralocorticoid aldosterone by the zona fasciculata saves sodium.
D. Glucocorticoids increased production causes Cushing's syndrome.

The correct answer is (C). Mineralocorticoids, such as aldosterone, act on the renal tubules to save sodium and water and lose potassium and hydrogen. Increased production of aldosterone by the zona glomerulosa causes retention of sodium and water, which can progress to alkalosis, edema, increased blood pressure, and muscle paralysis (Conn's syndrome). **Topic:** Endocrine System

77. All of the following are true of the testes endocrine function **except:**

A. Interstitial cells of Leydig are the source of testosterone
B. Seminiferous tubule is the source of spermatozoa.
C. Seminiferous tubule is the source of Sertoli cells.
D. Anterior pituitary LH is tropic on the Sertoli cell

The correct answer is (D). Anterior pituitary FSH acts on the Sertoli cells to facilitate the maturation of the spermatid and the secretion of inhibin. Anterior pituitary LH causes the Leydig cells to grow and secrete testosterone. **Topic:** Endocrine System

78. Similarities of the male and female endocrine control of reproduction are all of the following **except:**

A. Hypothalamus secretions act on the anterior pituitary.
B. Anterior pituitary secretions act directly on the gonads.
C. Gonads produce both gametes and steroids.
D. All of the above are true.

The correct answer is (D). The hypothalamus secretes releasing gonadotrophins to act on the anterior pituitary in both. The anterior pituitary responds with the secretion of stimulating hormones, which act directly on the gonads, testes or ovary, to produce gametes and to produce steroids. **Topic:** Endocrine System

79. All of the following are true of the ovarian cycle **except:**

    A. Ovarian cycle and the menstrual cycle are interrelated.

    B. Ovarian cycle consists of the follicular phase and proliferative phase.

    C. The luteal cells secrete estrogen and progesterone.

    D. Surge of LH is thought to cause the rupture of the follicle.

The correct answer is (B). The ovarian cycle is divided into two parts, the follicular phase and the secretory or luteal phase. **Topic:** Endocrine System

80. All of the following are true of the menstrual or uterine cycle **except:**

    A. Proliferative phase is influenced by estrogen from the graffian follicle.

    B. Luteal phase is influenced by corpus luteum of the uterus.

    C. If a pregnancy does not occur, the corpus luteum does not receive hCG.

    D. Hypothalmus regulates the hormones of reproduction.

The correct answer is (B). Day fourteen begins the secretory or luteal phase in the uterus. The endometrial lining now becomes more vascular and begins to secrete a clear fluid under the influence of estrogen and progesterone from the corpus luteum of the *ovary*. **Topic:** Endocrine System

81. Correct statements about contraception are all of the following **except:**

    A. Most female contraception consists of manipulation of hormone levels.

    B. Birth control pills contain low doses of an estrogen and/or progesterone.

    C. The two basic pill types are the combination pill and triphasic pill.

    D. Prevent ovulation by depressed levels of both gonadotropins.

The correct answer is (C). There are two basic types of hormone contraception. One type, the combination pill, combines both drugs in the same pill which is taken for twenty-one days, then no hormone is taken for seven days to allow for menstrual flow. Variations of this are the biphasic and triphasic pills, which vary the dose of the progesterone during the month. The second type of oral contraceptive, *progesterone only*, comes in two forms, pill or implant. **Topic:** Endocrine System

82. Correct statements about the placenta are all of the following **except**:

    A. Begins functioning at four weeks.

    B. Is a temporary endocrine structure.

    C. Hormone hCG is positive feedback to the corpus luteum of the ovary.

    D. The corpus luteum secretes estrogen, progesterone, and relaxin.

The correct answer is (A). The *hCG* secreted by the *placenta* can be detected in the blood as early as *six days* after conception and detected in the urine as early as fourteen days after conception. **Topic:** Endocrine System

83. All of the following are true of the pineal gland **except:**

   A. secretes melatonin
   B. roof of the 3rd ventricle, center of the brain
   C. highly permeable fenestrated capillaries like other endocrine glands
   D. secretions increase in the light

The correct answer is (D). The *pineal* gland is now known to secrete *melatonin*. It secretes the melatonin, synchronized with the amount of available light, increasing in the *dark* and decreasing in the light. **Topic:** Endocrine System

84. Pick the false statement or metabolic reaction.

   A. Local hormones synthesized and act where they are produced.
   B. Phospholipid, phospholipase A, arachidonic acid blocked by cortisol.
   C. Leukotrienes and cyclooxygenase are blocked by aspirin.
   D. Leukotrienes are involved in allergic response and inflammation.

The correct answer is (C). Arachidonic acid catalyzed by the enzyme cyclooxygenase forms prostaglandins, prostacyclin, and thromboxane. This pathway can be blocked by aspirin and other nonsteroidal anti-inflammatory drugs, which inhibit cyclooxygenase. However, arachidonic acid can still be catalyzed on another pathway by *lipoxygenases* to form the *leukotrienes*. **Topic:** Endocrine System

85. The following are true of the endocrine function of the small intestine **except:**

   A. Three main GI hormones, gastrin, CPK, and secretin.
   B. GIP is stimulated by glucose and fat in the duodenum.
   C. GIP functions to increase insulin by stimulation of the pancreatic B cells.
   D. VIP acts to stimulate intestinal secretion of electrolytes and water.

The correct answer is (A). Gastrin is secreted by the stomach. **Topic:** Endocrine System

86. The following is true of the male reproductive organs **except:**

   A. Seminiferous tubules have germinal epithelium.
   B. Interstitial cells produce testosterone.
   C. Vas deferens and duct of the seminal vesicle form the ejaculatory duct.
   D. All of the above are true.

The correct answer is (D). **Topic:** Reproductive System

87. Hormonal control of reproduction in the male and female are true **except:**

A. Releasing gonadotrophins from hypothalamus act on posterior pituitary.
B. Stimulating hormones are FSH and LH.
C. FSH acts on the Sertoli cells in the testes to mature the sperm, make inhibin.
D. FSH acts on granulosa cells to mature the eggs, make estrogen and inhibin.

The correct answer is (A). The hypothalamus secretes releasing gonadotrophins to act on the anterior pituitary in both the male and female. **Topic:** Reproductive System

88. The following are true of spermatogenesis **except:**

A. Spermatogenesis occurs in the seminiferous tubule germinal epithelium.
B. Spermatogonia mature into primary spermatocytes.
C. Secondary spermatocytes undergo meiosis I.
D. Maturation depends on androgen acting on the Sertoli cells.

The correct answer is (C). Spermatogenesis occurs in the seminiferous tubule, starting in the germinal epithelium after puberty. The long dormant primitive germ cells, spermatogonia, of the basal layer next to the basement membrane of the seminiferous tubule begin to divide mitotically. **Topic:** Reproductive System

89. The following are true of oogenesis **except:**

A. At birth ova are in the first meiotic division of prophase.
B. One ova completes meiosis I and produces the haploid secondary oocyte.
C. Secondary oocyte starts meiosis II, without DNA replication.
D. Completion of meiosis II upon fertilization produces a haploid ovum.

The correct answer is (B). Under the influence of FSH and LH, on about day six, one follicle grows rapidly and one ova completes meiosis I and produces the secondary oocyte, still diploid, and one polar body. **Topic:** Reproductive System

90. The following are true of the mature sperm and ova **except:**

A. The head contains the haploid number of chromosomes.
B. The midpiece contains a mitochondria, which spirals lengthwise.
C. Follicle cells provide nutrition to the oocyte in the oviduct.
D. When the oocyte is released at ovulation, it is in metaphase of meiosis I.

The correct answer is (D). When the oocyte is released at ovulation, it is in metaphase of meiosis II and it completes the meiosis only after fertilization. **Topic:** Reproductive System

91. The following are true of nonsexual reproduction **except:**

A. Multiple fission is the division of a cell into two equal daughter cells.

B. Budding is a mitotic process of very unequal cytoplasmic cell division.

C. Spore formation is a means of rapid increase in population

D. Natural parthenogenesis, or fatherless development, occurs in bees.

The correct answer is (A). Asexual reproduction is reproduction not involving the union of genetic material from two sources. Fission, binary, multiple, and budding, is the division of a cell into two or more daughter cells. Binary fission is the division of a cell into two equal daughter cells and multiple fission into several equal daughter cells. **Topic:** Reproductive System

92. The following are true of the fertilization stage of the zygote **except:**

A. Sperm in the vagina must mature before being capable of fertilization.

B. Sperm contact the corona radiata and the acrosomal reaction occurs.

C. Sperm penetrates the oocyte cell wall, the oocyte completes its maturation.

D. Female pronucleus fuses with the male pronucleus to complete fertilization.

The correct answer is (B). Fertilization usually occurs in the mid- to lateral fallopian tube, the ampulla. The sperm contact the zona pellucida and the acrosomal reaction occurs. **Topic:** Development

93. The following are true of the cleavage of the zygote **except:**

A. Diploid zygote replicate its DNA in preparation for mitosis.

B. Zygote undergoes mitosis to form 2 equal haploid daughter blastomeres.

C. First cleavage occurs at the 30-hour post fertilization stage.

D. Morula of 12–16 small cells forms by 60 hours or three days.

The correct answer is (B). The zygote nucleus undergoes mitosis to form 2 equal diploid daughter blastomeres, each with equal DNA from the male and female. **Topic:** Development

94. The following are true of the blastocyst stage of development **except:**

A. Blastocyst with fluid separates into inner and outer cell masses.

B. Accumulating fluid comes together in a cavity, the blastocele.

C. Inner cell mass becomes located at one pole and it is called the blastocyst.

D. Outer cell mass is the trophoblast and it gives rise to the placenta.

The correct answer is (C). The inner cell mass becomes located at one pole, and it is called the embryoblast because it gives rise to the tissues of the future embryo. **Topic:** Development

95. The following are true of the implantation of the blastocyst in the uterus **except:**

A. Trophoblastic cell enzymes begin to invade the uterine epithelium.
B. Blastocyst implanted superficially in the uterus about day six after ovulation.
C. Cytotrophoblast penetrates deeper into the endometrium to form lacuna.
D. Day eleven–twelve, the blastocyst is completely imbedded in the endometrium.

The correct answer is (C). The syncytiotrophoblast penetrates deeper into the endometrium forming vacuoles, which fuse to form lacuna and the uterine endometrium shows vascular congestion. **Topic:** Development

96. The following are true of the second week of the blastocyst development except:

A. Embryoblast differentiates into a bilaminar germ disc, or embryonic disc.
B. Amniotic cavity forms between ectoderm and cytotrophoblast.
C. Cytotrophoblast proliferates forming the extra embryonic mesoderm.
D. Ectodermal primitive streak appears.

The correct answer is (D). The prochordal plate is just forming in the entodermal disc at the end of the second week, and the ectodermal primitive streak appears in the third week. **Topic:** Development

97. All are true of the second month of the blastocyst development **except:**

A. Organogenesis, embryo most susceptible to congenital malformations.
B. Intermediate mesoderm becomes the somites.
C. Entodermal derivatives form the gut.
D. Entoderm gives rise to epithelial lining of respiratory tract, urinary bladder.

The correct answer is (B). The paraxial mesoderm, which becomes the somites, differentiates into segmental muscle, dermis and subcutaneous tissue, and the vertebral column. The intermediate mesoderm becomes the excretory units of the urinary system. **Topic:** Development

98. The following are true of the fetal membranes and placenta **except:**

A. Develop from the zygote and are therefore extraembryonic.
B. Chorion is thick over the embryo, becomes the fetal part of the placenta.
C. Chorion has inner entoderm and outer cytotrophoblast layers.
D. Amniotic cavity expands, the amnion and chorion fuse.

The correct answer is (C). The chorion is the lining of the chorionic cavity (extraembryonic coelom) that develops from the proliferation of the cytotrophoblast into mesoderm and then the coalescence of the spaces that appear in the mesoderm. It therefore has inner mesoderm and outer cytotrophoblast layers. **Topic:** Development

99. All are true of the fetal membranes and placenta **except:**

   A. Ectoderm lines a smaller sac, which becomes the secondary yolk sac.
   B. Yolk sac is folded up into the embryo to form the foregut, midgut, hindgut.
   C. Midgut communicates with the yolk sac via the vitelline duct.
   D. Buccopharyngeal membrane ruptures, foregut open to amniotic cavity.

The correct answer is (A). Heuser's membrane and the entodermal germ layer form the primitive yolk sac until the entoderm can make cells to line a smaller sac, which becomes the secondary yolk sac. **Topic:** Development

100. The following are true of the placenta **except:**

   A. The placenta also functions as an endocrine gland.
   B. The trophoblast gives rise to the fetal part of the placenta.
   C. Maternal part of the placenta formed by the thickened uterine endometrium.
   D. Villi are separated from the maternal blood lakes by only 1 cell layer.

The correct answer is (D). These villi project into the uterine decidua and after the fourth month are separated from the maternal blood lakes by only 2 cell layers, the syncytial layer and the vascular endothelial layer. **Topic:** Development

101. The following are true of the path of blood circulation for the fetus **except:**

   A. uterine spiral arteries, maternal blood, blood lakes, villi
   B. oxygenated blood, right atrium, foramen oval to the left atrium
   C. deoxygenated blood, chorionic plate, one umbilical vein, ductus venosus
   D. deoxygenated blood, right ventricle, pulmonary trunk, ductus arteriosus

The correct answer is (C). The oxygenated fetal blood flows through the chorionic plate into the one umbilical vein to the ductus venosus, which functions to bypass the liver, to the inferior vena cava. **Topic:** Development

102. The following are true of the neonatal circulation **except:**

   A. two umbilical arteries close first and within a few minutes
   B. ductus venosus closes allowing full flow through the ascending aorta
   C. ductus arteriosus closes, flow to right ventricle, now pulmonary trunk, lungs
   D. foramen ovale closes, because pressure higher in the left atrium

The correct answer is (B). The ductus venosus closes allowing full flow through the liver. **Topic:** Development

103. The following are true of multiple pregnancy **except:**

A. Identical and fraternal twins differ in the number of ovum fertilized.

B. Dizygotic twins occur if the inner cell mass divides during development.

C. Split of two cell zygote forms separate chorionic sac, amnion, and placenta.

D. Most multiple pregnancies are dizygotic.

The correct answer is (D). Most multiple pregnancies are dizygotic, which occurs when more than one ova is available and each is fertilized by a separate sperm. **Topic:** Development

104. The following are true of Mendelian genetics **except:**

A. Hand cross pollinate two true breeding strains, 1/4 F1 are recessive trait.

B. A genotype is the total combination of genes in an organism.

C. First law, any trait produced by at least a pair of alleles which segregate.

D. Punnett squares use a capital letter to represent the dominant trait.

The correct answer is (A). If the parent generation of two true breeding strains is cross pollinated by hand, the trait appearing in the F1 plants is the dominant trait and the trait not appearing is recessive. **Topic:** Genetics

105. The following are true of Mendel's second law **except:**

A. Second law is the law of independent assortment for linked alleles.

B. Crossing of dihybrids is a dihybrid cross.

C. RRYY and rryy, only two possible gametes per parent if the alleles sort independently.

D. Unlinked alleles are alleles not on the same chromosome.

The correct answer is (A). Mendel's second law states that the inheritance of any one pair of factors or alleles occurs independently of the simultaneous inheritance of any other pair. This is the law of independent assortment and studies two pairs of unlinked alleles. **Topic:** Genetics

106. The following are true of genetics **except:**

A. An inoperative allele is a non functioning allele.

B. The dominant allele may also be an inhibitor, preventing the expression.

C. If a dominant allele shows partial dominance, result is between two alleles.

D. Rare dominant or lethal-recessive dominant, must be homozygous to be expressed.

The correct answer is (D). The rare dominant or the lethal-recessive dominant have to be present to be expressed; they do not have to be homozygous, but they have to be homozygous to be lethal. **Topic:** Genetics

107. The following are true of polygenic traits **except:**

A. Phenotypic trait showing little variation is called a polygenic trait.
B. Pair and segregate and sort according to Mendel's laws.
C. Polygenic inheritance, alleles at more then one locus contribute to the same trait.
D. Selected alleles may be associated with undesirable effects on other systems.

The correct answer is (A). A phenotypic trait, such as skin color, that is not one definite quality or another but is somewhere along a continuing line, known as continuous variation, is called a polygenic trait.
Topic: Genetics

108. The following are true of paternity and inheritance **except:**

A. Four ABO blood type phenotypes, 3 alleles, and 6 different genotypes.
B. The child must receive one ABO allele from each parent.
C. If the child is type O, then the father can be AB.
D. The presence of RR or Rr makes a person Rh positive.

The correct answer is (C). The alleles are IaIa and IaIo for type A blood (A is dominant), IbIb and IbIo for type B blood (B is dominant), IaIb for type AB blood, and IoIo for type O blood. If the child is type O, it has alleles IoIo, then the father gave Io and the mother gave Io. If the suspected father is type AB, with alleles IaIb, he is excluded.
Topic: Genetics

109. The following are true of the distribution of living organisms **except:**

A. Biosphere is that part of the Earth that supports life.
B. Habitat is a place where plant or animal species naturally live and grow.
C. Biomes are more identified by their animals than their plants.
D. Adjacent biomes go through a transition zone and have indistinct borders.

The correct answer is (C). Biomes are vast, distinct, recognizable associations of plants and animals within a geographic area defined by the climate of that area. Biomes are more identified by their plants than their animals. **Topic:** The Animal Kingdom

110. The following are true of the interrelationships of animals **except:**

A. One species gains at no expense to another species is mutual symbiosis.
B. Food chain and food pyramid describe predator relationships..
C. One species gains at the expense of the other is a parasitic symbiosis.
D. Phytoplankton, kelp and seaweed are the primary producers of the ocean.

The correct answer is (C). When one species gains at the expense of the other, it is a parasitic symbiosis. In commensal symbiosis, one species gains but at no expense to the other species and in mutual symbiosis relationships, both species benefit as with the E coli bacteria in the human colon. **Topic:** The Animal Kingdom

111. The following are true of population dynamics **except:**

    A. Crude death rate is the number of deaths per year per 1,000 population.

    B. Population doubling time is 70 divided by the percent annual growth.

    C. Total fertility rate, live births per 1,000 women age group (15–44).

    D. 1983 population doubling time, world 38.89 yrs., Africa 23 yrs.

The correct answer is (C). The general fertility rate is the number of live births per 1,000 women in the reproductive age group (15–44). The total fertility rate is a prediction of the average number of children women will have over their reproductive lifetime. **Topic:** The Animal Kingdom

112. The following are true of the major environment habitats except:

    A. Blue, green, or brown water is rich in nutrients.

    B. Biomes follow latitude or altitude because of temperature variations.

    C. A salt water environment, the euphotic zone, receives light.

    D. Most wavelengths of light are absorbed in the upper 100 meters of water.

The correct answer is (A). Water devoid of particles and therefore of nutrition, is blue, while green, brown, or red water is rich in nutrients. **Topic:** The Animal Kingdom

113. The following are true of learning and conditioning **except:**

    A. Habituation is learning to respond to a specific stimulus.

    B. Classical conditioning is demonstrated by Pavlov's dog experiment.

    C. In operant conditioning, the response is followed by the stimulus.

    D. Operant conditioning illustrates the principle reward is reinforcing.

The correct answer is (A). Habituation is learning to *not* respond to a specific stimulus. As the stimulus is presented over and over, the response gradually lessens and may disappear. **Topic:** The Animal Kingdom

114. The following are true of evolution **except:**

    A. An observation provoked questions that led Darwin to his life's work.

    B. Convergent evolution is illustrated by the rabbit and the mara

    C. Darwin published his still available world journal, *Origin of Species*, in 1859.

    D. The thinking for the nineteenth century held the immutability of the species.

The correct answer is (C). Darwin published his journal, *The Voyage of the Beagle*, still available today. In 1859, he published *Origin of Species*, an abstract of a planned 6 volume work. **Topic:** Evolution

115. The following are true of the process of evolution **except:**

    A. Genetic makeup of the germ cells guarantees diversity.

    B. Natural selection was proposed by Darwin in his book *Origin of Species.*

    C. One species dependent on another illustrates coevolution .

    D. Two major themes of evolution are diversification and separation.

The correct answer is (D). Two of the major themes of evolution are diversification of organisms and adaptation of the organism. **Topic:** Evolution

116. The following are true of evolution and adaptive radiation **except:**

    A. Adaptive radiation, spread into new and differing environments, change.

    B. An example of adaptive radiation, finches on the Galapagos islands.

    C. Divergent evolution, adapting to new environment, become more similar.

    D. Divergence is represented visually in the phylogenetic tree.

The correct answer is (C). This is divergent evolution or divergence, which means that the species finds a new way of using the resources available, establishes a new niche that is favored by natural selection since the competition is less. As two species compete, natural selection would favor the most different of each population, such as, if the difference allowed them to eat a new food or survive a predator. **Topic:** Evolution

117. The following are true of evolutionary extinction **except:**

    A. Coming to an end or dying out of a species.

    B. Can occur due to lack of adaptation to the environment or to competition.

    C. Biotic population controls, population depressing factors of physical nature,

    D. Biotic controls are usually density dependent

The correct answer is (C). Biotic population controls are influences on a population by another living population. **Topic:** Evolution

118. The following are true of evolutionary homology **except:**

    A. Correspondence of structures of different organisms, common ancestor.

    B. Similarity in function and maybe appearance.

    C. Differences have arisen since the two separated from a common ancestor

    D. Wing of a bird and the forearm of the dog.

The correct answer is (B). Homology is the correspondence of structures of different organisms due to their common ancestor. The forelimb of a dog and the arm of a man are homologous structures, but are now used differently. The wing of a bird is also homologous with the forearm of the dog and the arm of a man but the bones in the wing are not all homologous with the arm and forearm bones. **Topic:** Evolution

Practice Test 1

| VERBAL REASONING | TIME—85 MINUTES | 65 QUESTIONS |

There are nine passages in the Verbal Reasoning test. Each passage is followed by several questions. After reading a passage, select the one best answer to each question. If you are not certain of an answer, eliminate the alternatives that you know to be incorrect and then select an answer from the remaining alternatives. Indicate your selection by blackening the corresponding circle on your answer sheet.

PASSAGE 1 (QUESTIONS 1-7)

There is no doubt that Americans today place a high priority on living a long and disease-free life. It is generally conceded that freedom from pain and debilitation ought to be looked upon as a natural right of all human beings. Achieving this goal is facilitated by the proper selection of health products and services.

Of all consumer goods and services, none is more essential to one's welfare than health care. There are several excellent consumer magazines distributed by product-testing agencies that may be helpful in choosing health care. Yet the array of products and medical facilities is huge, and the claims for the merits of each are confusing. Occasionally, we may visit a physician or dentist and receive specific care or advice, but few of us can afford professional counsel on all health matters.

Not only can we waste a great deal of money on ineffectual products and professionals, but our health, perhaps even our lives, may depend on getting proper treatment for disease and illness. There are times when self-treatment should not even be attempted. For example, some products—such as aspirin, laxatives, and antihistamines—are dangerous when used in excessive amounts, in the presence of certain physical disorders, or in combination with other medicines. In addition to the question of which products to select, there is always the question of whether any product should be selected without the consultation of a physician.

Obviously, people should not run to a physician for every little scrape, bruise, ache, or pain. If they did, our entire system of medical care would be swamped overnight and the doctors would be unable to take care of the more serious problems. How can we know then, which of the hundreds of different symptoms that can develop require the services of a physician? There are several circumstances under which a physician should always be consulted.

1. Severe symptoms. Any type of attack in which the symptoms are severe or alarming—such as severe abdominal or chest pain or bleeding—should obviously receive prompt medical attention.

2. Prolonged symptoms. Any symptoms—such as cough, headache, constipation, or fatigue—that persist day after day should be checked by a physician, even though the symptoms are minor. Serious chronic disorders are often revealed through persistent minor symptoms.

3. Repeated symptoms. Symptoms, even though minor, that recur time after time should be reported to a physician because, like prolonged symptoms, they may indicate a serious problem.

4. Unusual symptoms. Any symptoms that seem to be unusual, such as unusual bleeding, mental changes, weight gains or losses, digestive changes, or fatigue, call for a visit to a physician.

5. If in doubt, the safest action is to see a physician. If there is a serious problem, it can be corrected in its early stages; if there is no problem, then you have paid a very small price for your peace of mind.

1. The focus of this article is:

   A. the importance of selecting quality health care.
   B. determining when and when not to see a physician.
   C. holding down the cost of health care.
   D. maintaining consistency in quality of life.

2. After a careful reading of this selection, one might infer that visiting a physician for every little sickness would:

   A. bankrupt many Americans.
   B. cause too much time to be spent away from work.
   C. overburden the health-care profession.
   D. increase health-care insurance premiums.

3. The author alludes to the popularity of:

   A. false claims for medicines.
   B. the practice of quackery.
   C. self-treatment.
   D. obtaining free advice.

4. Most people can live a healthy and disease-free life:

   A. with the assistance of a caring physician.
   B. by trying and using a variety of self-treatments.
   C. by subscribing to and reading health-care magazines.
   D. with proper selection of health products and services.

5. There are many varieties of self-treatment medications available today; however, the author leads us to infer that:

    A. the misuse of such "innocent" medications can lead to addiction.

    B. one should read the directions and contraindications before use.

    C. a physician need not be consulted before using them.

    D. one must exercise care in selecting what to use and when to use it.

6. The determination of when to visit a doctor and when to practice self-treatment is quite difficult. The author gives an agenda for seeing a physician that includes:

    A. weight change.

    B. recurring symptoms.

    C. chest pain.

    D. all of the above.

7. One might conclude that competent health care is:

    A. readily available.

    B. becoming overly expensive.

    C. possible at the corner drug store.

    D. one's own responsibility.

PASSAGE 2 (QUESTIONS 8–17)

A crisis of morals and values confronts this nation and shows itself in many forms. The idealism of the young, their critical spirit, and their impatience with anything less than full justice and equal opportunity for everyone are not only admirable but a source of optimism and hope for the future. Some of their methods of expressing their impatience, however, do not always lead to a realization of their aims—they may, in fact, be self-defeating.

One of these by-products of social upheaval is the pervasive and widespread use of drugs for non-medicinal purposes, coinciding with an overuse of many drugs that have a very important role in medicine. Under present circumstances, it is understandable that an observer would first come to the conclusion that drugs were the primary problem. Only after considerable thought does it become apparent that the basic problem is the psychological and emotional state of those who look to drugs for a solution to their problems and thus postpone or avoid sound approaches toward their resolution. Hence, any analysis of the problem must focus on the individuals who use drugs. Until an individual can understand his or her drug need in terms of his or her own psychology, drug use for him or her will continue to be one of the symptoms that perpetuates its causes.

Almost every class entering high school or college today contains a higher percentage of students who have used illegal drugs than did the preceding class. The custom is spreading from high schools and colleges down to the middle schools and even grade schools. The use of marijuana and amphetamines, especially, is escalating apparently beyond control. Thousands of young people are demonstrating lack of judgment concerning drugs. They have some realization that these are dangerous substances, yet they take drugs anyway, risking their own health, their present and future mental functioning, the legal consequences if they are detected, and the further alienation from the adult world that drug use represents. And much of this is justified by the excuse that "Oh, older people just have closed minds about drugs!" Or: "Drug use makes one more open-minded!"

Definition of these two terms—closed-minded and open-minded— seems to be in order.

Open-mindedness is the capacity to look at issues in an unprejudiced way, to make up one's mind on the basis of evidence that is presented, and not to hold to previous points of view in the face of new evidence. A child is basically an open-minded individual, because he or she has no previous point of view to defend; he or she learns from what he or she sees and hears and experiences. On the other hand, the child is still in the process of learning the logic of adults. An adult would be called gullible and naive, rather than open-minded, if he or she believed everything he or she heard. To be truly open-minded, one must have some ability to use the rules of logic and reason and thus be able to judge new bits of data and discard those which obviously do not conform to the standards of logic upon which intellectual activity is based.

Closed-minded would be just the opposite. Thoughts and opinions would be set, whether with or without evidence and often with a measure of prejudice or unfavorable opinions or feelings formed beforehand or without knowledge.

8. Acknowledging that drug use is becoming more commonplace and less of a phenomenon, according to this article, where must we look first in an attempt to solve the drug problem?

   A. To those who sell drugs to young people.
   B. At making stronger laws to punish those who use drugs.
   C. At the psychological estate of those who look to drugs for comfort.
   D. At legalizing certain drugs in an effort to control their use.

9. This author makes the point that with each year:

   A. the number of drug users increases.
   B. more incoming college students have used illegal drugs.
   C. the effects of drug use are more pronounced.
   D. all of the above.

10. Among the drugs so popular with users of today is:

   A. uppers.
   B. prescription medicines.
   C. cocaine.
   D. crack.

11. One may infer from this reading that a drug user is attempting to:

   A. experience a release from stress.
   B. control a symptom of a psychological need.
   C. lose the need to make an effort in life.
   D. make a psychological breakthrough.

12. Many young people look at the objections to drug use as a(n):

   A. attempt to deprive them of rights.
   B. psychological independence.
   C. demonstration of control.
   D. indication of adult close-mindedness.

13. An indicator of close-mindedness is:

   A. accepting the opinions of others.
   B. stubbornness.
   C. attempting to understand.
   D. preformed ideas.

14. One who is open-minded would likely:

   A. not be prejudiced.
   B. listen and learn.
   C. be flexible.
   D. all of the above.

15. A child would be more likely to take everything that is said and done:

   A. as true.
   B. without regard to what he or she has been told.
   C. and not internalize it.
   D. and change to meet this new definition.

16. According to this selection, there are many dangers to the use of prescription drugs for non-medicinal purposes; these include:

   A. loss of sexual functioning.
   B. the passing on of deformed genes.
   C. future mental functioning.
   D. alienation of friends and family.

17. Based upon the definitions of open-mindedness and close-mindedness, the author infers that a drug user would be which of these and why?

   A. Open-minded, because there is prejudice against society.
   B. Close-minded, because there is the ability to take bits of data and make new judgments.
   C. Close-minded, without the ability to use rules of logic and judge new information.
   D. Open-minded, because the user applies rules of logic and judges new information.

PASSAGE 3 (QUESTIONS 18–27)

No material serves the body in as many vital functions as water. The importance of water to the body is so great that the loss of only 10 percent of the body's water can result in an individual's death. The body is more than 50 percent water, and many of the tissues of the body (such as blood) are as much as 90 percent water. Digestion, absorption, and the secretion of materials must take place in water. All chemical reactions of metabolism also require water. It provides the moisture in the cells of the lungs that enables the membranes to exchange oxygen and carbon dioxide. It is important in distributing heat uniformly throughout the body. It transports many vital substances throughout the body. And it also serves as a cushion for the brain and spinal cord.

How much water people require each day depends largely on the air temperature around them and the kind of physical activity they are engaged in. Water loss may range from 2½ quarts for a moderately active person to several times that much for a person working vigorously in the hot sun. The loss occurs primarily through the kidneys, lungs, digestive tract, and skin.

This water loss can be replenished by liquids and foods of all kinds. All foods—even dry bread—contain some water. Some water is produced within the body through the metabolic breakdown of stored nutrients. Since there are variables both in water needed and water available from different sources, it is not possible to state the specific amount of water a person should drink each day. In general, a person should drink a little more water than is sufficient to satisfy thirst. The slight excess beyond thirst provides for good kidney health.

Food supplies the nutrients for growth and replacement of worn or damaged cells, as well as for the manufacture of cellular products, such as enzymes and hormones. The overall composition of the body is about 59 percent water, 18 percent protein, 18 percent fat, and 4.3 percent mineral. At any one time, there is less than 1 percent carbohydrates in the makeup of the body. These substances that make up the body are not distributed equally in all organs. For example, the percentage of water varies from 90 to 92 percent in blood plasma to 72 to 78 percent in muscle, 45 percent in bone, and only 5 percent in tooth enamel. Proteins are found most abundantly in muscle. Fat tends to concentrate in the adipose (fat) cells under the skin and around the intestines. Carbohydrates are found mainly in the liver, muscles, and blood. As for the minerals, high levels of calcium and phosphorus form part of the bones and teeth, sodium and chlorine are found mainly in the body fluids (blood plasma and lymph), potassium is the main mineral in muscle, iron is essential to red blood cells, and magnesium is generally found throughout the body.

These are the primary minerals supplied to the body as food, but many other minerals are essential to the human body in proportionately smaller amounts. These minerals are termed "trace elements," and they, too, must be ingested with our food. Other chemicals (vitamins) are needed in very small amounts for various functions of the body to take place.

18. The focus of this selection is:

    A. to describe the body's need for water.

    B. cautioning against substituting items in the diet.

    C. the importance of certain elements to proper body functioning.

    D. the description of the body's need for a specific amount of water.

19. Among the specific functions of water in the body are:

    A. digestion, respiration, and secretion.

    B. absorption, energizing, and metabolism.

    C. respiration, energizing, and digestion.

    D. digestion, absorption, and secretion.

20. One might infer from the selection that water deprivation through dehydration is:

    A. undesirable.

    B. unhealthy.

    C. life-threatening.

    D. all of the above.

21. Based on the passage, which of the following would WEAKEN the body more?

    A. Substituting other liquids for water intake.
    B. Inactivity to preclude perspiration.
    C. extreme dieting with decreased liquid intake.
    D. Increasing the intake of carbohydrates.

22. Based upon the information in this article, the loss of 2½ quarts of water per day is normal, but more would be lost by a:

    A. stenographer in an air-conditioned office.
    B. construction worker outside in the summer.
    C. computer scientist working in a warehouse.
    D. housewife doing spring cleaning.

23. According to this selection, given the makeup of the body, the vital nutrients in addition to water are:

    A. minerals, carbohydrates, and glucose.
    B. glucose, vitamins, and fat.
    C. lymph, vitamins, and fat.
    D. minerals, carbohydrates, and proteins.

24. According to this article, water is found in the greatest proportion in the:

    A. blood.
    B. muscles.
    C. tissues.
    D. bones.

25. According to this article, the loss of water is remedied by:

    A. intake of liquids.
    B. intake of food.
    C. metabolism.
    D. all of the above.

26. The human body is a complicated machine that has a unique blend of:

    A. chemicals.
    B. vitamins.
    C. minerals.
    D. all of the above.

27. To assure the proper high level functioning of the kidneys, one should:

    A. drink a bit more water than necessary to satisfy thirst.
    B. ingest at least 2½ quarts of water per day.
    C. assure the intake of liquids and foods in proportionate amounts.
    D. maintain a mixture of various types of liquids daily.

PASSAGE 4 (QUESTIONS 28–33)

Aesthetic needs and impulses are not the specialized interest of a small group. Everyone seems to be concerned with what is beautiful, pleasing, or appropriate in the visual world. That is, we are interested in beauty wherever it may be found—in people, in nature, and in objects of daily use. Some artists do specialize, however, in making things that are beautiful or aesthetically satisfying in themselves, apart from any utility they may have. Objects created to be beautiful or intrinsically pleasing are nevertheless useful because they help to satisfy the aesthetic interests and requirements of modern people. In his earliest days, man may have been concerned about colors or shapes only to the extent that they were signs of danger or of opportunity. But, since his life depended on how accurately and intelligently he could see, vision was a matter of supreme importance. We still possess remarkable visual equipment and outstanding capacity for interpreting our optical experience. However, the conditions of contemporary life do not seem to demand as much of our perceptual capacities as we are equipped to supply. Hence, some forms of visual art appear to have evolved in complex cultures as a means of engaging our unused perceptual capacity. Perhaps aesthetic pleasure is, in fact, the satisfaction experienced in employing to the full our innate capacities for perception.

An elementary aesthetic pleasure might be called "the thrill of recognition." Obviously, recognition has always played an important role in human survival. Its significant role in all human affairs accounts for the popularity of art that is easily recognized, that provides a multitude of cues to its origin in reality. When we recognize something in a work of art, we are in a sense rehearsing our survival technique, sharpening our capacity to distinguish between friend and foe. It is only a short step from the ability to perform such discriminations to the ability to enjoy perception itself, suspending all the while any impulse to fight or flee. Rather, we learn to linger over visual events and thus to maximize our delight in them.

An artist whose lifelong effort was devoted to making the art of painting a source of pure visual delight was Georges Braque (1882–1963). An early associate of Pablo Picasso's in the creation of the intellectual austerities of Analytic Cubism, Braque employed the principles of Cubism to paint surfaces of immense sensuous appeal and decorative ingenuity. Braque's

work *The Round Table* shows his mastery with shape and texture and his droll wit in exploiting optical and pictorial conventions for pleasure and humor rather than reliable cognitive cues. One recognizes the room and the table easily enough with the top tilted forward to reveal a multitude of ordinary objects: a mandolin, a knife, fruit, a magazine, a paper, a pipe, an open book, and so on. The objects in themselves are unimportant; they have shapes and colors and textures that Braque can rearrange. He can show the top and side views of an object at the same time; he can paint opaque objects as if they were transparent; he can reverse the expected convergence of lines in perspective; he can exaggerate ornament with white lines, arbitrarily exchange light areas with shadow areas, or paint shadows a lighter and brighter color than the objects that cast them. The purpose of these "violations" and surprises is not to create a painting *of* something; rather, the painting must *be* something, a kind of organism that lives according to its own law. And that law seems to state that any twisting, slicing, distortion, or reversal of shape, color, and texture is justified if it can increase our delight in looking. The logic of the painting is based on the obligation to surprise or please the eye rather than to reproduce a set of relatively innocuous objects.

28. The focus of this selection is:

A. to explain why an artist paints.
B. an effort to expand the knowledge about the painter George Braque.
C. explaining what the painting *The Round Table* is all about.
D. exploring the development of sight beyond that needed to exist safely.

29. If the painting *The Round Table* is an example of Cubism, the reader might infer that Cubism is:

    A. a style of painting that does not adhere to reality.
    B. the shape of the painting.
    C. the type of paint and canvas used for the work of art.
    D. an indicator of the time period in which the work was completed.

30. As an artist appeals to the aesthetic senses, he addresses the viewer's sense of:

    A. the pleasing and sensible.
    B. reality and truth.
    C. what is sensible and gracious.
    D. beauty and pleasure.

31. Art—man's appeal to the aesthetic— may be beautiful, pleasant, and useful as evidenced by:

    A. the various uses for the art in the marketplace.
    B. their satisfaction of modern man.
    C. the growing popularity of art for the office.
    D. the efforts to appeal to both genders.

32. A close reading of this selection reveals that man has a history of using his sight for protection and learning; however, that same sense of sight can be used for:

    A. understanding one's fellow man.
    B. perception of color.
    C. interpreting our optical experience.
    D. discerning shapes.

33. The history of art reveals that:

    A. ancient man used it to communicate meaning.
    B. primitive forms existed in prehistoric times.
    C. man's unused perceptive ability is tapped.
    D. perception is unnecessary when confronted with aesthetics.

PASSAGE 5 (QUESTIONS 34–39)

Pocahontas was born around 1595, the daughter of Chief Powhatan. Chief Powhatan led the Powhatan Confederacy, which was a powerful grouping of about 200 Algonquin tribes (in the area now known as Virginia) along the James and York River systems. He had numerous children, but Pocahontas, then known as Matoaka ("playful one") seemed to have been his favorite. He apparently let her advise him in tribal matters to some degree.

Pocahontas was still a child, about 12 years old, when John Smith landed with the Jamestown settlers in Virginia in 1607. The settlers were disruptive to the Indians' way of life, doing things like stealing food, and they were in turn attacked. Pocahontas's act of saving John Smith's life was most likely an act staged by the Powhatan Indians to prove their strength, and a way of opening the door to diplomacy and trade between the two groups. It could also have been a type of dramatic "adoption" of John Smith for diplomatic reasons. (Please note that the act of saving his life may not have taken place at all; when John Smith wrote his memoirs, this incident was not included in the first version but was added later. He published memoirs during his lifetime to try to recruit new people to come to Virginia with him and was not above embellishing the truth to make a good tale, or so it was rumored.)

Still, Pocahontas did take a great interest in the new colony and people, and she frequently brought them food and tried to help them adapt to their new home. She was "untamed" to their way of thinking but good-spirited and well-liked. She learned their language and was able to keep both sides informed about the other's goings-on. It is certain she saved lives on both sides, preventing skirmishes. Her father disapproved of her intense interest in the English, and she was not allowed to visit them for a period of a few years, during most of her teens. There is speculation that she was married during part of this time to an Indian husband who died, but there is no proof either way.

In 1613, Pocahontas was kidnapped by the English in a political move against her father. She and her father had a falling-out, and she refused to negotiate for her own release. During this period of captivity, she was staying with the Rev. Alexander Whitaker and was instructed in the Christian faith. She accepted this doctrine and was baptized with the name "Rebecca." She had also been courted by the Englishman John Rolfe, and they were married in April 1614. This alliance finally brought peace between the colony and the Powhatans, which lasted for many years.

There was a son, named Thomas, born to the couple in 1615. The following year, they were invited back to England in recognition of Pocahontas's contributions to the welfare of the colony, and they set sail in 1616. Pocahontas was very well received, met the Queen, and enjoyed many parties in her honor. She also saw John Smith in London, for the first time in eight years.

Starting in late winter or early spring of 1616-1617, her health began to fail. The small family had plans to sail back to Virginia in March 1617, but Pocahontas died as they were to leave. She had contracted either tuberculosis or pneumonia and was buried in England. The grave site has since been lost. There are rumors that her son also died at this time, but many disbelieve this and think Thomas came back to Virginia.

34. The focus of this article is:

   A. dispelling myths about Pocahontas.
   B. how the Indians tricked the settlers.
   C. the life and times of Pocahontas.
   D. how the settlers tricked the Indians.

35. Indicators that Pocahontas may have saved John Smith's life are found in:

   A. Smith's diaries.
   B. legends handed down by the settlers.
   C. Indian folklore.
   D. records sent back to England.

36. If the story of Pocahontas saving the life of Smith is true, this author infers that:

   A. she was very young and unaware of what was happening.
   B. Smith may have staged the event.
   C. such a practice would not be unusual for that time in history.
   D. the Indians may have staged it for diplomatic purposes.

37. The life of Pocahontas, involved all of the following EXCEPT:

    A. a visit with the Queen of England.

    B. learning the English language.

    C. a long and happy life among the Virginia settlers.

    D. life as a princess of the Algonquin Indian tribe of Virginia.

38. Pocahontas may well have been "ahead of her time" because she:

    A. took a trip to England to meet John Smith.

    B. protected the Indians from the settlers.

    C. was made an honorary princess by the Queen of England.

    D. advised Chief Powhatan on matters regarding the entire tribe.

39. Peace between the Indians and the settlers was accomplished by:

    A. Smith's publication of his memoirs.

    B. the marriage of the Indian princess and a white man.

    C. the benevolent efforts of Pocahontas toward the settlers.

    D. the kidnapping of the Indian princess.

PASSAGE 6 (QUESTIONS 40–46)

The American Revolution changed the course of history and had a number of different causes. These causes included political differences. This included a struggle over issues involving power—control—the desire to dominate and to avoid being dominated. It was the arena of conflict over who would be the boss. Another cause was conflicting parties in England, especially the Whigs versus the Tories. With George II and George III, the Tories had gained ascendancy, and the former period of Whig domination was curtailed. The Tories and the King also wanted to assert their power over colonial affairs.

Additionally, there was an international cause of the war because of differences between the British and the French. The British victory in the Seven Years' War (French and Indian War) had opened the west to colonists, but this was resisted by British interests centered in Canada. An alliance with the Indians was seen as the basis for colonials gaining strength. Also, this struggle was not over, and the British were concerned with preparing for another war against France. British politicians opposed colonial politicians, and a power struggle over who would be in control of political processes in the colonies ensued. This became a struggle between the Tories, who gained their power by being loyal to the King and using his support, and the Separatists, who gained power by the support of lower-class colonists.

The Revolution had an economic cause, too. The struggle over wealth, profits, and all aspects of economic life such as trade and manufacturing, or mercantilism, ensued. Merchants, and others who believed in this theory, wanted profits from all trade to flow to the home country and for the colonies to be used as a source of raw materials, with income flowing back to the home country. Also, they did not want direct trade with other countries by colonies; rather, the preference was that all such trade should move through the home country. The owners of shipping also struggled with the merchants over terms of shipping and who would get the profits. In addition, the merchants and farmers struggled over prices and tariffs that established who profited. Manufacturers stood against both merchants and farmers in the same kind of struggle that occupied owners of plantations in the West Indies versus the North American colonies. This struggle was over the terms and nature of trade in sugar and molasses and where profits would be delivered. Merchants in India vied with the colonists in a struggle over profits from tea. Within the colonies, farmers stood against merchants and manufacturers in a struggle over profits that led to some supporting the crown and others wanting independence from the crown. Debtors struggled with creditors in an attempt to influence who would support Parliament and seek relief from debts.

There were social causes as well. This is the field in which people struggle over their place in society in its nonpolitical and noneconomic aspects, over who will get into the "social register" and be considered part of "high society" and that kind of thing. The struggle is often that of aristocrats of birth, generally having landed wealth, versus new wealthy merchants not having aristocratic titles. Both of these upper-class groups struggled against the artisans and middle-class merchants who formed the bulk of actual productive society for social acceptance. This was a struggle inside England, inside colonies, and between people in England and colonies. For instance, consider how Ben Franklin was treated when back in England versus when he was in the colonies.

There were intellectual causes for the revolution as well. This is the field in which struggle goes on over ideas. In this period, these were mostly religious ideas such as which church to have or keep or not keep as the official state church and whether there would be any official religion as there was in many colonies. Also, there was a struggle over the concept of the nature of man and man's inherent human rights. John Locke, for instance, was a part of this struggle. There was the conflict over views on the intellectual basis for justification of government and its role. And, thus, there was the beginning of struggle over ideas related to economics—Adam Smith versus the mercantile school.

For all of these reasons, there is no one way that historians can point to as one cause of the American Revolution.

40. The focus of this article is:

    A. separating from the mother country, England.

    B. to explain why there is no one cause of the Revolution.

    C. how the colonists broke away from England.

    D. the class system of England and the colonies.

41. Without the presence of economic factors, this selection indicates that there would have been:

    A. insufficient causes for the war to take place.

    B. amicable relations between the French and the English.

    C. sufficient causes in other areas to precipitate the Revolution.

    D. reason for the colonists to remain under the protection of the crown.

42. Based upon the presentation of material in this article, one might infer from this article that one of the major causes for the Revolution concerned:

   A. religion and the presentation of a state religion.
   B. the aristocracy against the newly rich.
   C. the influx of the French into the western United States.
   D. the exchange of goods and money.

43. The mention of Ben Franklin is used as a(n):

   A. anecdote.
   B. illustration.
   C. fact in point.
   D. parable.

44. The reader is able to infer from this selection that:

   A. the colonies—or "America"—were only a pawn in the struggles.
   B. England was looking for a reason to fight a war.
   C. France needed a reason to expand in the colonies.
   D. the religious struggle of the colonists had a place in the Revolution.

45. In this article, the author uses the term "mercantilism" to mean:

   A. trade of raw materials.
   B. trade and manufacturing.
   C. manufacturing and export.
   D. exchange of diplomacy for goods.

46. One might infer from this reading that the Indians:

   A. of North America were the reason for the American Revolution.
   B. benefited from the American Revolution.
   C. were not a factor at all in the cause of the war.
   D. played a minor part in the causes of the American Revolution.

PASSAGE 7 (QUESTIONS 47-52)

Polar molecules are molecules that have a concentration of negative charge on one end of the molecule and a concentration of positive charge on the other end. This is brought about by having the negative electrons within the atoms of the molecule shift toward those atoms that are most capable of attracting them. This shift produces an electrical force called a "molecular dipole." Other molecules that are polar will be attracted since each of them, in turn, has a positive and negative end. We know that positive attracts negative, therefore these molecules will line up so that this statement is observed.

Nonpolar molecules are molecules that do not have this concentration of positive or negative charge. That is because the shift of electrons occurs in a symmetrical (balanced) way so that there is, net-wise, no shift of electrons within the molecule, hence no concentration of negative electrons on one end of the molecule.

You can do a simple demonstration to show that molecules that are polar do have positive and negative areas within the molecule. You can take some buretts and fill them with different liquids such as water (polar), ethyl alcohol (polar), and carbon tetrachloride (nonpolar), and then take an amber rod and rub it with animal fur to impart a negative charge upon the rod. Open up the burette so that the liquid can begin flowing out of the burette in a stream. Bring the negatively charged rod close to the liquid stream and see what happens. What do you suppose will happen if the molecules are polar when the negatively charged rod is brought very close to the stream of liquid without actually touching it? What about the nonpolar carbon tetrachloride?

There are basically intermolecular forces in play to cause surface tension. Surface tension can be observed by placing the liquid in a constricted diameter tube. Because of the restriction in the diameter, the surface tension causes the liquid surface to "buckle" slightly. That can be done two ways. Either the surface can buckle upward, in which case we have a "convex" surface; or the surface can buckle downward, in which case we have a "concave" surface. These buckled surfaces are referred to as a "meniscus." We deal with them when we have to read a liquid level in a graduated cylinder, volumetric flask, burette, thermometer, or a barometric pressure instrument.

The intermolecular forces between molecules tend to pull the surface molecules toward the center of the liquid, since the surface molecules of the liquid have only molecules below them pulling downward toward the center of the liquid sample, whereas the molecules below the surface are pulled in all directions. This pulling downward of the surface molecules toward the center of the liquid sample causes the slight distortion of the surface known as surface tension.

47. The focus of this article is:

A. the creation of surface tension.
B. explaining magnetism.
C. the behavior of polar molecules.
D. describing the interaction of tension.

48. A molecular dipole occurs when:

A. negative electrons create an electrical attraction.
B. molecules become atoms.
C. molecules shift toward an attraction.
D. positive electrons shift.

49. The designation "polar molecule" describes:

A. separating the charges of a molecule.
B. a molecule with concentrated charges on either end.
C. the charge created with a mixture of molecules.
D. a union of positive and negative forces.

50. The reader can infer that when there is no concentration of negative electrons:

A. there is an absence of electrical force.
B. the electrical force is positive.
C. the electrical force is negative.
D. a nonpolar molecule exists.

51. A meniscus is formed:

A. when a surface buckles.
B. in the presence of a convex surface.
C. in the presence of a concave surface.
D. all of the above.

52. One can infer from this article that rubbing an animal's fur as a part of an experiment produces a:

A. surface tension.
B. positive charge.
C. negative charge.
D. balanced shift.

PASSAGE 8 (QUESTIONS 53-59)

Only within the past few decades have developmental psychologists turned to researching precisely how humans form personal value systems that provide our life with meaning, personal motivation, and choices. James Fowler refers to this construction process as faith development and contends that this creation of ultimate meaning is a universal human experience. Thus, the objects of our faith are deeply ingrained personal values that guide our lives. Fowler's Faith Development Theory suggests that the development of faith, or how we learn to know and value what we do, moves through successively progressive stages akin to those of cognitive, moral, and psychological growth.

The initial development of faith begins in infancy. This primal faith stage corresponds to what Erikson termed the trust/mistrust phase. Infants have their first experiences of trust with caretakers. These early images of trust/mistrust in self and others lay the foundation for the second stage of intuitive-projective faith that occurs between two and seven years of age. At this stage, children use language to interact with their environment and perform basic introspective tasks. Their imagination blossoms, providing a sense of unity between the environment and the initial formation of self-understanding. Identifications, aspirations, guidance, and reassurance result from this development, and imagination acts as the primary source of these early values and beliefs.

Fowler's third stage of faith development, called the mythic-literal phase, corresponds with Piaget's cognitive stage of concrete-operational thinking. Imagination becomes secondary to reality as the world becomes more predictable and orderly based on knowledge acquired through past and ongoing interactions. Faith grows from this ingrained thinking on polarities such as good and evil, self and others, and right and wrong. Distinct separations in ideas along these dimensions form a reliance from which children draw the rules, roles, and actions that govern their lives.

Formal operational thinking corresponds with synthetic-conventional faith development, the fourth Fowler stage. The self-consciousness of the teenage years enables the viewpoint of self as seen by others to emerge. The integration of these viewpoints with self-reflections represents the foundation of personal identity as something apart from, yet a part of, the world. However, individuals at this stage still lack the ability to inquire deeply into and to criticize aspects of this identity. Fowler suggests that the majority of adults never move beyond this stage.

Self-criticism and personal inquiry occur in the fifth stage of individuative-reflective faith. The beliefs, values, and commitments from which our faith is formed are ultimately based on personal reflection rather than mere information from significant others, and the responsibility for those choices is accepted as a personal self-decision. However, old values and beliefs are not casually discarded. Rather, they are reevaluated in terms of their current personal meaning and are then either further incorporated, altered and accepted, or discarded. New values and beliefs undergo virtually this same sort of examination.

An awareness that some polarities cannot be successfully incorporated occurs during the sixth stage of conjunctive faith.

This awareness presents itself as an ability to recognize that some aspects of self are unchangeable. This is further represented by an ability to embrace and learn from environmental differences, even though this knowledge does not necessarily alter our self-awareness.

The seventh and final stage of Fowler's Faith Development Theory, termed universalizing faith, is a strived-for condition rather than a universal doctrine. Characterized by some negation of self and personal subordination to some absolute power, as well as an enlarged vision of justice that calls us to transcend self, is reached by few, according to Fowler.

53. According to this selection, a personal value system involves:

    A. correct choices and moral values.
    B. education and experience.
    C. devotion to ideals and morals.
    D. faith, trust, and choices.

54. This author states that when man can perceive himself as able to change, grow, and learn, he has achieved:

    A. maturity.
    B. conjunctive faith.
    C. the last stage of personal development.
    D. responsibility.

55. The development of faith involves:

    A. moral changes.
    B. developing psychologically.
    C. cognitive growth.
    D. all of the above.

56. Being able to incorporate, alter, and accept indicates:

    A. a growing awareness of moral values.
    B. growing into maturity.
    C. inventory of personal values.
    D. reflection and self-criticism.

57. The viewpoint of self as seen by others involves:

    A. the development of personal identity as something apart from, yet a part of, the world.
    B. becoming what the world expects in terms of success and/or failure.
    C. living up to the expectations of society, including family and friends.
    D. securing the position in contemporary society that will guarantee the type of success to which one becomes accustomed.

58. When an individual is able to think in a concrete-operational manner:

    A. focus is less clear and goals much more difficult to construct.
    B. dealings with contemporary society become more strenuous.
    C. the imagination becomes the most important ingredient in life.
    D. the events of the world are more predictable, and imagination is secondary.

59. The focus of this article is:

    A. how to live without imagination.
    B. living in the modern world without goals.
    C. enjoying the "good life."
    D. man's ability and potential to grow and develop in trust.

PASSAGE 9 (QUESTIONS 60-65)

Komodo dragons will eat anything they can catch and overpower, including other Komodo dragons. Their favorite prey includes wild pigs, deer, and monkeys. Though Komodos can move quickly, they can do so only over short distances. So they hunt by ambush, waiting for prey to wander into range, then seizing it in their jaws. Younger Komodos are more mobile than adults, and they will actively hunt small mammals, nesting birds, and insects. Once prey is caught, the Komodo holds it in its claws and rips off chunks of flesh with its teeth. Komodos also eat carrion (dead flesh).

The habitat of the Komodo is the small Indonesian islands. The land upon which the Komodo dragon lives is hilly and sparsely covered with rain forest. The lowland areas consist mainly of open grassland and palm trees. Despite their small size, these islands support a wide range of subtropical plants and animals.

Komodo dragons, like most cold-blooded reptiles, sleep during the night. As the sun rises and warms their blood, they become active, awakening from their resting places among tree roots and rocks to set out in search of food. Despite their great size, Komodo dragons are quick moving and agile on the ground. They occasionally climb trees, gripping them with their large, powerful claws. They are also good swimmers, taking long, powerful strokes with their tails. When the usually solitary Komodos meet, they establish a clear hierarchy order based on size.

Komodo dragons mate in late June or July. During this period, males come into conflict with one another as they defend their territories. Five weeks after mating, the female digs a hole in the warm, moist earth and lays an average of a dozen eggs. The exact number and size of the eggs she lays will vary depending on the age and size of the female. She covers them and leaves them to incubate unattended, relying on the sun to keep them at the proper temperature.

The young dragons hatch eight months later. Barely eight inches long, they are in danger of being eaten by almost every predator on the islands, from snakes and birds of prey to larger Komodo dragons. The young that survive grow quickly, and after five years they will have reached six feet in length. Both males and females are mature enough to breed at around six years of age.

Here are a few facts about the Komodo:

SIZE
Length: males, 10 feet; females, slightly
    smaller
Weight: adults, 220–300 lbs.

BREEDING
Sexual maturity: six years
Breeding season: late June or July
No. of eggs: average of twelve
Incubation: eight months

LIFESTYLE
Habit: usually solitary, but come together to
    breed and feed on carrion
Diet: small mammals, wild pigs, deer, and
    monkeys
Life span: estimated at twenty years

RELATED SPECIES
The family of monitor lizards includes other
    giants, such as the 10-foot water
    monitor, as well as the tiny 8-inch
    Australian short-tailed monitor.

DISTRIBUTION
The Komodo dragon lives exclusively on the
    Indonesian islands of Komodo, Rintja,

Padar, Flores, Gili Mota, and Owadi Sami, north of Australia.

CONSERVATION

The population is stable at about 3,000. Because the Komodo dragon lives on uninhabited islands, it is currently in no danger from man.

DID YOU KNOW . . .

- the Komodo dragon was only discovered in 1912?
- an adult Komodo will eat an entire deer at one time—and then sleep for a week while digesting it?
- young Komodo dragons hatch fully formed from leathery, goose-sized eggs?
- unlike other large monitor lizards that have long, whiplike tails, the tail of the heavy-bodied Komodo dragon accounts for only half of its length?

60. The purpose of this article is to:

A. explain.
B. narrate.
C. describe.
D. inform.

61. The reader can infer from this article that Komodos have:

A. vegetarian instincts and live off of the jungle.
B. little or no contact with humans.
C. a monogamous relationship.
D. their young in litters.

62. According to this article, Komodos are quite agile despite their:

A. habitat's difficult terrain.
B. propensity to stay with their young.
C. large size.
D. enormous tails that are twice the size of their bodies.

63. The reader can infer that the Komodo gets its name from:

A. the scientist who discovered the species.
B. its place of origin.
C. a combination of the names of its ancestors.
D. its genetic makeup.

64. The author of this article infers that the Komodo dragons:

A. have overpopulated their area.
B. must be thinned out to avoid over population.
C. are in danger of extinction.
D. are in no danger of extinction.

65. The birth of Komodo dragons occurs:

A. after eight months of incubation.
B. from a large egg.
C. in warm, moist leaves.
D. all of the above.

PHYSICAL SCIENCES   TIME—100 MINUTES   77 QUESTIONS

Most questions in the Physical Sciences test are organized into groups, each preceded by a descriptive passage. After studying the passage, select the one best answer to each question in the group. Some questions are not based on a descriptive passage and are also independent of each other. You must also select the one best answer to these questions. If you are not certain of an answer, eliminate the alternatives that you know to be incorrect and then select an answer from the remaining alternatives. A periodic table is provided for your use. You may consult it whenever you wish.

1 H 1.0																	2 He 4.0
3 Li 6.9	4 Be 9.0											5 B 10.8	6 C 12.0	7 N 14.0	8 O 16.0	9 F 19.0	10 Ne 20.2
11 Na 23.0	12 Mg 24.3											13 Al 27.0	14 Si 28.1	15 P 31.0	16 S 32.1	17 Cl 35.5	18 Ar 39.9
19 K 39.1	20 Ca 40.1	21 Sc 45.0	22 Ti 47.9	23 V 50.9	24 Cr 52.0	25 Mn 54.9	26 Fe 55.8	27 Co 58.9	28 Ni 58.7	29 Cu 63.5	30 Zn 65.4	31 Ga 69.7	32 Ge 72.6	33 As 74.9	34 Se 79.0	35 Br 79.9	36 Kr 83.8
37 Rb 85.5	38 Sr 87.6	39 Y 88.9	40 Zr 91.2	41 Nb 92.9	42 Mo 95.9	43 Tc (98)	44 Ru 101.1	45 Rh 102.9	46 Pd 106.4	47 Ag 107.9	48 Cd 112.4	49 In 114.8	50 Sn 118.7	51 Sb 121.8	52 Te 127.6	53 I 126.9	54 Xe 131.3
55 Cs 132.9	56 Ba 137.3	57 La* 138.9	72 Hf 178.5	73 Ta 180.9	74 W 183.9	75 Re 186.2	76 Os 190.2	77 Ir 192.2	78 Pt 195.1	79 Au 197.0	80 Hg 200.6	81 Tl 204.4	82 Pb 207.2	83 Bi 209.0	84 Po (209)	85 At (210)	86 Rn (222)
87 Fr (223)	88 Ra 226.0	89 Ac† 227.0	104 Unq (261)	105 Unp (262)	106 Unh (263)	107 Uns (262)	108 Uno (265)	109 Une (267)									

*	58 Ce 140.1	59 Pr 140.9	60 Nd 144.2	61 Pm (145)	62 Sm 150.4	63 Eu 152.0	64 Gd 157.3	65 Tb 158.9	66 Dy 162.5	67 Ho 164.9	68 Er 167.3	69 Tm 168.9	70 Yb 173.0	71 Lu 175.0
†	90 Th 232.0	91 Pa (231)	92 U 238.0	93 Np (237)	94 Pu (244)	95 Am (243)	96 Cm (247)	97 Bk (247)	98 Cf (251)	99 Es (252)	100 Fm (257)	101 Md (258)	102 No (259)	103 Lr (260)

PASSAGE 1

In 1888, Henry Louis Le Châtelier formulated a principle governing chemical equilibrium. His principle states that if a system at equilibrium is subject to a change in conditions (concentration, temperature, or pressure), the system will change in a direction that will tend to restore a new set of equilibrium conditions. Examine the following equations that represent a chemical reaction (at equilibrium, in a closed container). The symbol $\Leftrightarrow$ in the equations listed below represents equilibrium (or a reversible reaction).

A. $4\,HCl_{(g)} + O_{2(g)} \Leftrightarrow 2\,Cl_{2\,(g)} + 2\,H_2O_{(g)}$
B. $CO_{(g)} + H_2O_{(g)} \Leftrightarrow CO_{2\,(g)} + H_{2\,(g)}$
C. $798.2\,kcal + 4\,Al_{(s)} + 3\,O_{2\,(g)} \Leftrightarrow 2\,Al_2O_{3\,(s)}$
D. $N_{2\,(g)} + 3\,H_{2\,(g)} \Leftrightarrow 2\,NH_{3\,(g)} + 92.2\,kJ$
E. $CO_{(g)} + 2\,H_{2(g)} \Leftrightarrow CH_3OH_{(g)} + 200.7\,J$
F. $N_2O_{4(g)} + 58.9\,kJ \Leftrightarrow 2\,NO_{2(g)}$

1. In equation A above, increasing the pressure on the system will have what effect on equilibrium?

   A. No effect.
   B. The equilibrium concentrations of both oxygen and chlorine will increase.
   C. The equilibrium concentrations of both chlorine and water will increase.
   D. The equilibrium concentrations of both hydrogen chloride and oxygen will increase.

2. In equation A above, adding more chlorine to the system will have what effect on equilibrium?

   A. The equilibrium concentration of water will decrease, and there will be no effect on either hydrogen chloride or oxygen concentration.
   B. The equilibrium concentrations of both hydrogen chloride and oxygen will increase.
   C. The equilibrium concentration of hydrogen chloride will increase and the equilibrium concentration of oxygen will decrease.
   D. No effect.

3. In equation B above, doubling the pressure will have what effect on the equilibrium concentration of carbon monoxide?

   A. No effect.
   B. It will double.
   C. It will be reduced by 50 percent.
   D. It will increase.

4. In equation B above, adding more carbon dioxide to the system will have what effect on equilibrium?

   A. The concentrations of the other three chemicals in the reaction will increase.
   B. The concentrations of both carbon monoxide and water will increase.
   C. The concentration of hydrogen will increase.
   D. The concentration of carbon monoxide will increase, but the concentration of water will decrease.

5. Increasing the temperature of reaction C above will have what effect on the equilibrium conditions?

A. Equilibrium will shift to favor the reactants.
B. The equilibrium concentration of oxygen will increase.
C. The equilibrium concentration of oxygen will decrease.
D. No effect.

6. If you are a chemical engineer, choose the correct combination of temperature and pressure that would *maximize* the production of ammonia ($NH_{3(g)}$) in reaction D above.

A. high temperature and high pressure
B. high temperature and low pressure
C. low temperature and low pressure
D. low temperature and high pressure

PASSAGE 2

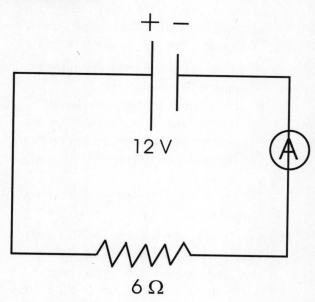

7. In the circuit above, a 6-ohm resistor is connected to a battery with no internal resistance whose terminal voltage is equal to 12 volts. If the resistance of the ammeter is zero, the current flowing through the ammeter will be:

A. 72 amps.
B. 2 amps.
C. 0.5 amps.
D. 6 amps.

8. Suppose you are told that the above battery has an electromotive force (*emf*) of 14 volts but the terminal voltage is still 12 volts. This would suggest that:

A. the current through the 6-ohm resistor would be greater.
B. the current through the ammeter would be greater.
C. the battery has an internal resistance.
D. there is something wrong: The *emf* cannot be greater than the terminal voltage.

9. Suppose you replace the 6-ohm resistor in the circuit with a 3-ohm resistor, keeping the same battery with an *emf* of 14 volts. You would observe that:

A. the current through the ammeter would be smaller.
B. the current through the 3-ohm resistor would be the same as the current through the 6-ohm resistor.
C. the terminal voltage of the battery is lower.
D. the terminal voltage of the battery is higher.

10. You now set up a circuit using a battery whose terminal voltage is 12 volts with zero internal resistance. You connect the 3-ohm and 6-ohm resistors to the battery in series with each other. The total resistance of the circuit will be:

A. 2 ohms.
B. 0.5 ohms.
C. 9 ohms.
D. 3 ohms.

11. The current through the 6-ohm resistor will be:

A. greater than the current through the 3-ohm resistor.
B. greater than the current through the battery.
C. equal to the current through the 3-ohm resistor.
D. less than the current coming out of the battery.

12. The voltage drop across the 6-ohm resistor will be:

A. less than the voltage drop across the 3-ohm resistor.
B. equal to the voltage drop across the 3-ohm resistor.
C. greater than the voltage drop across the 3-ohm resistor.
D. 12 volts.

PASSAGE 3

In many regards, learning chemistry is analogous to learning a foreign language, and the "language" of chemistry is known as nomenclature. The International Union of Pure and Applied Chemistry has begun to simplify a complex series of Greek and Latin prefixes and suffixes in the nomenclature of inorganic chemical names and has replaced many names such as ferrous and ferric and cuprous and cupric with a set of "easier" Roman numerals; however, a mastery of the nomenclature of polyatomic ions (radicals) is an imperative basic skill that leads to equation writing and balancing, and stoichiometric calculations. Answer the following nomenclature questions.

13. Name the following compound {$FeSO_4$}:

A. iron (I) sulfate
B. iron (I) sulfite
C. iron (II) sulfate
D. ferric sulfate

14. Which of the following formulas correctly represents the chemical calcium peroxide?

A. CaO
B. Ca_2O
C. CaO_2
D. Ca_2O_2

15. The chemical H_2SO_3 can be named hydrogen sulfite, and it has acidic properties. Name this compound as an acid.

A. hydrosulfurite acid
B. hydrosulfuric acid
C. sulfuric acid
D. sulfurous acid

16. Hydrates are compounds with water "trapped" within their chemical crystal structures, although not chemically bonded. The water can be "driven off" by heating, and the resulting chemical is then known as anhydrous. Name the following hydrate {$AuPO_4 \cdot 4H_2O$}.

    A. gold phosphate butahydrate
    B. aurous phosphate tetrahydrate
    C. gold (II) phosphate tetrahydrate
    D. gold (III) phosphate tetrahydrate

17. The chemical known as hydrophosphoric acid will have what formula?

    A. H_3P
    B. H_4P
    C. H_3PO_4
    D. HP

18. How many *total* oxygen atoms will be found in a molecule of aluminum nitrite?

    A. 2
    B. 6
    C. 9
    D. 12

19. At one time in the history of chemistry, the elements in the last row of the periodic table were known as the *inert gases*, because the elements were not known ever to combine with other elements to produce compounds. Gradually, under some unusual laboratory conditions, these elements were successfully combined with other elements (mainly halogens) to produce compounds. XeF_6 is one of these "noble" gas compounds. Name this compound.

    A. xenon fluorite
    B. xenon hexafluoride
    C. xenon hexafluorite
    D. xenon hexafluorate

20. The chemical HClO represents a weak acid with the following name:

    A. chlorous acid
    B. chloric acid
    C. hypochloric acid
    D. hypochlorous acid

Questions 21 through 25 are **NOT** based on a descriptive passage.

21. An old hockey puck of mass 0.16 kg is slapped so that its velocity is 50 m/sec. It slides 40 meters across the ice while coming to rest. How much work is done by friction on the puck?

    A. +4 Joule
    B. −60 Joule
    C. −200 Joule
    D. −340 Joule

22. A sample in a centrifuge moves in a circle of radius 15 cm. The centrifuge turns at 300 rpm. The sample experiences a horizontal acceleration of magnitude 12 g. The speed of the centrifuge is increased to 600 rpm. What is the new horizontal acceleration (magnitude and direction) of the sample?

    A. 25 g, away from center of circle.
    B. 25 g, toward the center of circle.
    C. 30 g, away from center of circle.
    D. 48 g, toward the center of circle.

23. The resistance of the filament of a light bulb is proportional to the absolute temperature of the filament. It is measured at 400 Kelvin to be R = 120Ω. It is measured at 500 Kelvin to be R = 150Ω. What is the temperature of the filament when the resistance is R = 900Ω?

   A. 270 Kelvin
   B. 600 Kelvin
   C. 625 Kelvin
   D. 3,000 Kelvin

24. For the system set up in the figure, what is the electrical force on the 1.5×10^{-5} Coulomb charge between the two charged plates?

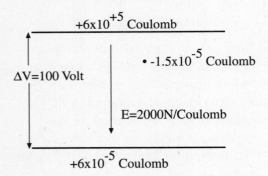

   A. 1.5×10^{-3} Newton, up
   B. 1.5×10^{-3} Newton, down
   C. 30×10^{-3} Newton, up
   D. 30×10^{-3} Newton, down

25. Consider an automobile head lamp that is powered by the battery of a car. The resistance of a light bulb filament increases as the temperature of the filament increases. When a bulb is turned on, the temperature starts at ordinary temperature and rises to a high temperature as the light bulb glows brightly. At what point in this process does the light bulb absorb the most power? (The voltage applied to the light bulb remains constant during the whole process.)

   A. At the instant the bulb is switched on.
   B. During the time when the filament is warming up to high temperature.
   C. When the bulb is at its highest temperature and glowing the most brightly.
   D. The power is not affected by the temperature of the filament.

PASSAGE 4

There are several methods of expressing the concentration of a solution, the most common of which are molarity (M) and molality (m). The molarity of a solution is the number of moles of solute in exactly one liter of total solution, and molality is described as the number of moles of solute in exactly 1 kilogram of solvent. Answer the following questions about solution concentrations. (The following values for molecular masses should be used.)

   Sodium chloride 58.5 g/mol
   Magnesium nitrate 148.0 g/mol
   Aluminum nitrate 213.0 g/mol
   Potassium carbonate 138.0 g/mol
   Lithium bromide 87.0 g/mol
   Iron II nitrate 180.0 g/mol

26. If 75.6 grams of NaCl are dissolved in enough water to make 2 liters of solution, calculate the final molarity:

A. 0.65 M
B. 1.6 M
C. 37.8 M
D. 29.3 M

27. How many grams of $Mg(NO_3)_2$ are needed to dissolve in enough water to make 250.0 ml of a 2.2 M solution?

A. 0.55 grams
B. 81.4 grams
C. 269.0 grams
D. 250.0 grams

28. If 75.0 grams of $Al(NO_3)_3$ are needed to dissolve in enough water to make a 0.75 M solution, calculate the solution's final volume:

A. 214.0 milliliters
B. 4.66 liters
C. 466.66 milliliters
D. 2.14 liters

29. 55.5 grams of K_2CO_3 are dissolved in enough water to make 500 milliliters of solution. If this solution is then diluted with an additional 1 liter of water, calculate the solution's final molarity:

A. 0.4 M
B. 0.8 M
C. 0.3 M
D. 3.0 M

30. How many grams of LiBr would be needed to dissolve in 250.0 milliliters of water to produce a 1.5 molal (m) solution?

A. 32.6 grams
B. 6.0 grams
C. 4.3 grams
D. 248.6 grams

31. $CCl_{4(l)}$ (carbon tetrachloride) has a specific gravity of 2.1. Assuming 15.0 grams of $Fe(NO_3)_2$ could dissolve in 0.75 liters of carbon tetrachloride, calculate the molality of the resulting solution:

A. It is impossible to calculate because the molecular mass of $CCl_{4(l)}$ is not specified.
B. 1.6 m
C. 0.08 m
D. 0.05 m

PASSAGE 5

A force of 20 Newtons is exerted on a 5 kg block for a distance of 10 m along a horizontal frictionless surface. The block travels for an additional 10 m without the force acting upon it. It then travels up a frictionless hill whose height is 4 m.

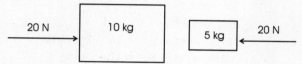

32. How much work is done by the force after the block has traveled its first 10 m?

A. 200 kg N
B. 200 N m
C. 50 kg m
D. zero

33. After the block has traveled its first 10 m, what is the change in its kinetic energy?

A. 0 J
B. 50 J
C. 100 J
D. 200 J

34. After the block has traveled its second 10 m, what is the change in velocity of the block?

   A. 0 m/s
   B. 4.47 m/s
   C. 6.32 m/s
   D. 8.94 m/s

35. As the block is traveling along its second 10 m, we can say that:

   A. the block is slowing down.
   B. the velocity of the block does not change.
   C. the block is doing work on the surface.
   D. its potential energy is changing.

36. After the block has gone to the top of the hill, we can say that:

   A. its potential energy is equal to its kinetic energy.
   B. its total energy is less than it was at the bottom of the hill.
   C. its total energy at the top is the same as it was on the bottom.
   D. it does not have enough energy to reach the top of the hill.

37. Suppose the block traveled over the top of the hill and back down the other side to the same level. We can say that the net work done by the block is:

   A. equal to the potential energy it had on the top of the hill.
   B. equal to the kinetic energy it had on the top of the hill.
   C. zero.
   D. It can't be determined. One needs to know the distance the block has traveled.

38. Suppose this block is now hauled from rest at the bottom of the hill up to the top of the hill by a machine in 10 s. What is the work done by the machine?

   A. 0 J
   B. 196 J
   C. 200 J
   D. 396 J

PASSAGE 6

The length of a column of mercury is 5 cm when immersed in ice water and 25 cm when immersed in boiling water. The column is immersed in a sugar solution and its length is 27 cm. The column is then immersed in a salt solution and its length is observed to be 4 cm.

39. What is the length of the mercury column at a temperature of 20°C?

   A. 5 cm
   B. 9 cm
   C. 21 cm
   D. 26 cm

40. What is the temperature of the sugar solution?

   A. 100°C
   B. 110°C
   C. 212°F
   D. 373K

41. What is the temperature of the salt solution?

   A. 23°F
   B. 5°C
   C. −10°C
   D. 270K

42. The temperature of the human body is 98.6°F. What is the temperature in C?

   A. 35°
   B. 36°
   C. 37°
   D. 38°

43. If the temperature of the atmosphere increases by 10°C, it also increases by:

   A. 10°F.
   B. 42°F.
   C. 10°K.
   D. 283K.

Questions 44 through 48 are **NOT** based on a descriptive passage.

44. The pressure and temperature of a gas are _____ related.

   A. directly
   B. inversely
   C. evenly
   D. none of the above

45. Which of the following has 18 neutrons?

   A. ^{35}Cl
   B. ^{40}Ar
   C. ^{85}Rb
   D. ^{19}F

46. The heat required to melt one gram of a solid at its melting point is known as its:

   A. heat of fusion.
   B. heat of solidification.
   C. heat of vaporization.
   D. heat of condensation.

47. Which of the following is true of isomers?

   A. They have the same structural and molecular formulas.
   B. They have the same molecular formulas, but different structural formulas.
   C. They have the same structural formulas, but different molecular formulas.
   D. They have the same structural and molecular formulas, but their masses vary.

48. Which of the following is false about the hydrogen bonds found in water?

   A. They create high surface tension.
   B. The result is a high vapor pressure.
   C. The specific heat of water is high.
   D. Water has a high boiling point.

PASSAGE 7

A train traveling at 20 m/s toward the east is traveling on the same track as another train traveling toward the west at 40 m/s. To avoid collision, the engineers on both trains blow their whistles to warn the other train. A passenger on the first train measures the frequency of his train's whistle as 1,200 Hz. A passenger on the second train measures the frequency of his whistle as 1,200 Hz. The speed of sound in air is 340 m/s.

49. The passenger on the first train would measure the frequency of the second train's whistle as:

   A. 1,200 Hz.
   B. 1,275 Hz.
   C. 1,341 Hz.
   D. 1,440 Hz.

50. The passenger on the second train would notice that the frequency of the first train's whistle was:

   A. lower than 1,200 Hz.

   B. equal to 1,200 Hz.

   C. higher than 1,200 Hz, but lower than the frequency of the second whistle heard by the passenger on the first train.

   D. higher than the frequency of the second whistle heard by the passenger on the first train.

51. A man standing by the side of the track in between both trains would notice that the:

   A. frequency of the first whistle is higher than the frequency of the second.

   B. frequency of both whistles is lower than 1,200 Hz.

   C. frequency of the second whistle is higher than the first.

   D. frequency of both whistles is the same.

52. The man standing by the side of the track would measure a beat frequency of:

   A. 0 Hz.

   B. 75 Hz.

   C. 85 Hz.

   D. 160 Hz.

53. The engineer of the first train hears the warning whistle and puts the engine in reverse so that it is now traveling toward the west at 20 m/s. The engineer of the second train is daydreaming and does not heed the warning. His train continues on its present path without any change. The passenger on the first train hears the frequency of the whistle of the second train as:

   A. lower than before, but higher than 1,200 Hz.

   B. lower than before and lower than 1,200 Hz.

   C. the same as the man standing by the side of the track.

   D. higher than before.

54. The man standing by the side of the track in between the two trains would now hear a beat frequency that is:

   A. zero.

   B. lower than before, but greater than the beat frequency now heard by the first passenger.

   C. lower than before, but not as great as the beat frequency now heard by the first passenger.

   D. higher than before.

PASSAGE 8

A balloon is filled with oxygen gas to a volume of 900 ml at sea level at standard pressure and 20 degrees Celsius temperature. The volume of the balloon is found to change under a variety of conditions.

55. Increasing the pressure to 800 torr will have what effect on the balloon's volume?

    A. The volume of the balloon will increase to 1 liter.

    B. The volume of the balloon will not change.

    C. The volume of the balloon will decrease to 855 ml.

    D. The volume of the balloon will decrease to 755 ml.

56. Doubling the temperature to 40 degrees Celsius, will have what effect on the balloon's volume?

    A. It will have no effect.

    B. The balloon will double in size.

    C. The balloon will increase in size slightly.

    D. The balloon will decrease in size slightly.

57. This balloon will rupture if its size expands to 1.5 liters. Assuming no change in temperature, the atmospheric pressure will have to change to what value to cause this rupture?

    A. The pressure would have to drop to 456 torr.

    B. The pressure would have to drop by 456 torr.

    C. The pressure would have to increase by 456 torr.

    D. The pressure would have to increase to 1.6 atmospheres.

58. How many grams of oxygen gas would be needed to fill the balloon to its 900 ml volume if the temperature was 15 degrees Celsius and the atmospheric pressure changed to 1.2 atmospheres?

    A. 0.046 grams

    B. 0.146 grams

    C. 1.46 grams

    D. 21.89 grams

59. Assume the same conditions as described in the previous question. However, the gas is changed to chlorine ($Cl_{2(g)}$). How many grams of chlorine will be needed?

    A. 0.046 grams

    B. 3.26 grams

    C. 1.63 grams

    D. 6.53 grams

60. The balloon is evacuated and 12.5 grams of nitrogen gas are pumped in. At what temperature will the balloon have a volume of 7.50 liters if the pressure changes to 900 torr?

    A. 239.5 degrees Celsius

    B. −33.5 degrees Celsius

    C. 33.5 degrees Celsius

    D. 4.18 degrees Celsius

PASSAGE 9

Beaker A contains 250.0 ml of a 0.01 M solution of acetic acid, and Beaker B contains 250.0 ml of a 0.005 M solution of HNO_2. The K_a value for acetic acid $= 1.8 \times 10^{-5}$ and the K_a for nitrous acid $= 4.5 \times 10^{-4}$.

61. Calculate the $[H^{+1}]$ concentration found in Beaker A:

    A. 0.001 M

    B. 0.005 M

    C. 0.00042 M

    D. 0.00084 M

62. Calculate the percent of ionization of acetic acid found in Beaker A:

A. 4.2%
B. 2.1%
C. 8.4%
D. unable to determine from information given.

63. Calculate the approximate pH of the acetic acid solution:

A. 4.2
B. 3.4
C. 0.6
D. 1.2

64. Calculate the approximate pOH of the acetic acid solution:

A. 9.8
B. 10.6
C. 13.4
D. 12.8

65. Calculate the $[H^+]$ concentration found in Beaker B:

A. 1.5×10^{-3}
B. 7.5×10^{-4}
C. 3.0×10^{-3}
D. 6.0×10^{-3}

PASSAGE 10

Radioactive isotopes in varying amounts are contained in a box. You have at your disposal instruments for measuring the type of particles emitted by the radioactive isotopes and the amount of isotopes remaining. You can also measure how fast a particular isotope decays and how the decay rate is affected by external factors such as temperature, pressure, and chemical reactions.

66. An atom of uranium 238 undergoes radioactive decay by emitting an alpha particle. After the uranium atom (atomic number 92) emits the alpha particle it is transmuted to an element with an atomic number of:

A. 90 and an atomic mass of 234.
B. 88 and an atomic mass of 236.
C. 93 and an atomic mass of 238.
D. 95 and an atomic mass of 242.

67. Carbon 14 (atomic number 6) used in radioactive dating undergoes beta decay. After it undergoes this radioactive decay we can say that:

A. the atomic number increases.
B. the atomic number decreases.
C. the atomic mass number increases.
D. the atomic mass number decreases.

68. Compared to an alpha particle, a beta particle has:

A. less mass and the same charge.
B. less mass and an opposite charge.
C. greater mass and the same charge.
D. greater mass and the opposite charge.

69. Starting with 1,000 g of an unknown element, you notice that 500 g has transmuted into a different element after 10 days. If you wait an additional 10 days, you would have:

A. none of the original element remaining.
B. 500 g of the original element remaining.
C. 250 g of the original element remaining.
D. There is insufficient information to determine how much would remain.

70. An isotope has a half-life of 6 hours. What fraction of the isotope would remain after one day (24 hours)?

    A. zero
    B. ½
    C. ⅛
    D. ¹⁄₁₆

71. You start with 64 g of a radioactive isotope. After 12 hours you notice that only 4 g of the isotope remain. What is the half-life of this isotope?

    A. 12 hours
    B. 6 hours
    C. 4 hours
    D. 3 hours

72. When gamma rays are emitted during radioactive decay this means that the atomic number of the isotope:

    A. remains the same and the atomic mass number increases.
    B. increases and the atomic mass number remains the same.
    C. remains the same and the atomic mass number remains the same.
    D. decreases and the atomic mass number decreases.

Questions 73 through 77 are **NOT** based on a descriptive passage.

73. When 75 mL of ethanol (ethyl alcohol) is diluted to a volume of 250 mL with water, what is the percent of ethanol by volume in the final solution?

    A. 30%
    B. 23%
    C. 75%
    D. >100%

74. All of the statements below are true of catalysts except:

    A. they are not used up in a reaction.
    B. they appear as neither reactant nor product.
    C. they raise the activation energy of the reaction.
    D. organic catalysts are called enzymes.

75. Except for the noble gases, the elements on the Periodic Table are:

    A. chemically fulfilled but electrically unfulfilled.
    B. chemically unfulfilled but electrically fulfilled.
    C. both chemically and electrically unfulfilled.
    D. both chemically and electrically fulfilled.

76. In the *E* configuration of geometric isomers, the substituted groups are found:

    A. on the same side of the double bond.
    B. on opposite sides of the double bond.
    C. at the ends of the molecule.
    D. in the middle of the molecule.

77. Which of the following is most likely not a role of proteins?

    A. building block of cells and cell parts
    B. hormone
    C. quick release of energy
    D. enzymes

| WRITING SAMPLE | 60 MINUTES | TWO TOPICS |

WRITING SAMPLE 1

A popular fear of Americans is that our nation will be "one large paved parking lot with border to border interstate highways connecting it."

Write a unified essay in which you perform the following tasks: explain what you think the statement means; describe specific situations in which there is evidence of a growing change in the countryside of this nation; discuss ways that the statement may not be necessarily true; provide evidence of what this means to today's society; conclude with a justification of the positive or negative implications.

WRITING SAMPLE 2

One of the great concerns of our government is violence on television and in movies, which is giving rise to violence in the streets.

Write a unified essay in which you perform the following tasks: explain what you think the statement means; describe specific situations in which there is evidence of a trend toward violence; dicusss ways that the statement may not be proven in regard to the effects of entertainment; provide evidence of what this means to today's society; conclude with a justification of the positive or negative implications.

BIOLOGICAL SCIENCE   TIME—100 MINUTES   77 QUESTIONS

Most questions in the Biological Sciences test are organized into groups, each preceded by a descriptive passage. After studying the passage, select the one best answer to each question in the group. Some questions are not based on a descriptive passage and are also independent of each other. You must also select the one best answer to these questions. If you are not certain of an answer, eliminate the alternatives that you know to be incorrect and then select an answer from the remaining alternatives.

PASSAGE 1 (QUESTIONS 1–8)

A variety of staining techniques are routinely used in the microbiology laboratory to identify bacteria. Some stains are simple stains while others are differential. Many of the basic dyes used bind to the bacterial cell due to its negatively charged surface. Other dyes may be repelled by the cell and can be used to produce a negative stain. The choice of technique depends on the type of information needed. The information is routinely used to help identify microorganisms, and it also helps determine appropriate therapeutic treatment.

1. The most widely used differential stain for bacteria is:

   A. the capsule stain.
   B. the Gram stain.
   C. the endospore stain.
   D. the flagella stain.

2. A negative stain:

   A. is used to develop photomicrographs of bacteria.
   B. can help determine whether a bacterium has a capsule.
   C. is conducted using methylene blue or some other basic dye.
   D. is used only on viruses during electron microscopy.

3. A differential stain is used to:

   A. distinguish between organisms based on cell wall composition.
   B. identify different components within a single cell.
   C. Both A and B are correct.
   D. Neither A nor B are correct.

4. An endospore stain is valuable because:

   A. it is the only way to visualize bacterial endospores.
   B. it is quick and cost-effective to run.
   C. it shows flagella in addition to endospores.
   D. it distinguishes between endospores and granules or vacuoles.

5. The reagents used in the Gram stain procedure include:

1. safranin
2. ethyl alcohol
3. gram's iodine
4. crystal violet

Which of the following indicates the correct order in which these reagents are used?

A. 1, 2, 3, 4
B. 4, 3, 2, 1
C. 4, 2, 3, 1
D. 1, 3, 2, 4

6. Which of the following would be a valid use of the results of the Gram stain procedure?

A. deciding what antibiotic to give a patient with acute meningitis while awaiting for culture results.
B. deciding whether the cause of meningitis is viral after Gram staining a specimen of cerebrospinal fluid.
C. deciding whether an organism is motile.
D. deciding whether combination therapy is required to prevent antibiotic resistance.

7. Interpretation of the Gram stain is based on:

A. cell wall composition and the color of the organism after staining.
B. the presence or absence of flagella after adding ethanol.
C. the ability of Gram's iodine to produce a golden color.
D. the fact that Gram-negative cells will appear colorless.

8. Staining procedures for eukaryotic cells differ from the Gram stain procedure because:

A. eukaryotes cannot be stained with basic dyes.
B. eukaryotic cells cannot be differentiated based on cell structure.
C. eukaryotes have no cell walls.
D. eukaryotes do not have cell walls with the same composition as those found in bacteria.

PASSAGE 2 (QUESTIONS 9–15)

Eukaryotic cells reproduce by mitosis or meiosis. Mitosis is the process used to produce additional somatic cells, since it creates genetic duplicates of the parent cell. Meiosis is used to make gametes that have a different genetic complement than that found in the parent cell. Mitosis and meiosis both involve division of the nucleus of the cell. Mitosis and meiosis can be divided into stages that are visually similar under the microscope, except that meiosis involves two distinct phases, meiosis I and meiosis II. While mitosis is essentially a cell-duplication process, meiosis involves an important reshuffling of genetic material that accounts for the inherited variation found in offspring.

9. A haploid cell with 12 chromosomes divides by _____ to produce daughter cells, each with _____ chromosomes.

A. mitosis, 24
B. mitosis, 12
C. meiosis, 12
D. meiosis, 24

10. A diploid cell with 12 chromosomes divides by _____ to produce gametes, each with _____ chromosomes.

    A. mitosis, 12
    B. mitosis, 6
    C. meiosis, 12
    D. meiosis, 6

11. Which of the following occur in meiosis but not in mitosis?

    I. Cytokinesis
    II. Anaphase I
    III. Crossing-over
    IV. Synapsis
    V. Formation of tetrads

    A. I, II, and III
    B. I, II, and IV
    C. None of these occurs in mitosis.
    D. II, III, IV, and V

12. Does cytokinesis always follow mitosis?

    A. Yes.
    B. Yes, in higher organisms such as angiosperms and chordates.
    C. No.
    D. None of the above choices are correct.

13. Crossing-over occurs during what stage of meiosis?

    A. prophase I
    B. prophase II
    C. metaphase I
    D. metaphase II

14. During what stage in meiosis do the homologous chromosomes separate?

    A. metaphase I
    B. metaphase II
    C. anaphase I
    D. anaphase II

15. Following meiosis, the division of a diploid parent cell ultimately produces _____ egg(s) in the female (oogenesis) and _____ sperm in the male (spermatogenesis).

    A. one, three
    B. one, four
    C. two, four
    D. four, four

PASSAGE 3 (QUESTIONS 16–21)

The local health department was notified of a husband, wife, and son who had become ill about 1 hour after eating dinner. All three had symptoms including nausea, vomiting, diarrhea, and fever. The three were treated and sent home. All three recovered within 48 hours of the onset of illness.

Table 1: Data on Food Eaten and Development of Food Poisoning

Food Eaten	Husband	Wife	Daughter	Son	Dog
Fish	x	x		x	x
Pasta	x	x	x	x	
Salad	x	x	x	x	
Wine	x	x		x	
Water	x	x	x	x	x
Ill	yes	yes	no	yes	yes

16. Which of the following was the likely cause of the illness?

    A. water
    B. pasta
    C. wine
    D. fish

17. If the dog had not become ill, what would be the likely conclusion?

    A. Dogs don't show the same signs and symptoms as people.
    B. The wine caused the illness.
    C. The fish caused the illness.
    D. The water caused the illness.

18. If the entire family and their dog had become ill, what would be the logical conclusion?

    A. The fish caused the illness.
    B. The pasta caused the illness.
    C. The salad caused the illness.
    D. The water caused the illness.

19. If the parents and children became ill but the dog did not, what would be the likely conclusion?

    A. The fish caused the illness.
    B. The pasta caused the illness.
    C. The wine caused the illness.
    D. The water caused the illness.

20. If the wife and son had consumed no wine, which of the following is the best conclusion?

    A. The wine caused the illness.
    B. The fish caused the illness.
    C. The pasta caused the illness.
    D. The water caused the illness.

21. If the dog became ill but the parents and children did not, what would be the best conclusion?

    A. The fish caused the illness.
    B. The pasta caused the illness.
    C. The combination of fish and water caused the illness.
    D. The food and water did not cause the illness.

Questions 22–26 are **NOT** based on a descriptive passage.

22. True associations of the tongue include all of the following EXCEPT:

    A. genioglossus, styloglossus, and hyoglossus muscles.
    B. thyroglossal duct cyst.
    C. cranial nerve XII (twelve) motor innervation.
    D. All of the above are true associations of the tongue.

23. Which salivary gland swells with a mumps infection?

    A. Parotid
    B. Submandibular
    C. Submaxillary
    D. Sublingual

24. True associations of the pancreas are all of the following EXCEPT:

    A. pancreatic duct, common bile duct, ampulla of Vater, sphincter of Oddi.
    B. endoplasmic reticulum, zymogen granules, enzymes, exocytosis.
    C. exocrine secretion of insulin and glucagon.
    D. secretin and CCK.

25. All of the following are true of carbohydrate digestion EXCEPT:

A. carbohydrates probably account for half of the calories eaten.

B. only monosaccharides and disaccharides can be absorbed.

C. brush border disaccharidases are maltase, lactase, and sucrase.

D. monosaccharides are glucose, galactose, and fructose.

26. All of the following are true of protein digestion EXCEPT:

A. gastric acid denatures the protein and activates the pepsinogen.

B. pepsin cleaves some of the peptide linkages leaving polypeptides.

C. exopeptidases, trypsin, and chymotrypsin cleave interior peptide bonds.

D. amino acids, dipeptides, and tripeptides are absorbed into mucosal cells.

PASSAGE 4 (QUESTIONS 27–32)

Genotype is the genetic makeup of the individual, while phenotype is what is expressed in appearance and in function. Some recessive traits are sex-linked, meaning that they are associated with the X chromosome. Consequently, the concept of dominant and recessive sex-linked traits holds true for females, who have two X chromosomes. However, since males have only one X chromosome and the sex-linked (or x-linked) trait is not carried on the Y chromosome, men who inherit a sex-linked trait express that trait phenotypically.

Sex-linked traits are sometimes very deleterious, and genetic counseling may be used to evaluate the probability of a couple having a child with a given trait.

27. Hannah, a woman with normal color vision, marries a man who is color blind. If Hannah is homozygous for normal color vision, what are the chances that this couple will have a son who is color blind?

A. 0%

B. 25%

C. 50%

D. 100%

28. Considering the example in the preceding question, what percentage or proportion of Hannah's daughters would be predicted to be color blind?

A. 0%

B. 25%

C. 50%

D. 75%

29. What is required for a female to exhibit a sex-linked trait phenotypically?

A. She must inherit the trait on both the X and Y chromosomes.

B. She must inherit the trait from both parents.

C. She will express the trait if either parent carried the defective gene.

D. Only males can express the trait.

30. John is color blind. He has two sisters, one who is color blind and one who has normal color vision. What is the genotype of John's mother?

A. She carries the gene for color blindness on one X chromosome.

B. She carries the gene for color blindness on both X chromosomes.

C. She carries no chromosomes for color blindness.

D. There is no way to determine her genotype.

31. Considering the situation presented in the previous question, what is the genotype of John's father?

    A. He carries the gene for color blindness on the X chromosome.
    B. He carries a gene for color blindness on both sex chromosomes.
    C. He carries no genes for color blindness.
    D. There is no way to determine his genotype.

32. If John marries a woman with normal color vision who is heterozygous for color blindness, what is the probability that one of their daughters will be color blind?

    A. 0%
    B. 25%
    C. 50%
    D. 100%

PASSAGE 5 (QUESTIONS 33–40)

The study of the human organism includes an examination of both anatomy and physiology. Different levels of organizational complexity exist within the human body and the comprehension of such concepts as complementarity of structure and function, hierarchical organization and homeostasis are critical to understanding the human as a whole. In addition to developing a knowledge of such concepts, it is necessary to learn the language or terminology of anatomy.

33. Which of the following best describes gross anatomy?

    A. It is the study of structures in one region of the body.
    B. It is the study of the structures of the body examined with the aid of microscope.
    C. It is the study of the large body structures visible with the naked eye.
    D. It is the study of individual systems of the body.

34. Which of the following is the best description of complementarity of structure and function?

    A. Anatomy and physiology are best studied together.
    B. Function always reflects structure; what a structure can do is dependent upon its form.
    C. Structure and function exist independently.
    D. Anatomy is the study of structure, and physiology is the study of function.

35. Which of the following is the appropriate order for increasing complexity of structure?

    A. subatomic particles, atoms, molecules, macromolecules, cells, tissues, organs, systems, organisms
    B. organisms, systems, organs, tissues, cells, macromolecules, molecules, atoms, subatomic particles
    C. epithelial, connective, muscular, nervous
    D. prokaryotic, eukaryotic, multicellular

36. Which of the following is not an example of a system?

    A. cardiovascular
    B. blood
    C. urinary
    D. reproductive

37. All living organisms share certain functional characteristics. Which of the following are characteristics of life?

    A. movement
    B. digestion
    C. reproduction
    D. All of the above are correct.

38. Homeostasis is a term coined by Walter Cannon to describe what condition of life?

    A. It is the ability of a living organism to maintain a dynamic equilibrium of internal conditions within a narrow range.
    B. It is the ability of a living organism to resist change.
    C. It is the ability of a living organism to control its external environment and internal environment.
    D. It is the ability of a living organism to communicate with its external environment.

39. Which of the following is an example of a positive feedback system?

    A. Increasing concentrations of glucose in the blood triggers the release of insulin driving the blood glucose levels down.
    B. Decreasing concentrations of glucose in the blood triggers the release of glucagon driving the blood glucose levels up.
    C. Pressure receptors in the birth canal respond to labor contractions causing the release of oxytocin, which increases the force of the contractions.
    D. Cerebrospinal fluid acidity increases, exciting the respiratory centers of the brain stem causing an increased respiration rate which decreases cerebrospinal fluid acidity.

40. A midsagittal section will divide the body into:

    A. equal superior and inferior portions.
    B. equal lateral portions.
    C. equal anterior and posterior portions.
    D. unequal lateral portions.

PASSAGE 6 (QUESTIONS 41–46)

Gas exchange is one the most fundamental and varied forms of interaction between animals and their environment. Carbon dioxide, a waste product of metabolism, must be released from the organism, and oxygen absorbed. While all forms of respiration depend ultimately on the diffusion of gases across a surface, the means of providing exposure of the exchange surface to fresh air or water can be as different as lungs are from gills. In fish, a counter current arrangement maximizes the contact between water with the greatest oxygen content and blood with the least. In the lungs of mammals, fresh air is moved into the lungs through the regular chest movements of inspiration.

41. Insects possess a(n) _____ system for gas exchange. The relative inefficiency of this arrangement puts an upper limit on their _____.

    A. endotracheal, rapidity of movement
    B. endotracheal, size
    C. tracheal, age
    D. tracheal, size

42. The counter current exchange system found in fish gills works by having the blood _____ the flow of water.

    A. move with
    B. move against
    C. near
    D. mix with

43. Gill-bearing aquatic and marine animals are at a respiratory disadvantage compared with terrestrial animals, because:

    A. water pressure compresses lungs and gills, reducing surface area.
    B. they must keep moving to obtain water rich in oxygen.
    C. the oxygen content of water is much lower than the oxygen content of the air.
    D. gills are ineffective at absorbing oxygen and much less efficient than lungs.

44. Breathing is regulated in mammals according to the:

    A. blood–carbon dioxide content.
    B. blood-oxygen content.
    C. oxygen requirements of the tissues and organs.
    D. amount of carbon dioxide in blood going through the heart.

45. Frogs use _____ pressure generated by muscles in the floor of the mouth to move air into their lungs; mammals rely on _____ pressure resulting from the movement of the rib muscles and diaphragm.

    A. positive, negative
    B. negative, positive
    C. partial, negative
    D. positive, partial

46. In swallowing food or drink, material is not aspirated (introduced) into the trachea because:

A. a flap of tissue, the glottis, closes the epiglottis opening into the trachea.

B. the esophagus is completely open to passage of food and liquid.

C. air pressure in the lungs opposes movement of material into the trachea.

D. the epiglottis seals the glottis.

Questions 47–51 are **NOT** based on a descriptive passage.

47. All of the following are true of fat digestion **except**:

A. various agents emulsify the fat so that fat can be near the brush border.

B. gastric lipase is present but less important than pancreatic lipase.

C. the micelle has a hydrophobic outside and a hydrophilic center.

D. cholesterol and triglycerides form chylomicrons to enter the lymphatics.

48. Qualities or properties of the sensory receptor include all of the following **except**:

A. generator potential above the threshold depolarizes.

B. specialized to receive only one stimulus type.

C. specialized depolarization produced for each type of stimulus.

D. they are transducers.

49. All of the following are true of the action potential of a neuron **except**:

A. sodium ions outside neuron greater than inside, resting potential −60mV.

B. ATP-driven sodium/potassium exchange pump actively maintains +40mV.

C. sodium rapidly enters cell achieving cell potential of +40mV.

D. all or none law observed.

50. All of the following associations are true of the neuronal synapse **except**:

A. the synaptic cleft, neurotransmitter chemicals, and diffusion.

B. neurotransmitter chemicals and postsynaptic depolarization only.

C. gate for one-way orderly conduction.

D. synapses are the same, neurotransmitters vary with type of nerve.

51. True associations of myelin are all of the following **except**:

A. nodes of Ranvier, saltatory conduction, and faster.

B. astrocytes, neurolemmal, and myelination.

C. oligodendrocyte, myelination, and central nervous system.

D. Schwann cell, oligodendrocyte, and myelination.

PASSAGE 7 (QUESTIONS 52–56)

The plasma membrane is a boundary that separates the living cell from its nonliving environment allowing the cell to selectively differentiate between exchanges with its environment. Early models deduced the nature of the plasma membrane by indirect evidence. Using this evidence, in 1935, J. F. Danielli and H. Davson proposed a model for the plasma membrane, several portions of which were supported by electron microscopy in the 1950s. In 1972, S. J. Singer and G. L. Nicholson proposed the model we currently accept.

52. Studies by Gorter and Grendel in 1925 supported the notion that the phospholipid content of the cell membrane was just enough to cover:

   A. one layer.
   B. two layers.
   C. three layers.
   D. None of the above is correct.

53. In addition to phospholipids, membranes isolated from red blood cells contained significant amounts of:

   A. nucleotides.
   B. protein.
   C. oligosaccharides.
   D. glycerol.

54. Early electron microscopy showed:

   A. the presence of proteins in the membranes.
   B. the phospholipid layer to contain large amounts of sugars.
   C. internal membranes similar to the plasma membrane.
   D. membrane molecules are soluble in water.

55. The fluid mosaic model was proposed by:

   A. Gorter and Grendel.
   B. Danielli and Davson.
   C. Singer and Nicholson.
   D. Overton.

56. Which of the following enter the cell the fastest?

   A. Cations
   B. Anions
   C. Lipid-soluble
   D. Lipid-insoluble

PASSAGE 8 (QUESTIONS 57–61)

Lipids are a varied group of biological molecules whose main identifying characteristic is their poor solubility in water. Among the simplest lipids are the fatty acids, which can be classified as saturated or unsaturated. Saturated fatty acids have only single bonds between carbon atoms, while unsaturated fatty acids have one or more double bonds. Both saturated and unsaturated fatty acids can be incorporated into more complex lipids. Examples of these are cephalins, triglycerides, and sphingolipids.

57. $CH_3(CH_2)_{14}COOH$ is an example of:

   A. an unsaturated fatty acid.
   B. a saturated fatty acid.
   C. a triglyceride.
   D. a lipoid.

58. Cholesterol is a:

   A. triglyceride.
   B. steroid.
   C. phospholipid.
   D. sphingolipid.

59. Compared to an unsaturated fatty acid, a saturated fatty acid has a melting point that is:

   A. higher than that of an unsaturated fatty acid.
   B. lower than that of an unsaturated fatty acid.
   C. sometimes higher and sometimes lower than that of an unsaturated fatty acid.
   D. None of the above is correct. Noncrystalline materials do not have characteristic melting points.

60. The addition of a sodium or potassium ion (using NaOH or KOH) to a fatty acid is called:

   A. esterification.
   B. hydrogenation.
   C. saponification.
   D. lipodosis.

61. Fatty acids interact with glycerol molecules to form:

   A. monoglycerides.
   B. phospholipids.
   C. triglycerides.
   D. All of the above are correct.

PASSAGE 9 (QUESTIONS 62–67)

The skeletal system provides a rigid framework that supports and anchors the soft tissues of the body. Its articulations provide a movable system of levers for locomotion, as well as producing the blood cells and serving as a reservoir for important ions. In addition, it provides protection for the more fragile, vital organs.

62. Two types of osseous tissue exist: spongy and compact. Which of the following best describes compact osseous tissue?

   A. Contains many cavities and red bone marrow.
   B. Appears very ordered, growing in organized cylinders called osteons.
   C. Appears somewhat random, contains trabeculae.
   D. None of the above is correct.

63. Bones are typically classified according to their shape. Which of the following is not a classification of bone?

   A. Long
   B. Short
   C. Square
   D. Irregular

64. Osteoid is the organic matrix of osseous tissue. Which of the following properties of bone is not due to the osteoid?

   A. Flexibility
   B. Rigidity
   C. Ability to withstand stretching and torsion
   D. Tensile strength

65. Which of the following are not bones of the cranium?

   A. Nasal and maxilla
   B. Parietal and temporal
   C. Sphenoid and ethmoid
   D. Occipital and frontal

66. The following is a list of major bones with their associated bone markings. Which bone is paired with inappropriate bone markings?

   A. Ulna—olecranon and coronoid processes, trochlear and radial notches, head and styloid process.

   B. Scapula—body, superior and inferior articular processes, spinous and transverse processes, pedicle, vertebral foramen, lamina.

   C. Femur—head and neck, greater and lesser trochanters, medial and lateral condyles, medial and lateral epicondyles, gluteal tuberosity, linea aspera.

   D. Humerus—head and neck, greater and lesser tubercles, capitulum and trochlea, medial and lateral epicondyles, deltoid tuberosity, radial and coronoid fossas, olecranon fossa.

67. The coccygeal bone of the pelvic girdle is actually composed of three fused bones. Which of the following is not a component of the coccygeal bone?

   A. Ischium
   B. Ilium
   C. Pubis
   D. Sacrum

PASSAGE 10 (QUESTIONS 68–72)

The rapid increases since 1850 in the number of people living has raised many scientific, political, and ethical questions and has provoked prolonged debate about the need for population control measures. As the table shows, while it took from the beginning of human history to 1850 for a population of one billion people to develop, it has taken less than an additional 150 years to increase that number to about five billion.

Date	Population (Millions)	Annual % Rate of Growth	Doubling Time (Years)
8000 BC	5	0.047	1,500
1650 AD	500	0.35	200
1850	1,000	0.875	80
1930	2,000	1.56	45
1960	3,000	1.9	37
1986	4,900	1.6	44

In the scientific discussion of population changes several terms are useful:

   I. *crude birth rate* (cbr) = number of live births per 1,000 individuals.

   II. *crude death rate* (cdr) = number of deaths per 1,000 individuals.

   III. *percent annual population growth* = (cbr-cdr) × 0.1. Here is an example of how to calculate the annual percent population growth: In 1986 the world population was 4.9 billion. The cbr was 27 live births per 1,000 individuals and the cdr was 11 deaths per 1,000 individuals. Therefore, (27 − 11) × 0.1 = 1.6%. With an expected increase in population of 1.6% × 4.94 billion people = 80 million people or 0.08 billion people.

   IV. *doubling time* = the number of years it will take a population to double in size. Doubling time is calculated as: doubling time in years = 70 divided by percent annual growth rate. In 1986, the doubling time was $\frac{70}{1.6}$, or 44 years.

68. In the example given above, in which the cbr was 27 and the cdr was 11, the percent annual population growth was calculated as 1.6%. If the cdr remains constant, how many more births would be needed per 1,000 individuals to raise the percent annual population growth rate from 1.6% to 1.9%?

A. 1
B. 2
C. 3
D. 4

69. If in the year 2020, the Earth's human population is 6 billion, with a percent annual population growth of 2.0%, how many years will it take for the population to double?

A. 20 years
B. 25 years
C. 30 years
D. 35 years

70. If the Earth's human population is 6 billion in the year 2020, and the doubling time is 30 years, at that rate of increase how many years will it take for the population to increase to 24 billion people?

A. 30 years
B. 45 years
C. 60 years
D. 120 years

71. What will the relationship be between cbr and cdr if there is to be zero population growth (ZPG)?

A. cbr = cdr
B. cbr is only slightly more than cdr
C. cdr > cbr
D. It cannot be determined from the above information.

72. If population growth for a particular region or country is considered, other factors must be introduced into calculations in order to accurately project population changes. Which of the following should also be taken into account?

I. epidemics and other events that greatly increase the number of deaths
II. birth control practices
III. emigration
IV. immigration

A. I and II
B. I, II, III, and IV
C. III and IV
D. I and III

Questions 73–77 are **NOT** based on a descriptive passage.

73. True statements about the brain are all of the following EXCEPT:

A. The pons functions to link the cerebellum with the higher conscious centers.
B. The limbic system alerts the cortex of incoming stimuli.
C. The limbic system is associated with emotional responses.
D. The nuclei of cranial nerves 5, 6, 7, and 8 are located in the pons.

74. The false statement about the central nervous system is which of the following?

A. The frontal lobe contains the primary motor cortex.
B. The frontal lobe contains the frontal association areas for analyzing and sorting.
C. The temporal lobe functions mainly in hearing.
D. All of the above are true.

246

75. The following associations of the peripheral nervous system are true EXCEPT:

A. the autonomic system is parasympathetic (PS) and sympathetic (S).
B. presynaptic fibers of both PS and S all secrete acetylcholine.
C. the sympathetic system is composed of cranial nerves and the sacral nerves.
D. The sympathetic presynaptic fibers are short.

76. All of the following are true of the peripheral nervous system EXCEPT:

A. spinal nerve, union of the dorsal and ventral nerve root, very short.
B. CN 7, supplies the muscles of mastication.
C. CN 6, lateral rectus extrinsic eye movement muscle.
D. CN 5, skin sensation around the nose and mouth.

77. True associations of the retina of the eye are all of the following EXCEPT:

A. pigmented layer of the choroid coat contains the visual receptors.
B. rods are the most numerous and depend upon vitamin A.
C. cones respond to more detail and to colors but respond poorly in dim light.
D. bipolar layer and ganglion layer are anterior to the rods and cone layer.

QUICK-SCORE ANSWERS

ANSWERS FOR PRACTICE TEST 1

Verbal Reasoning

1. B	23. D	45. B
2. C	24. A	46. D
3. C	25. D	47. C
4. D	26. D	48. C
5. D	27. A	49. B
6. D	28. D	50. D
7. D	29. A	51. D
8. C	30. D	52. C
9. D	31. B	53. D
10. B	32. C	54. B
11. B	33. C	55. D
12. D	34. A	56. D
13. D	35. A	57. A
14. D	36. D	58. D
15. A	37. C	59. D
16. C	38. D	60. D
17. C	39. B	61. B
18. C	40. B	62. C
19. D	41. C	63. B
20. D	42. D	64. D
21. C	43. B	65. D
22. B	44. D	

Physical Sciences

1. C	27. B	53. A
2. B	28. C	54. D
3. A	29. C	55. C
4. B	30. A	56. C
5. C	31. D	57. A
6. D	32. B	58. C
7. B	33. D	59. B
8. C	34. A	60. C
9. C	35. B	61. C
10. C	36. C	62. A
11. C	37. C	63. B
12. C	38. B	64. B
13. C	39. B	65. A
14. C	40. B	66. A
15. D	41. A	67. A
16. D	42. C	68. B
17. A	43. C	69. C
18. B	44. A	70. D
19. B	45. A	71. D
20. D	46. A	72. C
21. C	47. B	73. A
22. D	48. B	74. C
23. D	49. D	75. B
24. C	50. C	76. B
25. A	51. C	77. C
26. A	52. C	

Biological Sciences

1. B	27. A	53. B
2. B	28. A	54. C
3. C	29. B	55. C
4. D	30. A	56. C
5. B	31. A	57. B
6. A	32. C	58. B
7. A	33. C	59. A
8. D	34. B	60. C
9. B	35. A	61. D
10. D	36. B	62. B
11. D	37. D	63. C
12. C	38. A	64. B
13. A	39. C	65. A
14. C	40. B	66. B
15. B	41. D	67. D
16. D	42. B	68. C
17. B	43. C	69. D
18. D	44. A	70. C
19. B	45. A	71. A
20. B	46. D	72. C
21. D	47. C	73. B
22. D	48. C	74. D
23. A	49. B	75. C
24. C	50. B	76. B
25. B	51. B	77. A
26. C	52. B	

EXPLANATORY ANSWERS FOR PRACTICE TEST 1

VERBAL REASONING

PASSAGE 1

1. The correct answer is (B). The author attempts to point out the symptoms that demand a visit to the doctor and alludes to those that can be personally treated. Answer (A) is incorrect. While selecting quality health care is very important, there is no effort on the part of the author to deal with this subject. Answer (C) is incorrect. The author alludes to the importance of holding down the cost of health care, but focuses on care for the proper reasons. Answer (D) is incorrect; there is no mention of maintaining consistency in quality of life.

2. The correct answer is (C). The author makes the statement that "If they did, our entire system of medical care would be swamped overnight and the doctors would be unable to take care of the more serious problems." Answer (A) is incorrect; while this may be true, this is not indicated in this article. Answers (B) and (D) are incorrect. Although both are probably true, there is no evidence in this article to support either statement.

3. The correct answer is (C). The author points out that both money and time are saved by proper self-treatment. Answer (A) is incorrect. The false claims of medicines are mentioned but not considered popular. Answer (B) is incorrect. Quackery is not mentioned in this article. Answer (D) is incorrect; while this is popular and advisable, this is not the popular treatment described.

4. The correct answer is (D). The author makes this statement in the last sentence of paragraph one. Answer (A) is incorrect; while this may be a true statement, there is no mention of maintaining a healthy life with the assistance of a caring physician. Answer (B) is incorrect; the author actually alludes to the danger of using a variety of self-treatments. Answer (C) is incorrect; the author mentions the availability of health-care magazines.

5. The correct answer is (D). The author makes the statement in paragraph one—that one must exercise care in selecting and in use. Answer (A) is incorrect; there is no mention of addiction in the article even though this may be a true statement. Answer (B) is incorrect; while this is a valid statement it is not a part of this selection. Answer (C) is incorrect. The author indicates that quite often a physician should be consulted before using these medications.

6. The correct answer is (D). The last section of the article lists specifically the indicators presented in choices (A), (B), and (C).

7. The correct answer is (D). Throughout the article, the author implies the importance of taking the initiative and making personal decisions. Answer (A) is incorrect. While this may be a true statement, this is not supported in the article. Answer (B) is incorrect. This is possible; however, it is not supported in the article. Answer (C) is incorrect. There is self-medication available, but the competence in health care is not supported in the article.

Passage 2

8. The correct answer is (C). Paragraph two makes the statement that in order to understand drug use, one must attempt to understand the psychological needs of those who seek comfort in drugs. Answer (A) is incorrect. While seeking out those who sell drugs to young people is an admirable step in controlling drugs, the article does not mention this. Answer (B) is incorrect; making stronger laws to punish those who use drugs may be appropriate, but it is not the focus of this article. Answer (D) is incorrect. While there are those who applaud legalizing certain drugs in an effort to control their use, this is not mentioned in the article.

9. The correct answer is (D). There is evidence in paragraphs two and three to support that answers (A), (B), and (C) are correct. Therefore the correct choice is answer (D).

10. The correct answer is (B). Paragraph two makes the statement that "One of these by-products of social upheaval is the pervasive and widespread use of drugs for non-medicinal purposes, coinciding with an overuse of many drugs that have a very important role in medicine." Answer (A) is incorrect; while the use of "uppers" is important, this is not mentioned in the article. Answers (C) and (D) are incorrect for the same reason.

11. The correct answer is (B). Paragraph two makes the statement that drug use is a symptom of psychological need. Answer (A) is incorrect. While this may be one cause of drug use, this is not mentioned in the article. Answer (C) is incorrect; while this is often a by-product of drug use, this is not mentioned here. Answer (D) is incorrect; there is nothing in the article to support making a psychological breakthrough.

12. The correct answer is (D). The author of this selection makes this statement in paragraph three. Answer (A) is incorrect. Although this may be the feeling of some, there is no evidence in this article to support the statement. Answers (B) and (C) are incorrect. There are indications by the author that this may be the ultimate cause of drug use, but not an objection.

13. The correct answer is (D). The last paragraph of the selection contains this statement: ". . . feelings formed beforehand or without knowledge." Answer (A) is incorrect. Accepting the opinions of others is an indicator of open-mindedness. Answer (B) is incorrect. While stubbornness may be a part of close-mindedness, this is not evinced in this selection. Answer (C) is incorrect. Attempting to understand is evidence of open-mindedness.

14. The correct answer is (D). There is evidence in the next-to-last paragraph of all these factors mentioned in answers (A), (B), and (C).

15. The correct answer is (A). There is evidence in the next-to-last paragraph of the gullibility of a child. Answer (B) is incorrect. There may be truth in this statement, but this article does not support it. Answer (C) is incorrect. Most children do not internalize immediately, and there is no evidence to support this in the article. Answer (D) is incorrect. There is no evidence that children change to meet this new definition.

16. The correct answer is (C). In paragraph three of the selection, the author opines, ". . . risking their own health, their present and future mental functioning." Answers (A), (B), and (D) are incorrect; although these may be among the by-products, these are not reported in this article.

17. The correct answer is (C). A drug user does *not* apply the rules of logic. Answer (A) is incorrect. Prejudice is *not* a quality of the open-minded. Answer (B) is incorrect. Making new judgments is *not* a quality of the close-minded. Answer (D) is incorrect. Drug users, according to this article, do not apply rules of logic and judge new information.

PASSAGE 3

18. The correct answer is (C). One of the elements important to proper body functioning is water, which is described in this article as are other needs of the body. Answer (A) is incorrect because it mentions only water and its use by the body. Answer (B) is incorrect; there is no mention of this in the selection. Answer (D) is incorrect. The author specifically states that there is no way to determine the specific amount of water needed.

19. The correct answer is (D). Paragraph one states that digestion, absorption, and secretion are major functions of water in the body. Answers (A) and (C) are incorrect: respiration is not one of water's functions. Answer (B) is incorrect; energizing is not one of the functions of water.

20. The correct answer is (D). Answers (A), (B), and (C) are all implied through the course of the article selection.

21. The correct answer is (C). Decreasing the intake of water will weaken the body significantly. Answer (A) is incorrect; other liquids have a water base, which provides some of the water needed by the body. Answer (B) is incorrect; inactivity to preclude perspiration would not weaken the body as much as decreasing the intake of water. Answer (D) is incorrect. The intake of carbohydrates, which might be water-based, would not be as damaging.

22. The correct answer is (B). Working outside in the sun significantly increases the loss of water. Answer (A) is incorrect. An office worker engages in sedentary activities, which in an air-conditioned office, would not increase the loss of water. Answer (C) is incorrect. A computer scientist working in a warehouse would be sedentary, and water loss would not increase. Answer (D) is incorrect. While strenuous activity does increase water loss, this does not cause the *most* water loss of all the choices.

23. The correct answer is (D). The last paragraph of the selection lists these vital nutrients. Answer (A) is incorrect. Glucose is not mentioned. Answer (B) is incorrect; glucose is not mentioned, and vitamins and fat are allusions. Answer (C) is incorrect. Lymph is not an intake.

24. The correct answer is (A). The water content in plasma, part of the blood, is 90 to 92 percent. Answer (B) is incorrect. Muscle is 72 to 78 percent water. Answer (C) is incorrect. There is no indicator of the water content in tissue. Answer (D) is incorrect. Bone is 45 percent water.

25. The correct answer is (D). Answers (A) and (B) are correct; the author states that ". . . water loss can be replenished by liquids and foods of all kinds." Answer (C) is correct; the selection contains this information: "Some water is produced within the body through the metabolic breakdown of stored nutrients." Therefore, answer (D) is the correct choice.

26. The correct answer is (D). Answer (A) is correct. According to the author of this article, chemicals in trace amounts are vital for the body to function. Answers (B) and (C) are correct: vitamins are included with the minerals of the body.

27. The correct answer is (A). The excess of water intake beyond that needed to satisfy the thirst assures the high-level functioning of the kidneys. Answer (B) is incorrect. Determining the proper amount of water necessary per day is impossible because of the differences in human beings. Answer (C) is incorrect. While this is necessary for good health, it is not the assurance of proper kidney function. Answer (D) is incorrect; while this is a valid practice, it is not a necessity for high-level kidney functioning.

PASSAGE 4

28. The correct answer is (D). The author explains in the first paragraph and again in the last paragraph the importance of seeing beyond the obvious. Answer (A) is incorrect. There is an allusion to why Braque paints, but this is not the focus. Answer (B) is incorrect. The illustration of Georges Braque is used as an example. Answer (C) is incorrect. The painting *The Round Table* is only an example.

29. The correct answer is (A). The author of the selection indicates that the painting *The Round Table* has articles that are not pictured realistically. Answers (B) and (C) are incorrect. There is no evidence to support the shape of the painting or the type of paint and canvas used for the work of art. Answer (D) is incorrect. There is no indicator of the time period in which the work was completed.

30. The correct answer is (D). The first paragraph describes the appeal to the beautiful and pleasant. Answers (A) and (C) are incorrect. There is no mention of what is sensible. Answer (B) is incorrect. There is no support for art that is truthful.

31. The correct answer is (B). Paragraph one states that "Objects created to be beautiful or intrinsically pleasing are nevertheless useful because they help to satisfy the aesthetic interests and requirements of modern people." Answers (A) and (C) are incorrect. There is no mention of placing art in locations. Answer (D) is incorrect; there is no mention of gender appeal.

32. The correct answer is (C). At the end of paragraph one, the author states: "We still possess remarkable visual equipment and outstanding capacity for interpreting our optical experience." Answer (A) is incorrect. There is no evidence of the need or capacity for understanding one's fellow man. Answers (B) and (D) are both incorrect. While each may be a true statement, there is no evidence to support either of them.

33. The correct answer is (C). Paragraph one states that the history of art reveals that "some forms of visual art appear to have evolved in complex cultures as a means of engaging our unused perceptual capacity." Answer (A) is incorrect. There is no evidence to support the fact that ancient man used art to communicate meaning. Answer (B) is incorrect. While this is probably a true statement, there is no support in this selection for this theory. Answer (D) is incorrect. There is no evidence of this in the article.

PASSAGE 5

34. The correct answer is answer (A). The author clearly points out some of the stories about Pocahontas and her life, including several stories about her that cannot be proven. Answers (B) and (D) are incorrect; trickery of the settlers by the Indians is only mentioned briefly, and there are no references to the Indians being tricked by the settlers. Answer (C) is incorrect; while there are efforts to narrate some parts of the life of Pocahontas, there is no effort to talk about the times.

35. The correct answer is (A). The author states that the second version of Smith's diaries indicate that she saved Smith's life. Answers (B), (C), and (D) are incorrect. While these may well be true, there is no indicator of them in the selection.

36. The correct answer is (D). The author indicates that the Indians may have had two reasons for staging the event: either to "adopt" Smith and establish inroads with the settlers, or to establish better relations with the settlers. Answer (A) is incorrect. While the author tells us that Pocahontas was very young, we are *not* told that she was unaware of what was happening. Answer (B) is incorrect. There is an allusion to the fact that the event is not accurately reported; however, there is not an indication that Smith *staged* the event, meaning that it actually happened in a planned manner. Answer (C) is incorrect. While this may have been a usual undertaking, we are not given such information.

37. The correct answer is (C). Pocahontas died in England while still very young. The author indicates that she was twelve in 1607 and died in 1617, making her only twenty-two at the time of her death. Answers (A), (B), and (D) are all parts of her life as narrated by the author.

38. The correct answer is (D). Paragraph one gives the information that she was the "favorite" daughter and occasionally "advised" the chief. Answer (A) is incorrect; the trip to England was with her husband, and the meeting with Smith seems accidental. Answer (B) is incorrect; there is no evidence that she tried to protect the Indians, but rather befriended the settlers. Answer (C) is incorrect; there is no indication that she was made a princess by the Queen of England.

39. The correct answer is (B). According to this article, the marriage of Pocahontas and Rolfe brought about the peace. Answer (A) is incorrect; there is no indication of the effect of the publication of Smith's memoirs. Answer (C) is incorrect. The benevolent efforts of Pocahontas were made with no thought of return. Answer (D) is incorrect; the kidnapping of Pocahontas did not establish peace but led to her meeting with Rolfe, whom she would marry.

PASSAGE 6

40. The correct answer is (B). The opening paragraph and the closing paragraph outline that there is no *one* cause of the Revolution. Answer (A) is incorrect; while there is the underlying idea of separation, this is not the focus. This is obvious since we do not see this word used. Answer (C) is incorrect; there are a number of causes for the colonists to be unhappy and want to break away, but no evidence that they do break away. Answer (D) is incorrect. There is little mention of the class system.

41. The correct answer is (C). The inference of the conclusion of the article leaves the reader with the idea that the war was inevitable because of all of the causes. Answer (A) is incorrect because it contradicts the evidence in the conclusion. Answer (B) is incorrect. There is no evidence in the article to support amicable relations between the French and the English. Answer (D) is incorrect. There is no evidence for the colonists to remain under the protection of the crown.

42. The correct answer is (D). There are a number of causes with a base in the exchange of goods and money among colonists, the crown, the French, the farmers, and the merchants. Answer (A) is incorrect. There is only one cause that relates to religion and the presentation of a state religion. Answer (B) is incorrect. The class structure of the aristocracy against the newly rich is a minor part of the causes of the Revolution. Answer (C) is incorrect. The French immigration is almost a nonfactor.

43. The correct answer is (B). The sentence "For instance, consider how Ben Franklin was treated when back in England versus when he was in the colonies" is inserted into the article to illustrate the point that social acceptance was a factor in the Revolution. Answers (A) and (D) are incorrect. Both an anecdote and a parable are short stories that make a point. There is only a sentence here, not a story. Answer (C) is incorrect. In order to qualify as a fact in point, an illustration must give evidence to support its point. This requires more than one sentence.

44. The correct answer is (D). The mention of the "state religion" indicates that this is the correct answer. Answer (A) is only partially correct. There is some evidence that the colonies, or "America," were only a pawn in the struggles, but this is not the inference of this article. Answer (B) is incorrect. England was *not* looking for a reason to fight a war, but was not against fighting it either. Answer (C) is incorrect. France needed *no* reason to expand in the colonies.

45. The correct answer is (B). The statement, ". . . trade and manufacturing, or mercantilism, ensued" supports this statement. Answer (A) is only partially correct and therefore is not the proper choice. Answer (C) is incorrect. Manufacturing is correct; however, in this article export is not associated with mercantilism. Answer (D) is incorrect; the exchange of diplomacy for goods is not mentioned in this article.

46. The correct answer is (D). There is the statement in the article that "An alliance with the Indians was seen as the basis for colonials gaining strength." The strength of the colonists was one of the causes of the war; therefore, the Indians played a minor role. Answer (A) is incorrect. The Indians were not "the reason for the American Revolution." The author makes the point that there was no *single* reason. Answer (B) is incorrect. There is no evidence in this selection that the Indians benefited from the American Revolution. Answer (C) is incorrect. The alliance between the Indians and colonists was one of the minor causes according to this article.

PASSAGE 7

47. The correct answer is (C). The author of this article seeks to define, explain, and illustrate the behavior of polar molecules. Answer (A) is incorrect; surface tension is described, but that is not the purpose of the article. Answer (B) is incorrect; magnetism is not explained at all within this article. Answer (D) is incorrect. There is no evidence of an attempt to explain the interaction of tension.

48. The correct answer is (C). Paragraph one states that when ". . . the negative electrons within the atoms of the molecule shift toward those atoms that are most capable of attracting them. This shift produces an electrical force called a molecular dipole. Answer (A) is incorrect. The production is an electrical force, not an electrical attraction. Answer (B) is incorrect. Paragraph one states that ". . . the atoms of the molecule shift," implying that molecules do not become atoms. Answer (D) is incorrect. Negative, not positive, electrons shift.

49. The correct answer is (B). Paragraph one states: "Polar molecules are molecules that have a concentration of negative charge on one end of the molecule and a concentration of positive charge on the other end." Answer (A) is incorrect; the term "separating" is not used in this article. Answer (C) is incorrect. The electrical charge is created when the molecules shift, not mix. Answer (D) is incorrect; the statement in paragraph one describes a "shift," not a union.

50. The correct answer is (D). The author writes: "Nonpolar molecules are molecules that do *not* have this concentration of positive or negative charge." Answers (A), (B), and (C) are incorrect. A nonpolar molecule has *no* electrical force of any kind.

51. The correct answer is answer (D). The author states: "Either the surface can buckle upward, in which case we have a 'convex' surface; or the surface can buckle downward, in which case we have a 'concave' surface. These buckled surfaces are referred to as a 'meniscus.' " Answers (A), (B), and (C) are stated in this paragraph.

52. The correct answer is (C). The author states in this selection that rubbing ". . . with animal fur impart(s) a negative charge." Answer (A) is incorrect. The article states that surface tension is the movement of the surface in either a concave or convex manner. Answer (B) is incorrect. A negative charge is created. Answer (D) is incorrect. The balanced shift is the manner of concentration of molecules.

Passage 8

53. The correct answer is (D). Paragraph one indicates this. Answer (A) is incorrect. There is evidence in this article of the need for personal choices, but moral values are not a major issue. Answer (B) is incorrect. This selection mentions neither education nor experience. Answer (C) is incorrect. While these are intrinsic parts of a personal value system, this article does not deal with them.

54. The correct answer is (B). This statement is found in the next-to-the-last paragraph. Answer (A) is incorrect. There is no mention of maturity in this article. Answers (C) and (D) are incorrect. There is no support for these statements in this article.

55. The correct answer is (D). In the first paragraph, the author states: "Fowler's Faith Development Theory suggests that the development of faith, or how we learn to know and value that we do, moves through successively progressive stages akin to those of cognitive [Answer (C)], moral [Answer (A)], and psychological growth [Answer (B)]."

56. The correct answer is (D). Paragraph five indicatess that the ability to alter and accept or discard is evidence of reflection upon the past and self-criticism of the actions. Answer (A) is incorrect. The growing awareness of moral values, while an important part of the development of faith, is not mentioned by this author as a part of altering, accepting, and discarding. Answer (B) is incorrect. Growing into maturity, according to this author, is a result of the reflection and self-criticism. Answer (C) is incorrect. The author makes no mention of inventorying personal values.

57. The correct answer is (A). In paragraph four, the author states: "The integration of these viewpoints with self-reflections represents the foundation of personal identity as something apart from, yet a part of, the world." Answer (B) is incorrect. There is no indication of a requirement of satisfying worldly expectations as a part of faith development. Answer (C) is incorrect. While living up to the expectations of society, including family and friends, is admirable, this is not an ingredient of faith development, according to the author. Answer (D) is incorrect. Securing the position in contemporary society that will guarantee the type of success to which one becomes accustomed is desirable; however, according to the author, this is not one of the primary ingredients for faith development.

58. The correct answer is (D). In paragraph three, the author states that concrete-operational thinking demands less imagination while looking at the world in a realistic manner. Answer (A) is incorrect. Focus would be *more* clear with concrete thinking because the focus would be real. Answer (B) is incorrect. While using *less* imagination and being realistic would be, at times, difficult, this should not affect dealings with contemporary society, according to the writer. Answer (C) is incorrect. Concrete-operational thinking uses less imagination, not more.

59. The correct answer is (D). The focus of the article is on Fowler's theory of faith development. This involves man's ability and potential to grow and develop in trust, according to this selection. Answer (A) is incorrect. Fowler stresses living *with* imagination as a means of developing faith. Answer (B) is incorrect. Goal-setting and striving to meet those goals are also part of Fowler's formula. Answer (C) is incorrect. While the article alludes to enjoying life, there is no attempt to define the "good life."

PASSAGE 9

60. The correct answer is (D). The reader of this article is *informed* of the habits and definition of Komodos. There is no effort to explain the actions of the Komodo, which renders answer (A) incorrect. Answer (B) is incorrect; narration requires the telling of a story with a beginning, middle, and end. There is no effort at narration. Answer (C) is incorrect. While a portion of the article does describe the dragon and its work, there are few details, which makes the description incomplete.

61. The correct answer is (B). The author writes that Komodos live in uninhabited places. "Uninhabited" means a lack of inhabitants; therefore, there is little contact with humans. Answer (A) is incorrect. The author states that the Komodos are carnivorous, preferring to kill and eat living things. Answer (C) is incorrect. There is no mention in the article of a monogamous relationship, nor is there a reference to a nonmonogamous relationship. Answer (D) is incorrect; the article informs the reader that Komodos lay eggs.

62. The correct answer is (C). The author states this in paragraph three: "Despite their great size, Komodo dragons are quick moving and agile on the ground." Answer (A) is incorrect. The terrain of the Indonesian islands, according to this article, is *not* difficult. Answer (B) is incorrect. The inference is that the eggs hatch, and the young fend for themselves. Answer (D) is incorrect; the author carefully states that "the tail of the heavy-bodied Komodo dragon accounts for only half of its length."

63. The correct answer is (B). This article states that the name of one of the Indonesian islands inhabited by the dragon is called Komodo. Answer (A) is incorrect. There is no indication of the name of the scientist who discovered the species. Answer (C) is incorrect. There is no indication of a combination of the names of the ancestors of the Komodo. Answer (D) is incorrect. There is no mention of genetic makeup.

64. The correct answer is (D). The author states: "The population is stable at about 3,000. Because the Komodo dragon lives on uninhabited islands, it is currently in no danger from man." Answer (A) is incorrect. The sentence quoted above demonstrates that the area is not overpopulated. Answer (B) is incorrect. There is no mention of overpopulation. Answer (C) is incorrect. The sentence quoted above is counter to this statement.

65. The correct answer is (D). Answer (A) is correct, as stated by the author: "Incubation: eight months." Answer (B) is correct: "young Komodo dragons hatch, from leathery, goose-sized eggs fully formed." Answer (C) is correct: ". . . the female digs a hole in the warm, moist earth and lays an average of a dozen eggs." Because answers (A), (B), and (C) are correct, answer (D), "all of the above," is the correct choice.

PHYSICAL SCIENCES

PASSAGE 1

1. The correct answer is (C). In equilibrium problems dealing with changing pressures, count the total number of "compressible moles" (moles of gases) on the reactant side and then on the product side. In this reaction, there are 5 moles of gas on the reactant side (4 moles of hydrogen chloride and 1 mole of oxygen) compared to 4 moles of gas on the product side (2 moles each of chlorine and water). Increasing the pressure will shift the equilibrium to the side with fewer compressible moles. Therefore, the concentrations of both chlorine and water will increase.
   General Chemistry 9.9

2. The correct answer is (B). Adding additional chlorine will cause the following sequence of events to happen: With more chlorine in the reaction chamber, there will be additional Cl_2 molecules to react with the available water molecules, which will then force the reaction to "reverse," producing more hydrogen chloride and oxygen until a new set of equilibrium conditions is met. If you add more reactants, more products will be produced. In reversible reactions, adding more product produces more reactants (the case here).
   General Chemistry 9.9

3. The correct answer is (A). See the explanation of answer 1 above. Counting the moles of gas of both the reactants and the products in the equation gives an equal number of gas moles on either side. Therefore, increasing the pressure will favor neither side.   *General Chemistry 9.9*

4. The correct answer is (B). Adding more products to this reaction will shift equilibrium to the reactant side, thus increasing the concentrations of both carbon monoxide and water.
   General Chemistry 9.9

5. The correct answer is (C). This is an endothermic reaction. *Note:* Endothermic reactions can be noted in equations when the heat of reaction is:

   1. Written on the reactant side (as in this reaction)
   2. Expressed as a (+) Delta H value
   3. Included as a (+) value at the end of an equation

   Exothermic reactions can be noted in equations when the heat of reaction is:

   1. Written on the product side
   2. Expressed as a (−) Delta H value
   3. Included as a (−) value at the end of an equation.

   Since this is an endothermic reaction, increasing the temperature will force equilibrium to favor the products; therefore, the concentration of oxygen (a reactant) will decrease.
   General Chemistry 8.2, 9.9

---

* For more information, refer to this section in Peterson's *Gold Standard MCAT*.

6. The correct answer is (D). This is the *Haber Reaction*, which is important in chemical history for the production of ammonia used in chemical fertilizers. It is an exothermic reaction; therefore, lower temperatures will favor the product (ammonia). Counting the number of gas moles on each side of the equation gives 4 moles of reactant gases (1 mole of nitrogen and 3 moles of hydrogen) compared to 2 moles of product gas (ammonia). Therefore, an *increase* in pressure will favor the production of ammonia.
 * *General Chemistry 8.2, 9.9*

Passage 2

7. The correct answer is (B). By Ohm's law, V=IR so $I = \dfrac{V}{R} = \dfrac{12}{6} = 2$.
 * *Physics 10.1*

8. The correct answer is (C). The terminal voltage is the potential drop of the external circuit. The battery must raise the charge by this amount so that the charge can continue to circulate. Since the *emf* of the battery is greater than this amount, it must be doing extra work against a resistance to lift the charge. * *Physics 10.3*

9. The correct answer is (C). As the total resistance of the circuit is lower, the current running through the system is higher. This means that the voltage drop through the battery due to its internal resistance is higher and the terminal voltage is lower.
 * *Physics 10.1, 10.3*

10. The correct answer is (C). When resistors are connected in series, the total resistance is equal to the sum of the individual resistors. * *Physics 10.2*

11. The correct answer is (C). When resistors are connected in series, there is no branching of current. The current in all elements connected in series must be the same. * *Physics 10.2*

12. The correct answer is (C). By Ohm's law, V = IR. The current I is the same through each resistor; therefore, the voltage drop will be greater across the higher resistor. * *Physics 10.1, 10.2*

Passage 3

13. The correct answer is (C). At one point, this chemical was known as "ferrous sulfate;" however, the term "ferrous" has been replaced with the Roman numeral designation II, which represents the oxidation number of iron. The oxidation number for the sulfate ion is also 2 and the +2 assigned to the iron atom and the −2 assigned to the sulfate ion "cancel out."
 * *General Chemistry 1.6, 5.2*

14. The correct answer is (C). Peroxide is the $\{O_2^{-2}\}$ polyatomic ion, and the subscript 2 that appears in its formula cannot be canceled out in writing formulas. * *General Chemisty 1.6*

15. The correct answer is (D). In ternary compounds (compounds formed with 3 elements), a chemical name that contains the "ite" suffix contains an "ous" suffix in acid nomenclature. The prefix "hydro" is used in the nomenclature of binary acids.
 * *General Chemistry 6.1*

---

* For more information, refer to this section in Peterson's *Gold Standard MCAT*.

16. The correct answer is (D). Gold has an oxidation number of +3 in this example, which is "canceled out" by the −3 oxidation number, carried by the phosphate ion. "Tetra" is the correct prefix that is assigned to a hydrate containing 4 water molecules. "But" is the prefix assigned to an *organic* compound with 4 *carbons*.
   * *General Chemistry 1.6*

17. The correct answer is (A). The term "hydro" in the nomenclature of acids refers to a *binary* (only 2 elements) acid. Since phosphorous has an oxidation number of −3, the correct formula would be H_3P.
   * *General Chemistry 1.6, 3.3*

18. The correct answer is (B). Aluminum nitrite would have the formula $Al(NO_2)_3$, which would contain 6 oxygen atoms per molecule.
   * *General Chemistry 1.6*

19. The correct answer is (B). "Ide" is the correct suffix for a *binary* (containing only 2 elements) compound.
   * *General Chemistry 3.3, 5.2*

20. The correct answer is (D). This chemical can also be named hydrogen hypochlorite. When named as an acid, the "ite" ending changes to "ous," and the word "acid" is added to the end of the name.   * *General Chemistry 6.1*

21. The correct answer is (C). The work-energy theorem relates the change in kinetic energy to work done on the puck:

work on puck =

$$\frac{1}{2} mv^2_{final} - \frac{1}{2} mv^2_{initial}$$

Since the force of gravity is vertical, while the displacement of the puck is horizontal, the force of gravity does no work. Since the only horizontal force on the puck is the friction force, all of the work on the puck is done by friction:

work on puck = work by friction =

$$\frac{1}{2} mv^2_{final} - \frac{1}{2} mv^2_{initial}$$

or

work by friction =

$$0 - \frac{1}{2}(0.16kg)(50m^2 = -200 \, Joule$$

Since friction always exerts a force opposite to the velocity, the work done by friction is expected to be negative, as calculated.   * *Physics 3.2, 5.3*

22. The correct answer is (D). The acceleration of the sample is the centripetal acceleration, toward the center of the circle. The centripetal acceleration is given by:

$$a = \frac{v^2}{R} = \frac{(2\pi R/T)^2}{R^2} = \left(\frac{2\pi}{T}\right)^2 R$$

where v is the tangential velocity of the sample, R is the radius of its circle, and T is the time for one round trip, the period.

If the rotation rate doubles, then the time for one revolution is cut in half, so the quantity $(2\pi/T)^2$ is quadrupled. Since R does not change, the acceleration is quadrupled to 48 g.   * *Physics 1.1.2, 3.3*

---

* For more information, refer to this section in Peterson's *Gold Standard MCAT*.

23. The correct answer is (D). If R is proportional to the temperature, T, we can write: where α is a constant. From either measurement, we calculate:

$$\alpha = \frac{R}{T} = 0.3\frac{\Omega}{Kelvin}$$

Thus when R = 900Ω, we can calculate:

$$T = \frac{R}{\alpha} = \frac{900\Omega}{0.3\Omega/Kelvin} = 3,000 \; Kelvin$$

24. The correct answer is (C). The electric force $\vec{F}$ on a charge q is related to the electrical field $\vec{E}$ by $\vec{F} = q\vec{E}$.

In this case, since the charge is negative, the direction of the force is opposite to the electrical field direction. The force is directed up. The magnitude of the force is

:

$$F = (1.5 \times 10^{-5} \; Coulomb)$$

$$\left(2,000 \; \frac{Newton}{Coulomb}\right)$$

$$= 3 \times 10^{-2} \; Newton$$

$$= 30 \times 10^{-3} \; Newton$$

* Physics 9.1.3

25. The correct answer is (A). The power, P, absorbed by the filament is given by: $P = IV$, where I is the current through the filament and V is the potential difference across the filament. (V is also the voltage of the battery.) We also know the relation between current and voltage: $V = IR$, where R is the filament resistance. (In this case, the resistance is not constant.) We can write the power in terms of the constant voltage and the resistance by eliminating I:

$$P = \left(\frac{V}{R}\right)V = \frac{V^2}{R}$$

From this it is clear that for constant battery voltage, the power is greatest when the resistance is lowest. That is, the power is greatest at the instant the bulb is switched on.

* Physics 10.2

* For more information, refer to this section in Peterson's *Gold Standard MCAT*.

262

PASSAGE 4

Although the questions are directed at finding the concentrations of solutions, a knowledge and mastery of mole conversions and metric conversions and an understanding of the value for the density of water (1 gram/milliliter or 1 kilogram/liter) are imperative in solving these questions.

The following equation "manipulators" are handy in solving these problems:

A.	Molarity =	Moles of Solute	÷	Liters of Solution
B.	Moles of Solute =	Molarity	×	Liters of Solution
C.	Liters of Solution =	Moles of Solute	÷	Molarity
D.	Molality =	Moles of Solute	÷	Kilograms of Solvent
E.	Moles of Solute =	Molality	×	Kilograms of Solvent
F.	Kilograms of Solvent =	Moles of Solute	÷	Molality

26. The correct answer is (A). First convert to moles (75.6 ÷ 58.5) and use equation A. *Physics 5.3.1*

27. The correct answer is (B). Using equation B, solve for moles (2.2 × 0.25) and convert to grams by multiplying by the molecular mass (148.0). *Physics 5.3.1*

28. The correct answer is (C). First convert to moles (75.0 ÷ 213.0) and then solve for *liters* using equation C. A metric conversion is then needed to convert to ml. *Physics 5.3.1*

29. The correct answer is (C). The addition of more water does not change the number of moles of solute, only the final volume. First solve for moles of solute (55.5 ÷ 138.0) and then use equation A—remember that the final volume will be 1.5 liters. *Physics 5.3.1*

30. The correct answer is (A). Using equation E above, first solve for moles (.250 × 1.5) and then convert to grams by multiplying by the molecular mass (87.0). *Physics 5.3.1*

31. The correct answer is (D). First find the mass of the solvent ($CCl_{4(1)}$) by multiplying the S.G. (2.1) × the volume (750 ml) = 1,575 grams or 1.575 (1.6)

kilograms. Now convert grams of solute to moles (15.0 ÷ 180.0) and use equation D above.
Physics 5.3.1, 6.1.1

PASSAGE 5

32. The correct answer is (B). Work is equal to force × distance. The unit of work is Newton-meters or Joules. *Physics 5.1*

33. The correct answer is (D). If work is done on an object, there is a change in its total energy. Since it is moving on a horizontal surface, there is no change in its potential energy, so all the work goes into changing its kinetic energy. *Physics 5.3(2)*

34. The correct answer is (A). During the second 10 m there is no force acting on the block, there is no friction, and there is no change in its potential energy. Therefore, its kinetic energy and thus its velocity do not change. *Physics 4.2, 5.3*

35. The correct answer is (B). Since there is no energy change, there is no change in velocity. *Physics 4.2, 5.3*

---

* For more information, refer to this section in Peterson's *Gold Standard MCAT*.

36. The correct answer is (C). As the block is traveling up the hill, there is no outside work done on the block, and the block is not doing any work on the environment (such as work against friction). As the block travels up the hill, energy is transformed from kinetic to potential, but the total amount of energy remains constant.
Physics 5.5

37. The correct answer is (C). No energy is lost by the block, so its total energy remains constant and no work has been extracted from the system.
Physics 5.1, 5.3

38. The correct answer is (B). The work done is equal to the change in potential energy.

P.E. = mgh; P.E.
$$= (5kg)(9.8m/s^2)(4m)$$
$$= 196\,J.$$
Physics 5.4

PASSAGE 6

39. The correct answer is (B). The freezing point of water is 0°C and the boiling point is 100°C. The difference between the freezing and boiling point of water is 100°C. Over that 100° range, the mercury column increases in length by 20 cm, or 0.2 cm/°C. For a temperature of 20°C, the length will be 5 cm + 20°C × 0.2 cm/°C = 9 cm.

40. The correct answer is (B). Since the mercury column is 2 cm longer than it would be at 100°C, the solution must be hotter by 10°C (10°C × 0.2 cm/°C = 2 cm).

41. The correct answer is (A). One cm of mercury represents 5°C or 9° Fahrenheit. This will be below the freezing point of water.

42. The correct answer is (C). The conversion between Celsius and Fahrenheit is:

$$C = \frac{5}{9}(F-32).$$
General Chemistry 7.5, Biology 13.1

43. The correct answer is (C). A degree Celsius is equal to a degree Kelvin, only the zero points are different. A change of 10°C is equal to a change of 10° Kelvin.   *General Chemistry 7.5*

44. The correct answer is (A). As the temperature of a gas increases, so does the pressure.
General Chemistry 4.1.5, 4.1.6

45. The correct answer is (A). Chlorine of atomic number 17 and a mass of 35 has 18 neutrons.   *Physics 12.4*

46. The correct answer is (A). The heat of fusion is the amount of heat put in whereas the heat of solidification is the amount of heat removed.
General Chemistry 8.7

47. The correct answer is (B). Isomers are defined in this way.
Organic Chemistry 2.1

48. The correct answer is (B). Water actually has a low vapor pressure.
General Chemistry 4.2, 4.3.2

---

* For more information, refer to this section in Peterson's *Gold Standard MCAT*.

PASSAGE 7

49. The correct answer is (D). The Doppler shift is determined by:

$$f' = \frac{(f_0 \times v \pm v_R)}{(v \pm v_S)}$$

where v is the speed of sound in air, v_R is the velocity of the receiver (+ if it is moving toward the source and − if it is moving away), and v_S is the velocity of the source (− if it is moving toward the receiver and + if it is moving away). f_0 is the frequency of the sound heard by an observer at rest with respect to the source; in this case the passenger is listening to his own train whistle.
Physics 8.5, 8.5.1

50. The correct answer is (C). The frequency of the first train's whistle as heard by the passenger on the second train is 1,425 Hz, as determined by the above formula. *Physics 8.5, 8.5.1*

51. The correct answer is (C). In this case the velocity of the receiver is zero. The highest frequency will be the whistle that is approaching him with the greatest velocity. *Physics 8.5*

52. The correct answer is (C). The beat frequency is the difference in frequency of two coherent sound sources. He hears the frequency of the whistle traveling east as 1,275 Hz and the whistle traveling west as 1,360 Hz. The difference is 85 Hz.
Physics 8.4, 8.5, 8.5.1

53. The correct answer is (A).

$$f' = 1,200\frac{340-20}{340-40}$$

The frequency he hears is 1,280 Hz.
Physics 8.5, 8.5.1

54. The correct answer is (D). The first train is now moving away from him, so he hears a lower frequency (1,130 Hz), and the beat frequency increases to 230 Hz. *Physics 8.4, 8.5, 8.5.1*

PASSAGE 8

55. The correct answer is (C). Increasing the pressure will decrease the balloon's volume by a ratio of 760/800. (Standard pressure is 760 torr.)
General Chemistry 4.1.1, 4.1.4

56. The correct answer is (C). Gas volume changes in proportion to changes in *absolute* temperature (degrees Kelvin). Changing the temperature from 20 to 40 degrees Celsius is actually changing the temperature from 293 degrees Kelvin to 313 degrees Kelvin. Thus, the balloon will increase by a ratio of 313/293, establishing a new volume of about 961.4 ml (a slight increase).
General Chemistry 4.1.3

57. The correct answer is (A). A decrease in pressure will cause the balloon to expand to its "rupture point." Changing the pressure by a ratio of 0.9 liters/1.5 liters will create this rupture. 760 torr × (0.9/1.5) = 456 torr.
General Chemistry 4.1.4

---

* For more information, refer to this section in Peterson's *Gold Standard MCAT.*

58. The correct answer is (C). Use the *ideal gas equation* (PV = nRT) to solve this problem. Remember to change temperature to degrees Kelvin. For example, if the problem is solved using pressure in atmospheres (1.2), volume in liters (0.9), and temperature in degrees Kelvin (288), we would select a value of 0.0821 as our ideal gas constant "R." To solve for moles, the equation is manipulated to give $n = \dfrac{(PV)}{(RT)}$ and the above values are substituted. The answer "n" (.046) is a value for *moles*. Multiplying this value by 32.0 (the molecular mass of oxygen gas) gives the correct answer 1.46 grams.
* *General Chemistry 4.1.6*

59. The correct answer is (B). The same number of moles (.046) will be needed. However, the molecular mass of chlorine gas is 71.0. So, multiplying 71.0 × 0.046 gives the correct answer (3.26 grams). * *General Chemistry 4.1.6*

60. The correct answer is (C). Again, the PV = nRT equation is used, this time solving for (T) temperature. $[T = \dfrac{(PV)}{nR}]$. After substituting the values into the equation, an answer of 239.5 degrees Kelvin is obtained. Subtracting 273 from that answer converts the result into degrees Celsius. * *General Chemistry 4.1.6*

PASSAGE 9

61. The correct answer is (C). These problems involve the dissociation of weak acids. For strong acids, the hydrogen ion concentration (which is used to find the pH) is the same as the starting molarity, since the acid dissociates 100%. Therefore, for a strong acid

HX, the dissociation equation would look like HX → H^+ + X^-, and the value for the concentration of $[H^+]$ and $[X^-]$ would be exactly the same value as the starting value for [HX]. However, for weak acids, only a small percent of the initial concentration dissociates into $[H^+]$ and $[X^-]$. The equilibrium expression, which is called the ionization or acid constant (K_i) or (K_a), is a value that permits calculation of this small degree of dissociation.

$$K_a = \frac{[H^+][X^-]}{[HX]} \text{ (the small amount of weak acid dissociated)}$$

Since the percent of dissociation is usually very small, the denominator is usually assumed to be the initial concentration of HX.

To solve this problem, the K_a of acetic acid (often shown as HOAc) is:

$$1.8 \times 10^{-5} = \frac{[H^+][OAc^-]}{0.01}$$

(the starting molarity of the HOAc)

Since $[H^+] = [OAc^-]$ in the balanced equation, we can replace their product with x^2.

Now we have

$$1.8 \times 10^{-5} = \frac{x^2}{0.01}$$
$$x^2 = 1.8 \times 10^{-7}$$
$$x = 4.2 \times 10^{-4}$$

* *General Chemistry 6.1, 6.6*

62. The correct answer is (A). The percent dissociation is the molarity of the dissociated ion divided by the starting molarity × 100 (to convert to percentage)—or, in this case,

$$\left(\frac{0.00042}{0.01}\right) \times 100$$

---

* For more information, refer to this section in Peterson's *Gold Standard MCAT*.

63. The correct answer is (B). The pH is calculated by finding the −log of the $[H^+]$ concentration that was found in question 61. 0.00042 M pH = 3.4.
  General Chemistry 6.6, 6.6.1

64. The correct answer is (B). The pOH can be calculated using the formula:

pH + pOH = 14

Therefore pOH = 14 − pH (3.4) = 10.6
  General Chemistry 6.5

65. The correct answer is (A). Using the K_a value for nitrous acid, the problem will be solved using the following steps:

$$4.5 \times 10^{-4} = \frac{x^2}{0.005}$$
$$x^2 = 4.5 \times 10^{-4} \times 0.005$$
$$x^2 = 2.25 \times 10^{-6}$$
$$x = 1.5 \times 10^{-3}$$

  General Chemistry 6.6, 6.6.1

PASSAGE 10

66. The correct answer is (A). An alpha particle is a helium nucleus with atomic number 2 and atomic mass number 4. When this is emitted, the mother isotope atomic number and atomic mass number must go down by 2 and 4, respectively. *Physics 12.3, 12.4*

67. The correct answer is (A). A beta particle is an electron. A neutron in the nucleus decays to form a proton and an electron. The proton remains in the nucleus, and the electron (beta particle) is emitted. Therefore, the atomic number has increased by 1, and the atomic mass number will remain the same. *Physics 12.3, 12.4*

68. The correct answer is (B). A beta particle (an electron) has much less mass and a negative charge compared with the alpha particle (helium nucleus), which is positively charged.
  Physics 12.1, 12.3

69. The correct answer is (C). One half of the isotope has transmuted in 10 days; therefore, the half-life is equal to 10 days. Every time a half-life elapses, one half of the remainder is transmuted. After 10 more days, one half of the remaining 500 g transmutes, leaving you with 250 g. *Physics 12.4*

70. The correct answer is (D). After 24 hours, 4 half-lives have elapsed. What remains is $\left(\frac{1}{2}\right) \times \left(\frac{1}{2}\right) \times \left(\frac{1}{2}\right) \times \left(\frac{1}{2}\right)$, which is equal to $\frac{1}{16}$.
  Physics 12.4

71. The correct answer is (D). 4 g is ¹⁄₁₆ of 64 g. ¹⁄₁₆ represents four half-lives. Since 12 hours is equal to four half-lives, one half-life is 3 hours. *Physics 12.4*

72. The correct answer is (C). Gamma rays are emitted when the nucleus drops from an excited state to a lower state. Gamma rays are high-energy electromagnetic radiation and have no mass and no charge. *Physics 12.3*

73. The correct answer is (A). 75 mL divided by the new volume, 250 mL, equals 30%. *General Chemistry 1.4*

74. The correct answer is (C). Catalysts lower the activation energy of the reaction, thus providing a lower energy pathway. *General Chemistry 9.7*

---

* For more information, refer to this section in Peterson's *Gold Standard MCAT.*

75. The correct answer is (B). The atoms on the chart have the same number of electrons as they do protons, but, except for the inert gases, not all their energy levels are complete.
General Chemisty 2.3

76. The correct answer is (B). The definition of the *E* configuration places the substituted groups on opposite sides of the double bond.
Organic Chemistry 4.1

77. The correct answer is (C). Quick release of energy is a role of carbohydrates.   *Biology 1.1, 4.1, 4.4, 6.3*

BIOLOGICAL SCIENCE

PASSAGE 1

1. The correct answer is (B). The Gram stain is used to identify Gram-positive vs. Gram-negative cells, based on the cell wall composition of the organism.
Biology 2.2

2. The correct answer is (B). The capsule cannot be observed with the Gram stain. A negative stain is repelled by the bacterial cell, and creates a dark background. Consequently, it is possible to better observe the actual size and shape of an organism, including observation of a capsule, if present.
Biology 2.2

3. The correct answer is (C). These two answers comprise the basic definition of a differential stain for bacteria.
Biology 2.2

4. The correct answer is (D). Although endospores are often visible with the Gram stain, an endospore stain is required to make this distinction.
Biology 2.2

5. The correct answer is (B). Any other order will produce erroneous results.
Biology 2.2

6. The correct answer is (A). Since antibiotics have a spectrum of activity based on their mode of action, it is helpful to know cell wall composition and the morphology of the organism until culture results are available. The latter may take several days.
Biology 2.2

7. The correct answer is (A). Red cells indicate a Gram negative cell wall and purple cells indicate a Gram-positive cell wall.   *Biology 2.2*

8. The correct answer is (D). Also, for eukaryotes having no cell wall, different methods are needed because the alcohol in the Gram stain interacts with the lipids in the cell membrane, rendering the Gram procedure ineffective.   *Biology 2.2, 2.3*

PASSAGE 2

9. The correct answer is (B). A haploid cell cannot divide except by mitosis, and mitosis always produces daughter cells with the same number of chromosomes as the parent cell. The resulting process would not double the number of chromosomes as (A) suggests. This would occur in diploid cells just prior to mitosis in somatic cells. Haploid somatic cells are commonly found in organisms such as mosses.
* Biology 1.3, 14.2

10. The correct answer is (D). Meiosis is reduction division, and the key to knowing this is the word gamete, a reference to a sex cell that is produced by meiosis. The number of chromosomes in the parent cell is cut in half, from the diploid number to the haploid number. Here, the diploid parent cell had 12 individual chromosomes found as six pairs, and each haploid gamete, following meiosis II, received one chromosome from each pair giving a total of six individual, unpaired chromosomes per new cell. ** Biology 14.2*

11. The correct answer is (D). Cytokinesis is the actual physical division of the parent cell into two daughter cells that happens in both mitosis and meiosis. The other phenomena are unique to meiosis. Anaphase I is the unraveling of the separated chromosome pairs toward the end of meiosis I. Crossing-over is the exchange of end pieces of homologous chromosomes as they come together as tetrads during synapsis of meiosis I. ** Biology 1.3, 14.2*

12. The correct answer is (C). Mitosis is actually the process of nuclear division. It is usually, but not always, followed by cytokinesis (parent cells split into two physically distinct, and new daughter cells). Skeletal muscle cells, for example, frequently have more than one nucleus. The multinucleate state arises because mitosis was not followed by cytokinesis. There is nothing unique about the higher plants or animals in this respect. ** Biology 1.3, 5.2*

13. The correct answer is (A). Crossing-over must occur early in meiosis (during meiosis I) if recombined chromosomes are to be distributed to all gametes. ** Biology 14.2*

14. The correct answer is (C). The homologous chromosomes part during the anaphase stage of meiosis I. Meiosis II would be too late for proper and equal allocation of the recombined chromosomes to the gametes. Metaphase I is a coming together and does not relate to separation as does anaphase. ** Biology 14.2*

15. The correct answer is (B). From each parent cell, oogenesis produces one haploid ovum, and three polar bodies while spermatogenesis results in the formation of four sperm. ** Biology 14.2*

---

* For more information, refer to this section in Peterson's *Gold Standard MCAT*.

PASSAGE 3

16. The correct answer is (D). The daughter had no fish and no wine. However, the dog also had no wine, but did eat the fish. The husband, wife, and son also ate the fish. All but the daughter got sick, and their common factor was fish consumption.

17. The correct answer is (B). The dog and the daughter did not consume wine.

18. The correct answer is (D). All consumed the water.

19. The correct answer is (B). The pasta and salad would be the likely culprits, but salad is not given as a choice.

20. The correct answer is (B). The fish is still the common item consumed by all who became ill.

21. The correct answer is (D). If the husband, wife, daughter, son, and dog have all eaten the same foods and drunk the same liquids and only the dog became ill, it is not likely that any of these items in Table 1 contributed to the dog's illness.

22. The correct answer is (D).
* *Biology 6.1, 9.2*

23. The correct answer is (A). The parotid gland swells and the opening into the mouth is red in mumps and other infections of the parotid.   * *Biology 9.2*

24. The correct answer is (C). The endocrine secretions of the pancreatic islet cells are insulin and glucagon.
* *Biology 6.3.4, 9.3, 9.4.2*

25. The correct answer is (B). Only monosaccharides can be absorbed.
* *Biology 9.5, Organic Chemistry 12.3.2*

26. The correct answer is (C). Endopeptidases, trypsin, chymotrypsin, and elastase cleave interior peptide bonds, and the exopeptidases, aminopeptidases, and carboxypeptidases, cleave the amino and carboxy ends of the polypeptides.   * *Biology 9.3, 9.5*

PASSAGE 4

27. The correct answer is (A). Hannah is homozygous dominant. Therefore, she can only pass the normal trait, color vision, to her sons. The father contributes the Y chromosome to the male offspring. The Y chromosome does not carry a gene for color vision.
* *Biology 15.1, 15.3*

28. The correct answer is (A). All female offspring would be heterozygous for the trait of color blindness. None of the children would be color blind.
* *Biology 15.1, 15.3*

29. The correct answer is (B). Since sex-linked traits behave like dominant recessive traits, a female who is homozygous for such a trait would express it.   * *Biology 15.1, 15.3*

30. The correct answer is (A). Both male and female children inherit an X chromosome from their mother. The color blind sister must have two recessive genes, one on each X chromosome.   * *Biology 15.1, 15.3*

31. The correct answer is (A). Only the X chromosome carries this sex-linked trait.   * *Biology 15.1, 15.3*

32. The correct answer is (C). Of all of the daughters they could produce, there is a 50:50 chance that each one would have normal color vision.
* *Biology 15.1, 15.3*

* For more information, refer to this section in Peterson's *Gold Standard MCAT*.

PASSAGE 5

33. The correct answer is (C). (A) is regional anatomy and (D) is systemic anatomy, and both are considered specific methods of gross anatomy. (B) is microscopic anatomy.
   * Biology 6–14

34. The correct answer is (B). The insepa-rable nature of structure and function dictates that anatomy and physiology are appropriately studied together.
   * Biology 6.2, 6.3, 6.4

35. The correct answer is (A). (B) is a decreasing order of complexity, (C) is a list of tissue types, and (D) is different types of life forms.
   * Biology 1.1, 14.5; General Chemistry 1.2; Organic Chemistry 12.2; Physics 12.1

36. The correct answer is (B). Blood is considered a part of the cardiovascular system.   ** Biology 7.1, 10.1, 14.1*

37. The correct answer is (D). Functional characteristics also include maintenance of boundaries, responsiveness, excre-tion, metabolism, and growth.
   * Biology 2.1, 16.4

38. The correct answer is (A). Living organisms cannot completely resist change nor control their external environment. Communication with the environment is considered a necessary component of homeostasis.
   * Biology 6.1, 7.1, 10.1, 12.1, 13.1

39. The correct answer is (C). (A), (B), and (D) are all examples of negative feedback.   ** Biology 6.3.6*

40. The correct answer is (B). Transverse sections divide the body into superior and inferior portions, frontal sections divide the body into anterior and posterior portions, and although a sagittal section does divide the body into lateral portions, it is only the midsagittal that divides it into equal portions.

PASSAGE 6

41. The correct answer is (D). Insects employ air sacs to help in moving air in and out of the body, but the system is still very inefficient when compared to lungs or gills. This limitation makes the giant ants or other insects of science fiction biological impossibilities. Endotracheal means "inside trachea," which is where the gases move.

42. The correct answer is (B). The counter-current system found in fish gills works by having the blood in the gill filaments (which is lower in O_2 and higher in CO_2) flow in the opposite direction as the water (higher in O_2 and lower in CO_2) crossing the filaments. Diffusion is enhanced by having the most oxygen-depleted blood opposite the most oxygen-rich water (and the reverse for carbon dioxide). Choice (C) is the next most nearly-correct answer, but does not indicate what is special about the countercurrent arrangement. Moving with the flow of water would negate the possibility of this taking place and would, therefore, not lead to mixing.
   * Biology 10.3

---

* For more information, refer to this section in Peterson's *Gold Standard MCAT.*

43. The correct answer is (C). Air is 20% oxygen by volume, while water has only a fraction of that oxygen content. Answer (D) is incorrect, since gills are good at extracting as much as 80% of the oxygen from water. Choice (B) has been found to be incorrect in many instances, and the animals compensate for the compression mentioned in (A) by equalization of pressure in their bodies during rare visitations to different depths.
General Chemistry 1.1, 5.1.1

44. The correct answer is (A). In the brain, a breathing center monitors the carbon dioxide levels in the blood, not oxygen as had previously been thought.
Biology 12.4.1

45. The correct answer is (A). Frogs in effect "swallow" air, pushing it into their lungs by forcing air from their mouths with the mouth and nostrils shut. Mammals expand the volume inside their chest cavity by raising the ribs and dropping (contracting) the diaphragm, thereby reducing the pressure in the lungs to that below atmospheric pressure. Air moves into the lungs, as expected, from a region of higher (external) pressure to a region of lower (internal) air pressure. Exhaling is achieved by reversing the process.
Biology 12.4

46. The correct answer is (D). The flap of tissue is the epiglottis. The opening itself is the glottis. During inhaling, choice (C) would bring material into the lungs and is wrong. *Biology 9.2*

47. The correct answer is (C). Micelles are formed by the interaction of the bile salts and the small lipid droplets. The micelle has a hydrophilic outside and a hydrophobic center. *Biology 9.4.1*

48. The correct answer is (C). The action potential is a self-propagating wave of membrane depolarization and is the same as in all neurons.
Biology 5.1.2, 6.1.1, 6.2, 6.2.1, 6.2.2, 6.2.3, 6.2.4

49. The correct answer is (B). The depolarized state is brief—as sodium enters rapidly and potassium leaves the cell slowly, the electrical balance, or the resting potential (-60mV), is restored, repolarizing the neuron even though the ion concentrations are not the same as before depolarization.
Biology 5.1.1, 5.1.2, 5.1.3

50. The correct answer is (B). The neurotransmitter in the cleft is rapidly taken up again by the presynaptic membrane to end the transmission and conserve the chemicals for repackaging.
Biology 5.1

51. The correct answer is (B). The Schwann cell without myelin, providing only support, is called a neurolemmal cell and the fiber is known as an unmyelinated fiber. *Biology 5.1, 5.1.2*

PASSAGE 7

52. The correct answer is (B). The chemical analysis of membranes isolated from red blood cells by Gorter and Grendel showed just enough phospholipid content to cover the cell twice, thus the conclusion that the plasma membrane was a bilayered structure.
Biology 1.1

* For more information, refer to this section in Peterson's *Gold Standard MCAT*.

53. The correct answer is (B). Nucleotides are one of the building blocks of DNA, not the membrane. Oligosaccharides are small polymers of sugar and are used to help transport proteins in concert with the Golgi apparatus, and glycerol is the backbone molecule of lipids. The membrane was found to contain proteins.   *Biology 1.1*

54. The correct answer is (C). Early electron microscopy was not sufficient to distinguish proteins in the membrane; chemical analysis showed this much earlier. Sugars are not found in the membrane, and the entire membrane is not soluble in water. Upon examining internal organelles with the electron microscope, researchers discovered that the internal membranes looked similar to the plasma membrane.
   Biology 1.1, 1.2.1

55. The correct answer is (C). The model proposed by Singer and Nicholson was called the fluid mosaic model.
   Biology 1.1

56. The correct answer is (C). Cations and anions are too general an answer to have any validity here, and since the membrane is made of a phospholipid bilayer, lipids and lipid-soluble substances will cross it fastest.
   Biology 1.1, Organic Chemistry 12.4.1

PASSAGE 8

57. The correct answer is (B). The molecule has all single bonds making it saturated and is the simplest of lipids.
   Organic Chemistry 12.4

58. The correct answer is (B). Cholesterol is a member of the steroid class of lipids, which all have a ring structure.
   Organic Chemistry 12.4.1

59. The correct answer is (A). Saturated fats have a more linear structure with a tighter arrangement of molecules allowing greater intermolecular attractions. More energy is required to overcome these attractions.
   Organic Chemistry 12.4

60. The correct answer is (C). This is the process by which soap is made.
   Organic Chemistry 9.4.1

61. The correct answer is (D). All of the molecules presented contain glycerol.
   Organic Chemistyr 9.4.1, 12.5

PASSAGE 9

62. The correct answer is (B). (A) and (C) are characteristics associated with spongy bone.   *Biology 5.4.4, 11.3, 11.3.1*

63. The correct answer is (C). The other classification by shape is flat.
   Biology 11.3.1

64. The correct answer is (B). Hydroxyapatite (mineral salt) is responsible for the rigidity.   *Biology 5.4.4*

65. The correct answer is (A). Although nasal and maxilla are bones of the skull, they do not produce a portion of the cranial cavity and are classified as facial bones.   *Biology 11.3*

66. The correct answer is (B). These are bone markings of a typical vertebra.
   Biology 11.3

67. The correct answer is (D). The sacrum is a plate composed of five fused vertebrae and is a part of the pelvic girdle, but is not part of the coccygeal bone.

---

* For more information, refer to this section in Peterson's *Gold Standard MCAT.*

PASSAGE 10

68. The correct answer is (C). Three more births per 1,000 individuals, increasing the cbr from 27 to 30, would increase the rate of growth from 1.6% to 1.9%. This is easy to figure, since the rate is simply the difference between the cbr and cdr, stated as a percentage. Algebraically, the answer can be calculated as follows:

$$(x - 11)0.1 = 1.9$$

$$x - 11 = \frac{1.9}{0.1}$$

$$x = 19 + 11$$

$$x = 30$$

69. The correct answer is (D). Using formula IV in the passage,
$\frac{70}{2} = 35$ years.

70. The correct answer is (C). With an initial population of 6 billion, in 30 years time (one doubling time) the number of people will grow to 12 billion. After another doubling time of 30 years, the population will grow from 12 to 24 billion. Thus the total time to go from 6 billion to 24 billion people is 30 years + 30 years, or 60 years total.

71. The correct answer is (A). When cbr = cdr, the percent annual population growth will be zero. Answer (C), cdr > cbr, will result in a percent annual population growth of less than zero.

72. The correct answer is (C). In considering only part of the Earth, as opposed to the entire Earth, migration of people (immigration and emigration) must be taken into account. Factors I and II are already taken into account in the cdr and cbr, respectively.

73. The correct answer is (B). The limbic system includes the limbic lobe as well as associated subcortical nuclei and is associated with emotional responses and the integration of olfactory information with visceral and somatic information. *Biology 6.1*

74. The correct answer is (D). The frontal lobe contains the primary motor cortex and frontal association areas for analyzing and sorting sensory information. The temporal lobe is at the lateral lower side of the brain and functions mainly in hearing, but has some visual processing. *Biology 6.1*

75. The correct answer is (C). The sympathetic motor outflow is from the thoracic and lumbar spinal segments (not cranial or sacral nerves), functioning to prepare the body for flight or fight by increasing heart rate, respiratory rate, and increasing blood flow to the muscles and brain.
Biology 6.1, 6.1.4, 6.1.5

76. The correct answer is (B). CN 7, facial motor and sensory nerve, supplies the muscles of facial expression and taste sensation of anterior two-thirds of the tongue. *Biology 6.1*

77. The correct answer is (A). The pigmented layer of the choroid coat, on the most posterior surface, serves to absorb excess light that would blur vision if allowed to reflect.
Biology 6.2.4

---

* For more information, refer to this section in Peterson's *Gold Standard MCAT.*

Practice Test 2

There are nine passages in the Verbal Reasoning test. Each passage is followed by several questions. After reading a passage, select the one best answer to each question. If you are not certain of an answer, eliminate the alternatives that you know to be incorrect and then select an answer from the remaining alternatives. Indicate your selection by blackening the corresponding circle on your answer sheet.

PASSAGE 1 (QUESTIONS 1–10)

Censorship was hardly a concern of educators, although it was an obvious concern for librarians, until recently. Before World War II, censorship rarely surfaced in schools, although some works—such as John Steinbeck's *Of Mice and Men*, and *The Grapes of Wrath*—did cause some discussion in the newspapers of the time. When students began to read the books, the furor spread into the school. Following World War II, Norman Mailer published *The Naked and the Dead*, and J. D. Salinger wrote *Catcher in the Rye*, which described the society of that day as overly permissive, lax, and even immoral. Youth and young adults were caught up in that description. Most of the objections were aimed at the writers and publishers and certainly, some were aimed at the bookstores stocking the books. Few high school teachers taught the controversial books for many years; even fewer librarians would stock them. But both teachers and librarians became aware anew that they needed to be more careful about books they allowed students to read for extra credit and for book reports.

Paperback books offered little of the intellectual or pedagogical value to teachers before World War II. After the war, many teachers blithely assumed that paperbacks had not changed, and given the often lurid covers, teachers seemed to have a point, though it was more superficial than real. Teachers and parents continued to object to student use of paperbacks even after the publication of *The Bible* and Plato's *Dialogues* and *Four Tragedies* of Shakespeare proved that paperbacks had merit. Students discovered even earlier that paperbacks were handy to stick into a purse or pocket, and the titles were appealing, not stodgy, as were most textbooks. Paperbacks came to schools, censors not withstanding, and these cheap and ubiquitous books created problems galore for teachers.

Perhaps as important, until about 1967, young-adult books were generally safe, pure, and simplistic, devoid of the reality that young people faced daily—violence, pregnancy, premarital sex, profanity, alcohol, drugs, tobacco, abortion, runaways, alienation, the generation gap, suicide, death, prejudice, poverty, class distinction,

275

divorce, and the list goes on. The looming topics were sports, going to the prom, getting a car for the Friday-night date, and the first kiss. Young people read them for fun, knowing that they were nothing more than escape reading and had little relationship to reality or to anything of real significance.

Then, in 1967, Ann Head's *Mr. and Mrs. Bo Jo Jones* and S. E. Hinton's *The Outsiders* appeared, and the face of young-adult literature changed and could not go back to the good-old-pure days.

The books that followed were not always great or honest, but a surprising number were. English teachers and librarians who had accepted the possibility of censorship with adult authors popular with their students—Steinbeck, Fitzgerald, and Hemingway, for example—now learned that the once-safe young-adult novel was no longer "safe." Censorship attacks soon began. Many of the works were denounced.

Since 1963, the enactment of censorship in communities and schools has increased. Teachers and librarians eager to promote reading as a means of learning about life found themselves expected to sit quietly while the censors trod all over them. In 1982, a survey of high school libraries found that 34 percent of them reported a challenge to at least one book, compared to 30 percent in 1977. A 1986 Canadian survey was no better.

So it was that schools found themselves embroiled in an emotional and pedagogical dilemma that was the stuff of which novels were made, but it was also very real to the people represented in the daily newspapers' accounts of challenges and students caught in the middle. Censorship became a real part of the American education system affecting the youth and young adults not only of the 1980s, but stretching into the 1990s as well.

1. Based upon the material presented in this selection, the reader should conclude that:

   A. too much attention has been given to subjects that are real in the lives of students today.
   B. focusing on the problems students face is not what students want.
   C. school personnel are diligent in selecting only books that present material about life today.
   D. local reaction to the subject material of books in schools has grown radically during the past thirty years.

2. The author's mention of Steinbeck's works is intended to:

   A. remind the reader to avoid these works as questionable.
   B. portray Steinbeck as an innovative writer whose works are generally appealing.
   C. illustrate what "bad" books really are and warn students to shun them.
   D. present works that are familiar as an example of what censorship really is.

3. The fact that some censors insist that all young adult books must be examined by parents, teachers, and librarians with the ultimate decision made by those not in education would most directly challenge the assumption:

   A. of freedom of the press.
   B. that young people can choose for themselves.
   C. that subject matter is changing and must be closely watched.
   D. that parents should not be involved in education.

4. On the basis of statements made in the passage, one is justified in concluding that the:

A. teachers and librarians have given over the choice of reading material to students.

B. school administrators have refused to allow parents and community leaders to have a say in library holdings.

C. authors of today fear writing about matters of concern to youth because of the reality of censorship.

D. censorship of books for school libraries will continue to grow even though new authors are writing about new subjects.

5. The author's presentation of the rise in the publication of paperbacks is intended to:

A. show that students prefer this informal presentation.

B. indicate the questionable topics for which paperbacks were first known.

C. illustrate why censorship became important as the paperbacks' popularity grew.

D. show the increased availability of books because of the decrease in price.

6. Based upon the passage, which of the following would likely characterize the young-adult novel?

I. Plots about teen issues of pregnancy, abortion, and adoption.

II. Plots about drug and alcohol abuse.

III. Issues of divorce, suicide, and prejudice.

A. II only.

B. III only.

C. I and II only.

D. II and III only.

7. According to this article, information contained in the modern young-adult novel is considered:

A. old-fashioned, good, and pure.

B. absolutely honest and forthright.

C. surprisingly great and honest.

D. more superficial than real.

8. The fact that some teachers and librarians choose to include the paperback young-adult novels on reading lists would most directly challenge the assumption that:

A. educators more than parents and community leaders know the needs and preferences of students.

B. taking a chance with censorship is a popular trend in education today.

C. censorship should be a priority concern before books are purchased and/or recommended to students.

D. students will read the books that are available to them in the school setting.

9. The word pedagogical is used to illustrate to the reader the:

   A. appeal to the intellectual offered by the paperback.
   B. dearth of appropriate subject matter chosen for the books.
   C. emotional appeal to young people of the literature presented.
   D. lack of teaching value in the paperbooks available before World War II.

10. To illustrate a difference between the paperbacks available immediately after World War II and those available today, the author describes:

   A. unattractive titles.
   B. questionable authors.
   C. cheap construction.
   D. subject matter.

PASSAGE 2 (QUESTIONS 11–18)

The past two decades have seen a revolution in our expectations about college students. Rising standards of academic performance in primary and secondary schools, the baby boom after the war, the slowness with which major American universities have expanded their size—all have resulted in increasing selectivity by the admissions officers of the most prestigious American colleges and universities. Furthermore, once a student is admitted to college, higher admission standards have meant that more could be demanded of him or her; students who a generation ago would have done "A" work now find themselves doing only "C" work with the same effort. The sheer volume of required reading and writing has increased enormously; in addition, the quality of work expected has grown by leaps and bounds. Finally, for a growing number of young Americans, college is but a stepping-stone to professional and graduate school after college, and, as a result, consistent academic performance in college increasingly becomes a prerequisite for admission to a desirable business school, medical school, law school or graduate school.

Not only have academic pressures mounted in the past generation, but these pressures have become more and more cognitive. What matters, increasingly, to admissions committees and college graders is the kind of highly intellectual, abstract reasoning ability that enables a student to do well on college boards, graduate records exams, and other admission tests, and—once he or she is in college or graduate school—to turn out consistently high grades that will enable him or her to overcome the next academic hurdle. And while such intellectual and cognitive talents are highly rewarded, colleges increasingly frown upon emotional, nonintellectual, and passionate forms of expression.

In contrast to these cognitive demands, there are extremely few countervailing pressures to become more feeling, morally responsible, courageous, artistically perceptive, emotionally balanced, or interpersonally subtle human beings. On the contrary, the most visible pressures on today's students are in many ways anti-emotional, impersonal, quantitative, and numerical.

Increasingly, then, one of the major pressures on American students is a demand to perform well academically, to postpone and delay emotional satisfactions until they are older, to refine and sharpen continually their cognitive abilities. As a result, students today probably work harder than students in any other previous generation; a bad course or a bad year means to many of them that they will not get into graduate school. Taking a year off increasingly means running the danger of losing opportunities for grants and/or scholarships as well as having to reenter with more demanding requirements.

Thus, while the systematic quest for cognitive competence occupies much of the time and effort of the preprofessional student at today's selective colleges, this pursuit does little to inform the student about life's wider purposes. One of the peculiar characteristics of professional competence is that even when competence is attained, all the other really important questions remain unanswered: what life is all about; what really matters; what to stand for; how much to stand for; what is meaningful, relevant, and important; what is meaningless, valueless, and false. Thus, for many students, the pursuit of professional competence may be illusory. How students search for significance and relevance of course varies enormously from individual to individual.

11. According to the article, which of the following are some of the virtues of the quest for cognitive competence?

   A. Students become informed about life's wider purposes.
   B. Cognitive demands provide for consistently high grades.
   C. Students learn to postpone many of life's experiences and demands until later in life.
   D. Pressures are anti-emotional.

12. The author states that mounting academic pressures have given students the capacity to achieve in all of the following areas EXCEPT:

   A. intellectualism.
   B. reasoning.
   C. logic.
   D. practicality.

13. The selectivity of college admissions offices has come about as a direct result of:

   I.   the population explosion of the postwar baby boomers.
   II. rising standards of private college preparatory schools.
   III. rapidly expanding size and offerings of colleges and universities.

   A. I only.
   B. II only.
   C. III only.
   D. I and II only.

14. From this selection, one may infer that the author's tone is:

   A. melancholy.
   B. involved.
   C. detached.
   D. sentimental.

15. The conclusion of this article implies that:

   A. individuals should approach their choice of a vocation with great care.
   B. one's choice of profession should be determined by one's personal goals.
   C. the completion of a college program ensures one financial security.
   D. being intellectual is not enough in today's world.

16. One might assume from this reading that colleges and universities are beginning to look at:

   A. the whole student for admissions purposes.

   B. grades more closely than assessment tests.

   C. assessment tests more closely than grades.

   D. health records and personal information.

17. In discussing the pressures placed upon today's college student, what does the author state about them?

   A. Most pressures are social.

   B. Few of the pressures are practical.

   C. The pressures have become energizing and increase the student's vitality.

   D. The pressures have become increasingly more cognitive.

18. Based upon the material contained in this article, the cognitive dependence discussed by the author would have to be:

   A. evidence of an advanced ability in a given subject.

   B. the primary focus upon grades and test results.

   C. the belief that all of life depends upon who one really is.

   D. one's dependence upon social and moral intuition.

PASSAGE 3 (QUESTIONS 19–24)

Every society contains pressures and demands that its members simply take for granted. Thus, the pressure for extremely high levels of cognitive efficiency seems to most of us a necessary and an even desirable aspect of modern society. The pressure has to do with the sheer quantity, variety, and intensity of external stimulations, imagery, and excitation to which most Americans are subjected. For lack of a better label, this condition is one of increasing "stimulus-flooding."

Many people have, at some point in their lives, had the experience of being so overcome by external stimulations and internal feelings that they gradually find themselves growing numb and unfeeling. Medical students, for example, commonly report that after their first and often intense reactions to the cadaver in the dissecting room, they simply "stop feeling anything" with regard to the object of their dissection. Or, we have all had the experience of listening to so much good music, seeing so many fine paintings, being so overwhelmed by excellent cooking that we find ourselves simply unable to respond further to new stimuli. Similarly, at moments of extreme psychic pain and anguish, most individuals "go numb," no longer perceiving the full implications of a catastrophic situation or no longer experiencing the full range of their own feelings.

This psychological numbing operates at a great variety of levels for modern society. Our experience from childhood onward with the constantly flickering images and sounds of television, films, radio, newspapers, paperbacks, neon signs, advertisements, and sound trucks, numbs us to many of the sights and sounds of our civilization. The exposure to many intelligent political creeds, superstitions, religions, and faiths numbs us to validity and the special spiritual and intellectual values of each one; we move along values and ideologies as in a two-dimensional landscape.

In all of these respects, modern society confronts the difficult problems of keeping stimulation from without to a manageable level, while at the same time protecting itself against being overwhelmed by its own inner responses to the stimuli from the outer world. Defenses or barriers against both internal and external stimulations are, of course, essential in order for us to preserve our intactness and integrity as personalities. From earliest childhood, children develop thresholds of responsiveness and barriers against stimulation in order to protect themselves against being overwhelmed by inner or outer excitement. Similarly in adulthood, comparable barriers, thresholds, and defense are necessary, especially when we find ourselves in situations of intense stimulation.

Thus, in at least a minority of Americans, the normal capacity to defend oneself against undue stimulations and inner excitation is exaggerated and automatized, so that it not only protects but walls off the individual from inner and outer experience. In such individuals, there develops an acute sense of being trapped in their own shells, unable to break through their defenses to make contact with experience or with other people, a sense of being excessively armored, separated from their own activities as by an invisible screen, estranged from their own feelings and from potentially emotion-arousing experiences in the world. Presumably, most of us have had some inkling of this feeling of inner deadness and outer flatness, especially in times of great fatigue, let-down, or depression. The world seems cold and two-dimensional: food and life have lost their savor; our activities consist of merely going through the motions, our experiences lack vividness, three-dimensionality, and intensity. Above all, we feel trapped or shut in our own subjectivity.

The pressure for cognitive professional competence leads to a search for meaning in other areas of life; the feeling and fear of psychological numbing leads to a pursuit, even a cult of experiences for their own sake. Each of us paves our road with such experiences.

19. In addition to cognitive accomplishments—arriving at a place of comfortable performance—most human beings need to be aware of their:

    A. potential tendency to over-perform and burn out.
    B. barriers or walls—internal and external—which may numb them.
    C. need to push for greater accomplishments in life.
    D. capacity for social pressure as well.

20. The illustration of the medical students and their experience with the cadaver is used by the author to indicate that :

    A. when we are continually exposed to the same stimuli we tend to learn to take them for granted.
    B. most anything can lose its "shock" value.
    C. stimulus repetition causes a failure to recognize it as anything but ordinary.
    D. all of the above.

21. The word *stimuli* as used in this article indicates:

    A. those external forces or objects of which we become aware.

    B. things that make us react sharply.

    C. life-changing forces.

    D. a willingness to not be shocked by anything.

22. The inference of the author is that care should be exercised to avoid numbing our feelings by:

    A. overexposure to the same stimuli for a lengthy period of time.

    B. looking only at shocking things that make us fear.

    C. looking only into bland subjects that cause us to be bored.

    D. underexposure to fine arts.

23. Causes of numbness to stimuli include:

    A. boredom with the things at hand.

    B. depression, tiredness, and disappointment.

    C. too many requirements at hand.

    D. inadequate experience.

24. The author gives a graphic description of an individual desensitized to stimuli as being:

    A. immobilized and untalkative.

    B. nonproductive and sleepy.

    C. possessed of a feeling of entrapment.

    D. noncommunicative.

PASSAGE 4 (QUESTIONS 25–34)

Exercise physiologists show that physical exercise, if sufficiently intensive and regular, can control the various phenomena of aging—such as the decrease in muscle mass, diminished oxygen intake, reduced heat production, and the fall in total body quantity. (Physical exercises can also increase overall cerebral activities.) Exercises stimulate the neural controls of metabolism, respiration, blood circulation, digestion, and the activities of the glands of internal secretion. A correct combination of alert mental activity and physical exercise is at present the best method of preserving, for as long as possible, at a high level, the activity of the brain cells.

This control of the phenomena of aging—desire for longevity—should begin as early as possible, before one has completed his/her physical development (between fourteen and twenty-two years of age). It is considerably more difficult to control premature biological aging when it has already set in. A regular exercise program contributes to vitality and healthful good looks throughout the middle years. A person who has maintained a successful personal fitness program can enjoy middle and later years to the fullest. This is why the habits of physical exercise and total fitness should be formed from earliest childhood.

Total fitness is produced when someone engages in balanced activities, strengthening all body systems, particularly the cardiovascular system, the respiratory system, the nervous system, and the muscular system. But it is very important to realize that total fitness is produced by optimum intensity and duration of physical activity. The amount and duration of physical activity required is different for every person.

Contrary to some common thought, involvement in exercise programs and sports will not develop bulky muscles. A program that would overdevelop specific muscles would be unhealthy for males or females. Exercise improves the figure by "normalizing" it and causing it to become better proportioned. If the arms or legs are too heavy, exercise works toward slimming; if too thin, exercise develops them.

The likelihood of maintaining a physical fitness program depends on how interesting it is to you. In order for people to continue an activity program throughout the years, it must maintain their interest. Most of the well-publicized physical fitness programs that stress exercises, machines, or rely on an athletic club need great motivation from a person to be maintained throughout life. The best way for an exercise program to be fun is to take part in an individual activity or dual sport. But one cannot receive satisfaction out of a sport that he/she is not in condition to perform. Consequently, an individual must have a general conditioning program that is routine (usually three days a week) and that can be maintained easily to stay in condition for any sport.

An individual, while in school or college, should develop skills in several different activities to participate in throughout life. Five major factors should be considered as one plans physical fitness activities for later life. The individual should develop: (1) muscular strength, (2) muscular endurance, (3) circulatory endurance, (4) flexibility, and (5) skill (coordination). Physical education courses should help the individual to gain knowledge in activities and sports that develop and maintain these factors.

The concepts of exercise, but not the principles, have changed drastically in recent years. Modern total fitness programs are the result of laboratory studies that have added greatly to our knowledge. Exercise is accepted today as being essential to counterbalance our overly sedentary lifestyle. Now, the question becomes: "How much and what kind of exercise?" The body needs oxygen and the rhythmic physical activity that supplies the body with oxygen. During exercise, the blood is richer in oxygen and nutrients and it more effectively eliminates wastes from the muscles and other organs. Activities that promote such efficient body functioning include walking, running, swimming, cycling, dancing, skiing, and tennis. Also, for exercise to be effective, it must be routine and done at one's individual capacity.

25. On the basis of this article, one could infer that the main purpose of exercise and physical activity is:

   A. to stop the aging process.
   B. to keep physical development ongoing.
   C. to maintain efficient body functioning.
   D. to keep weight at a minimal level.

26. The human body benefits in many ways from physical exercise, with special benefit to the _____ system:

   A. digestive
   B. skeletal
   C. cardiovascular
   D. all of the above.

27. When selecting the mode of physical activity in which to engage, one should make the paramount concern:

    A. the convenience of a gym or workout facility.
    B. the expense involved in outfitting for the activity.
    C. a partner with whom to engage.
    D. whether the activity is interesting and fun.

28. One of the valuable and interesting products of continued physical activity is:

    A. increased cerebral activity.
    B. fewer chronic illnesses.
    C. less need for vitamins or other medication.
    D. weight maintenance.

29. If this article and its statements are true, then we might infer that an individual who exercises regularly from youth onward might expect:

    A. sustained sexual potency in later life.
    B. a longer and more productive life than those who do not so engage.
    C. the regeneration of skin cells to prohibit drying.
    D. thinness that lasts into later life.

30. From a reading of this article, one might assume that the physical activity to which the author alludes might include:

    A. golf, bowling, and individual exercise.
    B. baseball, swimming, and weight training.
    C. swimming, diving, and surfing.
    D. ice skating, scuba diving, and golf.

31. If one elects *not* to participate in physical activity until quite late in life, there would be the problem of:

    A. no appropriate activities.
    B. lack of equipment.
    C. aging having already set in.
    D. difficulty in finding a gym.

32. A careful reading of this article reveals that physical exercise is:

    A. not as important for males as it is for females.
    B. more difficult for females than males.
    C. less difficult for females than males.
    D. equally important and difficult for females and males.

33. According to the author's criteria, the standard for setting up and maintaining an exercise program should be:

    A. age, gender, location, and finances.
    B. gender, location, finances, and preference.
    C. location, finances, preference, and age.
    D. finances, interest, age, and gender.

34. One of the common myths, according to the author, is that physical exercise:

    A. is only to control weight.
    B. builds bulky muscles.
    C. makes one less vital.
    D. decreases brain power.

PASSAGE 5 (QUESTIONS 35-41)

For years, classified U.S. military satellites have been recording flashes from meteors in the Earth's atmosphere. System operators, more interested in tracking enemy missiles, have paid them little heed, but now the Air Force Space Command is allowing the records of past meteor sightings to be released to scientists, who say they offer a powerful new tool for counting the number of small asteroids raining down on the planet.

The value of these military satellites is that they can easily watch for meteors around the world, even over vast stretches of ocean. And unlike telescopes, they can detect meteors during the day. The satellites "see all the time, essentially 100 percent of Earth's surface," says one of those included with the project. "That capability has just not existed in the scientific community."

Infrared sensors on early-warning satellites routinely detect the explosions of asteroids as the objects scream into the atmosphere. With energy equivalents of up to 20 kilotons of TNT, some of the explosions seen to date match the power of the atom bomb dropped on Hiroshima in World War II. Between 1975 and 1992, satellites recorded 136 such events—and those were only a portion of the explosions that occurred. The satellites are designed to track missiles, not asteroids, and the computers that sift through the data are programmed to weed out signals from meteors. "Unless an operator is looking at his screen, sees this thing happening, and then records it, it gets tossed," says a former physicist who is now a consultant with the space program.

Along with a California congressman, this physicist is leading a campaign to have the satellites keep this data routinely. All it would take, he says, is reprogramming the computers to note the meteor sightings. The brightness of the flash could be programmed in several levels to indicate the size of the comparable force.

The satellites can detect objects the size of a marble as they burn up in the atmosphere, though the computers would likely be programmed to record only the largest events. Most of the explosions seen so far have occurred at altitudes of 18 to 31 miles and are "pretty much evenly distributed around the globe," he says. Based on the amount of energy released, scientists guess that some of the incoming asteroids have been as large as 200 feet in diameter when they broke up. The large number of meteors recorded supports recent ground-based observations suggesting that many more asteroids are crossing Earth's path than once believed—perhaps ten or even 100 times more.

Keeping mum for years about such an exciting research tool has not been easy, according to those who worked on the design of the early-warning satellites. Only recently has permission been obtained from the Air Force's Space Command to make the existing meteor data public. While this is frustrating to those involved in the project, there is a growing awareness of the importance of the mission to the military, as well as to the civilian population. Neither of these should be compromised for the other.

35. According to this article, which of the following would be the best reason for recording this data?

A. Knowing the frequency of these occurrences would help mankind determine the best places to live.

B. Being able to understand the density of the earth's atmosphere would give scientists data for determining the possibility of life on other planets.

C. The data recorded would give information to study in order to determine if and when there might be a danger to the earth and its inhabitants.

D. With the data available, scientists could determine reasons for an increase or a decrease in activity.

36. A reader could infer that the capability of satellites to track meteor flashes has been kept a secret because:

A. the purpose of the satellites is military in nature.

B. Americans might become frightened if they knew about the flashes.

C. meteor flashes can be extremely dangerous.

D. scientists were not interested in small flashes.

37. The equipment available for recording explosions in space can:

A. measure explosions the size of an atomic bomb.

B. detect an explosion the size of a marble.

C. track missiles in space.

D. all of the above.

38. One might conclude from this passage that the author of the selection:

A. feels no need to know how many asteroids enter the earth's atmosphere.

B. is interested in finding uses for the data recorded by satellites in outer space that might hasten peace.

C. is ambivalent about the matter of satellites used for military purposes.

D. supports reprogramming to record asteroid data.

39. According to the article, explosions in space:

A. occur with programmable regularity.

B. vary in altitude from 18 to 31 miles.

C. cause electrical problems in parts of the world.

D. might impact civilized areas.

40. The opinion of scientists, according to this author, has changed to indicate that:

A. more asteroids cross the Earth's path than previously thought.

B. military use of satellites is unfortunate.

C. multiple uses of asteroid data might advance disease control.

D. weeding out signals from meteors actually has no validity.

41. The power of the explosions is illustrated by:

A. the data recorded between 1975 and 1992.

B. the comparison with the atomic bomb.

C. 136 records of such events recorded.

D. all of the above.

PASSAGE 6 (QUESTIONS 42-47)

The years prior to and including those of the Romantic Movement are notable for the beginnings of really serious attempts to improve and correct the spoken language—in other words, to set up a standard of pronunciation. In 1772, William Kendrick published the first dictionary that indicated vowel sounds, and he was quickly copied by both English and American lexicographers. Because many of these men felt that words should be pronounced as they were spelled, there was a tendency to reestablish older pronunciations, especially in respect to unaccented syllables. This was especially true in America, which was establishing an English of its own. Americans rebelled against the pronunciations of Samuel Johnson, long the accepted English authority. Although Johnson's dictionary had indicated no pronunciations, his poetry through its meter made clear which pronunciations he regarded as standard. Thus in his poem "The Vanity of Human Wishes," the following words obviously are to be pronounced with only two syllables: *venturous, treacherous, powerful, general, history, quivering, flattering,* and *slippery.* Yet, with the possible exception of *general,* they were three-syllable words in America.

It was not until the Romantic Age that Greek began to affect the English language directly. Many new philosophic and scientific names were being added to the language. Combining two or more words or roots from Latin or Greek gave the language such words as *barometer* and *thermometer.* Another method of creating new words was adding Greek combining forms, prefixes, and suffixes—such as *micro-* (small), *macro-* (large), *tele-* (far), *per-* (maximum), *-oid* (like), *-ic* (smaller), and *-ous* (larger)—to words already in use. In this manner, words like *microscope, macrocosm, telepathy, peroxide, paratoid, sulphuric,* and *sulphurous* were produced.

Partly as a result of the interest of the romanticists in the Middle Ages, words belonging to the past were reintroduced into the language. The imitation of older ballads revived some archaic words found in such poems. Coleridge uses *eftsoons* for *again, I wis* (from the Middle English *iwis*) for *certainly,* and *een* for *eye.* Keats uses *faeries,* the archaic spelling of *fairies, fay* in place of *faith,* and *sooth* to mean *smooth.* These words, not only old but odd, were scarcely likely to be adopted in conversation, but they served to acquaint readers with the language of England's past. In their search for color, the romanticists also included slang and dialect terms, and although these forms are sparsely used in comparison with their use in literature today, they began to find acceptance in writing. Many of the romanticists like to coin their own words; sometimes, as with *fuzzgig* and *critickasting,* these bordered on the ridiculous.

The romantic writers were concerned with bringing naturalness and simplicity back into the language. Consequently, some of them felt that borrowed or foreign words should be eliminated from the language because they corrupted the mother tongue. This discrimination against foreign words was not widespread, for English had become quite stabilized.

42. The focus of this article is:

    A. the explanation of unusual words used by English writers.

    B. the futility of learning specific words in a new language.

    C. the changing English language during the Romantic Movement.

    D. a language that is in stasis.

43. The author alludes to all of the following EXCEPT:

    A. pronunciation differences.

    B. borrowing words.

    C. poets' use of archaisms.

    D. coining of words.

44. The effect of the Greek language on the English language involves:

    A. philosophic differences.

    B. reintroducing archaic terms into the "modern" language.

    C. increasing the number of syllables in most words.

    D. the field of science.

45. There is evidence in this article to support the theory that:

    A. making English the official language of business is important.

    B. more people speak and read English than any other language.

    C. English is an inferior language.

    D. Americans pronounce certain words with more syllables than others do.

46. One of the ways to create new words is to:

    A. use prefixes.

    B. use suffixes.

    C. use word combinations.

    D. all of the above.

47. The author points out that Romantics use many different forms of language in order to put _____ into their writing:

    A. meaning

    B. color

    C. life

    D. action

PASSAGE 7 (QUESTIONS 48–53)

Most Americans were only slightly surprised when then President Richard M. Nixon declared in February 1970 that "drug misuse is a growing national problem" in which "hundreds of thousands of Americans—young and old alike—endanger their health through the inappropriate use of drugs of all kinds." Recently, the rate of increase in drug consumption has been so great that one federal official estimated that the use of *all* drugs will increase a hundredfold in the next ten years. According to a doctor, "they are practically replacing the function of the virtues in striving for a sane and well-ordered life." Americans are now consuming 1.05 billion gallons of alcoholic beverages each year; pharmacy shelves are brimming with tranquilizers and "uppers," three-fourths of which were unknown in 1950; and stories of the 12-year-old heroin addict and the 16-year-old marijuana dealer are now commonplace. Indeed, many elementary school children are selling drugs and the campuses of elementary and middle schools are profitable sites for the drug dealer of today.

Since drugs have been characterized as any "substance that has an effect on the body or mind," the idea of "drug abuse" is worth defining. Dr. Sidney Cohen, of the

National Institute of Mental Health, writes that "it is the persistent and usually excessive self-administration of any drug which has resulted in psychological or physical dependence, or which deviates from approved social patterns of the culture." The more-serious problem of "addiction" begins when an individual has so "lost the power of self-control with reference to a drug" that the user or society is harmed. Neither state is desirable for the individual or, because he or she is rarely a hermit, for the rest of us.

In any discussion of the "national drug problem," experts usually point first to alcohol. About forty-four out of every 1,000 adults in this country are alcoholics, and up to one half of all arrests each year are for "chronic drunkenness." Other statistics indicate that more than 50 percent of the annual deaths and injuries from automobile accidents across the nation either involve or result from alcohol. Heavy alcohol use is also known to cause permanent brain damage and cirrhosis of the liver, which is the sixth leading cause of death among Americans.

The other side of the picture, of course, is that most people use alcohol safely, understand its benefits as a depressant, and have the judgment and experience to avoid its hazards. The same may be said for other socially approved drugs, such as aspirin, coffee, and cigarettes: the majority of their users do not get into trouble with them. Where clear dangers of misuse exist, they are restricted by law to adults.

In the 1930s, most of the drugs abused today were unknown to the American public. Well over half of all prescriptions filled were based on aspirin, phenacetin, and caffeine, which were combined with codeine, quinine, or belladonna to treat serious ailments. Since then, the achievements of the "miracle" drugs have been worthy of their name, and killers like pneumonia, influenza, diphtheria, whooping cough, and polio have lost their threat. However, the medical laboratories have also succeeded in isolating heroin from the opium poppy, in synthesizing and therefore enabling mass production of the "active" ingredients in many natural mind-drugs like marijuana, in inventing LSD-25 and other hallucinogens, and in creating the stimulants and sedatives that are now consumed by the billions across the nation. The sale of all of these to the general public is either illegal or medically restricted, yet the consumption of these has increased so greatly in the past twenty years that their abuse now constitutes the "national drug problem."

48. The main idea of this article is to:

    A. inform.
    B. describe.
    C. narrate.
    D. tempt.

49. The statement that "according to a doctor, 'they are practically replacing the function of the virtues in striving for a sane and well-ordered life'" refers to the likelihood that drugs:

    A. have a virtuous place in society.
    B. can improve one's life.
    C. have no place in society.
    D. have the potential to change the goals for which people strive.

50. The author of this article introduces alcohol as a drug in order to illustrate that:

   A. alcohol is more harmless than narcotics.

   B. alcohol is just a beginning to real drug use.

   C. it is better to use alcohol than other drugs.

   D. more Americans use drugs than they think they do.

51. The author describes an addiction as:

   A. excessive self-administration of drugs.

   B. psychological dependence on drugs.

   C. physical dependence on drugs.

   D. all of the above.

52. One might infer from reading this article that:

   A. only Americans have a problem with drugs.

   B. illegal sale and use of drugs are a national problem.

   C. drug use begins with alcohol.

   D. the idea of erasing drugs is possible.

53. If the reader accepts the author's premise on the prediction for the next ten years, one might expect society to be:

   A. more permissive about drug use.

   B. less permissive about drug use.

   C. experiencing greater drug use.

   D. experiencing less drug use.

PASSAGE 8 (QUESTIONS 54–59)

A quack may be defined as a boastful pretender to medical skill. A quack is anyone who promises medical benefits that cannot be delivered. Quacks may attempt to go beyond the limits of medical science or the limits of their own training.

While quackery knows no seasons, the popular targets of quackery shift with the major causes of disability. Faithfully tagging behind public awareness of major health concerns are the ''sure cures'' and ''money-saving self-treatments'' of the quacks. There are several major forms of quackery about which a person should be well informed.

Despite the intensive efforts of government agencies to control cancer quackery, millions of dollars are still being spent every year on worthless cancer treatments. Cancer quackery is one of the most tragic of all rackets because many persons with early, curable cancers waste vital time waiting for a worthless remedy to cure their cancer. By the time they seek ethical treatment using standard methods, their cancers have already progressed to an incurable stage. Early treatment by a competent ethical physician can often result in complete cure of a cancer.

There are many examples of cases in which cancer patients have lost valuable time because of quacks. One actual case history is given here.

In this case, a chiropractor was ultimately convicted of second-degree murder in the death of a child he promised to cure of cancer, and is now serving a term of five years to life imprisonment. The patient (later, victim) was an eight-year-old whose mother became concerned about a slight swelling over her daughter's left eye. When the child was taken to UCLA Medical Center, exploratory surgery revealed a tumorous mass in the left orbit, which was diagnosed as an extremely malignant and fast-growing form of cancer. An examination also revealed that there was no evidence of the spread of the cancer to any other part of her body. The parents were told that it was necessary to remove the eye and all the surrounding tissue in the eye orbit. The parents consented to the surgery. But, before it was performed, they met a couple who claimed their own son had been cured of a brain tumor without surgery by the chiropractor. Consulted by phone, the chiropractor gave the parents absolute assurances he could help their daughter (without having seen the child or her medical records). His diagnosis for the cause of the cancer was a "chemical imbalance" that surgery would only make worse. Upon his insistence, the daughter was taken out of the UCLA hospital where, he claimed, the physicians would only use her as a guinea pig and "get their money." His own fee: $500 in advance, plus $200 to $300 per month for medicine! The daughter was immediately examined by the chiropractor and diagnosed as having hypochronic anemia, inflammation of the gallbladder, possible kidney disease, and hyperthyroidism—but no mention of cancer. Treatment included 124 pills (vitamins, food supplements, laxatives) daily, 150 drops of an iodine solution in a glass of water each hour for 11 hours a day, a 2-quart enema every other day, daily musculoskeletal adjustments in his office, and instructions for the parents to manipulate the ball of the daughter's foot daily with sufficient pressure to cause her to cry (which the parents refused to perform).

After over three weeks of "care," the tumor had enlarged to the size of a tennis ball and had pushed the eye out of the socket and down along the nose. The parents discharged the chiropractor and brought their daughter back to UCLA, where her condition was now recognized as hopeless. Four months later, she died.

Cancer quacks often claim to use an effective treatment that is exclusively their own and unavailable to other physicians.

54. The focus of this article is:

    A. cures for cancer.
    B. finding less-expensive treatment.
    C. securing alternative medicines.
    D. the futility of quackery.

55. According to this article, quackery is:

    A. widespread.
    B. changing.
    C. rarely successful.
    D. all of the above.

56. One might infer that when a patient decides to use a physician who is a quack, that patient:

    A. has the chance for a unique treatment.
    B. has a greater chance for successful treatment.
    C. takes responsibility for whatever may happen to him.
    D. undertakes treatment with drugs that are experimental.

57. One might infer that the story of the child with the tumor is used to illustrate that:

    A. promising medical results that cannot be delivered is quackery.
    B. chiropractors are not "real" doctors.
    C. prescribing and advising by telephone is not real "doctoring."
    D. just because a physician promises a certain result does not mean it will happen.

58. With the evidence given here, the reader will conclude that:

    A. quackery is not widespread in the world today.

    B. patients need to be well advised in the choice of a doctor.

    C. medicine taken in large doses can be fatal.

    D. following directions given by telephone is not a good idea.

59. The article implies that officials are attempting to:

    A. license those who are promising more than they can deliver.

    B. test and market the drugs used as alternative medicines.

    C. remind patients of the availability of less-expensive treatments.

    D. reduce the prevalence of quackery.

PASSAGE 9 (QUESTIONS 60–65)

In recent years, early childhood education has been the focus of considerable interest and attention. New programs, curriculum changes, ideas, and empirical data have accumulated at a rapid rate. Early childhood education is thriving and expanding. Within a relatively short span of time, early childhood education has become a major area of emphasis.

In the past decade, the scope and definition of early childhood education have changed considerably. Recently constructed theories offer novel concepts and new approaches to problems. Methods and tools of early childhood education have experienced change. Among the new developments are the widening interest in child-care centers, the emphasis on environmental influences, the cognitive and affective bases for learning, and the establishment of child-development centers. Among current trends in early childhood education, the following are most significant.

The high incidence of mothers working outside the home, beginning in the past two decades and continuously increasing, has created the need for institutions for younger children. Large governmental funding of projects in early childhood education has given impetus to the downward trend, and Title I kindergartens and Head Start programs have emphasized the value of an early start in education. Research supported by federal funds shows that the early years are the most critical for learning and development and that young children can learn much more during this period than was previously expected of them. These factors have drawn national attention to the importance of early childhood education and have caused many states to implement programs of kindergartens and nursery schools. Publicly supported programs of education for three-, four-, and five-year-old children will soon be a part of every state system, and there is a real possibility that public education will reach even younger children.

Since mothers working outside the home have created a pressing need for child-care centers and other preschool arrangements for young children, private institutions and child-care centers have flourished. Many allegedly offer learning experiences or kindergartens, and because there is in many states no educational control over such institutions, quantity is not matched with quality. While some of these centers and organizations strive for excellence, many are substandard and have uneducated teachers who are inadequate to undertake the responsibilities of teaching young children. Only when early childhood education is regulated by state legislation with properly prepared and qualified teachers will the quality of early education be consistent.

Nursery schools for three- and four-year-olds and kindergartens for five-year-olds have traditionally been directed toward either the social development of a child in a permissive atmosphere or toward an intellectual approach with structured learning. Education is now moving away from these narrow views of one or two facets of development to an emphasis on the total development of each individual. All areas—social, emotional, intellectual, and physical—are equally important. No one or two areas can be overemphasized at the expense of the others. The terms "nursery school" or "kindergarten" evoke previously held concepts of their functions, while the term "child-development center" places the emphasis on the total child. This newer term promotes an awareness of the goals of early childhood education. The concept of an educational center places the function of such a center in the proper perspective and enables it to acquire the broad scope necessary to meet all the needs of young children.

Head Start programs all over the country have successfully shown positive results concerning the extent of development that occurs when children are given proper experiences during the period of their greatest growth and development. In these and other experimental programs, children show gains in intelligence quotients over pretest and posttest periods. Studies show that "fixed intelligence" is no longer an absolute concept in education. They have reached the conclusion that intelligence is environmentally modifiable; that, with vital educational experiences in a controlled environment, IQ scores can be raised as much as twenty points. Their studies point to early childhood as the crucial period for intellectual development. These studies have added impetus to the trend of more formal educational programs for younger children.

60. The focus of this selection is:

    A. the importance of state funding for education.

    B. the involvement of the federal government in education.

    C. a decade of education degeneration.

    D. the importance of early intervention for child development.

61. According to the author, the development of a child in the early years will improve the child:

    A. intellectually, emotionally, and physically.

    B. emotionally, physically, and mentally.

    C. physically, mentally, and socially.

    D. all of the above.

62. The IQ of an individual measures an important part of one's development. According to this selection, what effect can the proper early education have on one's IQ?

    A. The IQ can be modified.

    B. The effects on the IQ are inconsequential.

    C. The IQ is not an important part of early education.

    D. One's environment has no effect on IQ.

63. The differences in day care, kindergarten, and child-development centers are:

A. so insignificant that they are inconsequential.
B. determined by the licensing and training of personnel.
C. a matter of semantics.
D. determined by the type of training offered to children.

64. The rise in population of day care, kindergartens, and child-development centers has been caused in part by:

A. the need to socialize children earlier.
B. the popularity of educating at an early age.
C. the rise in women employed.
D. the need for more years of education.

65. Given the advantages of early education, one might infer that without such benefits:

A. young children would learn what they need at home.
B. parents would have the responsibility of preparing their children.
C. federal and state funds would be saved for use in other ways.
D. many children would enter first grade unprepared.

Most questions in the Physical Sciences test are organized into groups, each preceded by a descriptive passage. After studying the passage, select the one best answer to each question in the group. Some questions are not based on a descriptive passage and are also independent of each other. You must also select the one best answer to these questions. If you are not certain of an answer, eliminate the alternatives that you know to be incorrect and then select an answer from the remaining alternatives. A periodic table is provided for your use. You may consult it whenever you wish.

1 H 1.0																	2 He 4.0
3 Li 6.9	4 Be 9.0											5 B 10.8	6 C 12.0	7 N 14.0	8 O 16.0	9 F 19.0	10 Ne 20.2
11 Na 23.0	12 Mg 24.3											13 Al 27.0	14 Si 28.1	15 P 31.0	16 S 32.1	17 Cl 35.5	18 Ar 39.9
19 K 39.1	20 Ca 40.1	21 Sc 45.0	22 Ti 47.9	23 V 50.9	24 Cr 52.0	25 Mn 54.9	26 Fe 55.8	27 Co 58.9	28 Ni 58.7	29 Cu 63.5	30 Zn 65.4	31 Ga 69.7	32 Ge 72.6	33 As 74.9	34 Se 79.0	35 Br 79.9	36 Kr 83.8
37 Rb 85.5	38 Sr 87.6	39 Y 88.9	40 Zr 91.2	41 Nb 92.9	42 Mo 95.9	43 Tc (98)	44 Ru 101.1	45 Rh 102.9	46 Pd 106.4	47 Ag 107.9	48 Cd 112.4	49 In 114.8	50 Sn 118.7	51 Sb 121.8	52 Te 127.6	53 I 126.9	54 Xe 131.3
55 Cs 132.9	56 Ba 137.3	57 La* 138.9	72 Hf 178.5	73 Ta 180.9	74 W 183.9	75 Re 186.2	76 Os 190.2	77 Ir 192.2	78 Pt 195.1	79 Au 197.0	80 Hg 200.6	81 Tl 204.4	82 Pb 207.2	83 Bi 209.0	84 Po (209)	85 At (210)	86 Rn (222)
87 Fr (223)	88 Ra 226.0	89 Ac† 227.0	104 Unq (261)	105 Unp (262)	106 Unh (263)	107 Uns (262)	108 Uno (265)	109 Une (267)									

*	58 Ce 140.1	59 Pr 140.9	60 Nd 144.2	61 Pm (145)	62 Sm 150.4	63 Eu 152.0	64 Gd 157.3	65 Tb 158.9	66 Dy 162.5	67 Ho 164.9	68 Er 167.3	69 Tm 168.9	70 Yb 173.0	71 Lu 175.0
†	90 Th 232.0	91 Pa (231)	92 U 238.0	93 Np (237)	94 Pu (244)	95 Am (243)	96 Cm (247)	97 Bk (247)	98 Cf (251)	99 Es (252)	100 Fm (257)	101 Md (258)	102 No (259)	103 Lr (260)

PASSAGE 1

Examine the following table which compares subatomic particles of several common elements and/or ions.

Symbol	Atomic Number	Atomic Mass	Proton Count	Neutron Count	Electron Count	Ion or Isotope?
K	19	39.0	19	20	19	Isotope
Al	13			14	13	Isotope
Ba^{+2}	56	137.0	56			Ion
		31.0	15		15	Isotope
F^{-1}	9			10		Ion
	12	24.0		12	10	

1. In the table above, to correctly complete the line describing the atomic "arrangement" for Al:

   A. Atomic Mass = 13, Proton Count = 13.
   B. Atomic Mass = 14, Proton Count = 13.
   C. Atomic Mass = 27, Proton Count = 13.
   D. Atomic Mass = 27, Proton Count = 14.

2. In the line describing the Ba^{+2} ion, the correct number of electrons should be:

   A. 56.
   B. 54.
   C. 58.
   D. 137.

3. In the line that shows an unknown species with an atomic mass of 31.0, the correct sequence of entries for Symbol, Atomic Number, and Neutron Count should be:

   A. [P] [15] [16].
   B. [P] [16] [16].
   C. [P^{-3}] [12] [16].
   D. [P] [16] [15].

4. In the line describing the arrangement of the F^{-1} ion, the correct number of protons should be:

   A. 10.
   B. 9.
   C. 8.
   D. 18.

5. The correct "symbol" that should be assigned to the species represented in the final line of the table should be:

   A. Mg.
   B. Ne.
   C. Mg^{+2}.
   D. Cr^{+2}.

6. The correct atomic mass that should be inserted into the box describing F^{-1} in the table is:

   A. 9.
   B. 10.
   C. 18.
   D. 19.

7. In an atom of a stable, "neutral" element, which of the following subatomic particles will be equal?

    A. electrons = protons = neutrons
    B. electrons = protons
    C. protons = neutrons
    D. electrons = neutrons

PASSAGE 2

A cannon is stationed on the top of a cliff 10.0 meters high. It can shoot an artillery shell with a muzzle velocity of 100.0 m/s. It is initially positioned so that the shell leaves the barrel horizontally. At the precise moment that a shell is fired from the cannon, a soldier drops a shell off the edge of the cliff.

8. How does the initial vertical velocity of the two shells compare?

    A. The shell fired from the cannon has a greater initial vertical velocity.
    B. The initial vertical velocities of the two shells are both equal to zero.
    C. The initial vertical velocities of the two shells are equal, but not equal to zero.
    D. They cannot be determined, as the masses of the two shells have not been given.

9. Assuming no loss to friction, how do the travel times of the two shells compare?

    A. The shell fired from the cannon will take a longer time, as it was traveling a longer distance.
    B. The shell fired from the cannon will take a shorter time, as it was traveling faster.
    C. Both shells will hit the ground at the same time.
    D. The heavier shells will hit the ground first.

10. Which shell will have the greater kinetic energy when it hits the ground?

    A. The shell fired from the cannon, assuming they both have equal masses.
    B. The shell dropped by the soldier, assuming they both have equal masses.
    C. They will both be equal, assuming they both have equal masses.
    D. They will both be equal no matter what their respective masses are.

11. The cannon is now raised so that it makes an angle of 30° above the horizontal. Assuming no air resistance, the time the shell takes to reach the ground, as compared to the horizontal position, is:

    A. equal to the time it took when shot from a horizontal position.
    B. greater than the time it took when shot from a horizontal position.
    C. less than the time it took when shot from a horizontal position.
    D. equal to the time the shell took when it was dropped from rest.

12. The angle of the cannon is increased from a horizontal position of 0° to a vertical position of 90°. As the cannon is shot from progressively greater angles, one can say that:

A. the time of flight will be greater and the range greater.

B. the time of flight will be smaller and the range greater.

C. the range will increase and then decrease.

D. the time of flight will increase and then decrease.

13. The cannon is fired from a horizontal position and an identical shell is fired from a vertical position. When the two shells hit the ground, one can say that:

A. the kinetic energy of the horizontal shell is greater.

B. the kinetic energy of the vertical shell is greater.

C. the kinetic energies of the two shells are equal.

D. their respective kinetic energies depend upon the angle it makes with the ground.

PASSAGE 3

Basic chemical reactions can be classified into several categories—including composition, decomposition, single replacement, and double replacement (metathecal). A *balanced* chemical equation is the representation of these chemical reactions and requires not only the mastery of formula writing, but understanding these four basic types of reactions. Answer the following questions regarding balanced chemical equations; assume all balancing coefficients will be integers, i.e., no fractional coefficients.

Note: In all situations, assume that the reaction *is possible*.

14. If sodium chloride is allowed to react with aluminum nitrate, which of the following products will be produced?

A. $NaNO_2 + AlCl_3$

B. $NaNO_3 + AlCl_2$

C. $NaNO + AlCl$

D. $NaNO_3 + AlCl_3$

15. If calcium reacts with phosphoric acid, what is the correct balancing coefficient that will be placed in front of the calcium phosphate in the final balanced equation?

A. 1

B. 2

C. 3

D. 6

16. In the reaction involving magnesium hydroxide with iron (III) chloride, the number assigned to balance the product iron (III) hydroxide will be what?

A. 1

B. 2

C. 3

D. 6

17. Assume the same reaction in the previous question. What will be the correct balancing coefficient placed in front of magnesium chloride in the final balanced equation?

A. 1

B. 2

C. 3

D. 6

18. Another type of chemical reaction is known as "oxidation" (or, simply, burning). When a hydrocarbon is burned, it is, in reality, combining with oxygen, and the products will be carbon dioxide and water. If the chemical propane {C_3H_8} is burned in a stream of oxygen, what will be the balancing numbers assigned to oxygen, carbon dioxide, and water (in that order) in the final equation?

A. 10 3 4
B. 5 3 4
C. 5 6 4
D. 5 3 8

19. A type of double replacement reaction is known as neutralization, and most chemistry students know that an acid mixed with a base will result in the formation of a salt and water. If phosphorous acid is mixed with calcium hydroxide, predict the formula, along with the correct balancing coefficient, that will be assigned to the resulting salt produced:

A. $2Ca_3(PO_3)_2$
B. $1Ca_3(PO_3)_2$
C. $2CaPO_3$
D. $1Ca_3(PO_4)_2$

20. Xenon hexafluoride is a fairly unstable compound that decomposes readily into its component elements. After writing a balanced equation for this decomposition, what balancing coefficient will be assigned to fluorine in the final balanced equation?

A. 1
B. 2
C. 3
D. 6

Questions 21 through 25 are **NOT** based on a descriptive passage.

21. A hot air balloon has volume of 80 cubic meters, and mass of 300 kg. The density of the air surrounding the balloon is 1 kg/m^3. What is the buoyant force on the balloon by the air? (let the gravitational field be g = 10 m/sec^2.)

A. 800 Newtons
B. 3,000 Newtons
C. 24,000 Newtons
D. 960,000 Newtons

22. 6.1 moles of boiling hot tea sits in an insulated coffee cup. After 0.1 mole of tea boils off, what is the temperature of the remaining water?

Note:
The specific heat capacity of the tea is
$$15 \frac{cal}{mole\ kelvin}.$$

The latent heat of vaporization is
$$9000 \frac{cal}{mole}.$$

The latent heat of fusion is 1800 $\frac{cal}{mole}$.

A. 2 Kelvin, increase
B. 2 Kelvin, decrease
C. 10 Kelvin, increase
D. 10 Kelvin, decrease

23. The graphs shown represent experimental data for four devices (labeled 1, 2, 3, and 4). The potential difference across a device and the current through it were measured. (Positive currents flow from left to right through the device, and negative currents flow from right to left. Positive potentials have higher potential on the left.) Which of the devices obey Ohm's law?

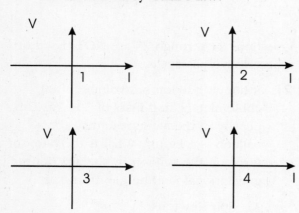

A. 1 and 2
B. 2 and 4
C. 1 and 3
D. 1, 3, and 4

24. Sinusoidal AC voltage is applied to a water heater. The plot of voltage across the heater as a function of time is shown. Also shown is a plot of the current through the water heater as a function of time. What is the average power being absorbed by the heater?

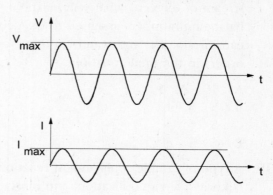

A. $P = \dfrac{I_{max}V_{max}}{2}$ Watts

B. $P = \dfrac{I_{max}V_{max}}{\sqrt{2}}$ Watts

C. $P = \sqrt{2}I_{max}V_{max}$ Watts

D. $P = 2I_{max}V_{max}$ Watts

25. A truck loses its brakes while traveling at 30 m/sec. The driver steers it up a hill and coasts to a stop. Ignore friction and calculate how high the truck rises before it stops:

A. 1.4 m
B. 3.0 m
C. 46.0 m
D. 450.0 m

PASSAGE 4

Stoichiometry is defined as the quantitative measurement of the amounts of elements and/or compounds involved in a chemical change. The chemical change is written in the form of a balanced chemical equation that represents accurately the ratios in which the chemicals react. Examine the following balanced chemical reactions in the equations below:

A. $2\ KClO_3 \Rightarrow 2\ KCl + 3\ O_2$

B. $2\ C_2H_4 + 7\ O_2 \Rightarrow 4\ CO_2 + 6\ H_2O$

C. $MgCl_2 + 2\ NaOH \Rightarrow Mg(OH)_2 + 2\ NaCl$

D. $2\ Al + 3\ H_2SO_4 \Rightarrow 3\ H_2 + Al_2(SO_4)_3$

E. $Ca + Cl_2 \Rightarrow CaCl_2$

Note: Use these values for atomic/molecular masses in the following problems.

Potassium chlorate 122.5 g/mol
Potassium chloride 74.5 g/mol
Ethene 28.0 g/mol
Oxygen 32.0 g/mol
Carbon dioxide 44.0 g/mol
Water 18.0 g/mol
Magnesium chloride 95.0 g/mol
Sodium hydroxide 40.0 g/mol
Magnesium hydroxide 58.0 g/mol
Sodium chloride 58.5 g/mol
Aluminum 27.0 g/mol
Sulfuric acid 98.0 g/mol
Hydrogen 2.0 g/mol
Aluminum sulfate 342.0 g/mol
Calcium 40.0 g/mol
Chlorine 71.0 g/mol
Calcium chloride 111.0 g/mol
Carbon 12.0 g/mol

26. Based on reaction A in the previous column, if 3.4 moles of potassium chlorate would decompose completely, how many moles and grams of oxygen will be produced?

    A. 5.1 moles, 163.2 grams
    B. 3.0 moles, 96.0 grams
    C. 5.1 moles, 81.6 grams
    D. 2.0 moles, 64.0 grams

27. Based on equation B in the previous column, how many grams of oxygen are needed to react completely with 4.0 moles of ethene?

    A. 14.0 grams
    B. 448.0 grams
    C. 224.0 grams
    D. 128.0 grams

28. Based on equation C in the previous column, how many grams of sodium hydroxide will be needed to produce 58.5 grams of sodium chloride?

    A. 80.0 grams
    B. 40.0 grams
    C. 20.0 grams
    D. 160.0 grams

29. See equation D in the previous column. Given 100 grams of aluminum and an unlimited supply of sulfuric acid, how many moles of hydrogen gas will be liberated?

    A. 100 moles
    B. 6.0 moles
    C. 11.1 moles
    D. 5.55 moles

30. Based on the previous question, what volume will the hydrogen gas occupy (assume S.T.P. conditions)?

    A. 22.4 liters
    B. 44.8 liters
    C. 124.32 liters
    D. 134.4 liters

31. See equation E on page 301. If 75.0 grams of calcium are combined with 75.0 grams of chlorine, how many grams of calcium chloride will be produced?

    A. 75.0 grams
    B. 1.87 grams
    C. 207.57 grams
    D. 117.66 grams

PASSAGE 5

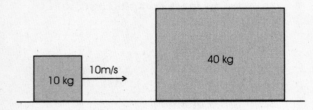

32. A block of mass 10 kg moving to the right with a velocity of 10 m/s collides with a block of mass 40 kg at rest. The two blocks stick together and move off as a unit. This type of collision is known as a(n):

    A. elastic collision.
    B. inelastic collision.
    C. partially elastic collision.
    D. momentous collision.

33. In the above problem, after the two blocks collide and move off together, their velocity will be:

    A. 10 m/s.
    B. 5 m/s.
    C. 2 m/s.
    D. zero.

34. The total momentum of the system before they collide is:

    A. 500 kg m/s.
    B. 250 kg m/s.
    C. 100 kg m/s.
    D. zero.

35. The total momentum of the system after they collide is:

    A. smaller than the total momentum before they collide and in the same direction.
    B. equal in magnitude to the momentum before they collide but in the opposite direction.
    C. the same in both magnitude and direction to the momentum before they collide.
    D. zero.

36. If the two blocks do not stick together after they collide, but instead undergo a perfectly elastic collision, we can say that:

    A. the velocities of the two blocks would still be the same as if they had stuck together.
    B. the 10 kg block would be moving toward the left, and the 40 kg block would be at rest.
    C. they would both be moving toward the right, but with different velocities.
    D. the 10 kg block would be moving toward the right, and the 40 kg block would be moving toward the left.

PASSAGE 6

A container filled with ice at −10°C is placed upon a hot iron block of equal mass at a temperature of 300°C. The system is completely insulated from its surroundings.

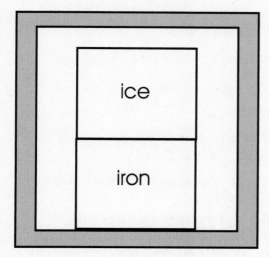

37. One will notice that, as time goes by, the:

A. temperature of both the iron and the ice will remain constant.
B. temperature of the iron will decrease and the temperature of the ice will increase.
C. temperature of the iron will increase and the temperature of the ice will decrease.
D. temperature of both the iron and the ice will decrease.

38. You notice that the change in temperature of the ice is smaller than the change in temperature of the iron. This implies that the:

A. specific heat of the ice is greater than that of the iron.
B. specific heat of the ice is smaller than that of the iron.
C. iron is at a much higher temperature than the ice.
D. system is not completely insulated and heat is leaking through.

39. As the temperature of the iron decreases, one will notice that the:

A. temperature of the ice will continue to increase even after it starts to melt.
B. temperature of the ice will increase until it starts to melt and then remain constant.
C. temperature of the ice will remain constant.
D. temperature of the iron will decrease until the ice starts to melt and then remain constant.

40. After the system has come to equilibrium we can say:

A. the temperature of the whole system will be uniform.
B. the heat lost by the iron will equal the heat gained by the ice.
C. the change in temperature of the water will have been equal to the change in temperature of the iron.
D. both A and B.

41. As the ice melts the:

    A. temperature of the ice remains constant and the temperature of the iron decreases.

    B. temperature of the ice remains constant and the temperature of the iron remains constant.

    C. temperature of the ice increases and the temperature of the iron decreases.

    D. temperature of the ice increases and the temperature of the iron remains the same.

42. Suppose the mass of the iron block is doubled while its initial temperature remains the same. We can say that when the system reaches equilibrium the:

    A. heat lost by the iron will have been equal to twice the heat gained by the water.

    B. heat lost by the iron will have been equal to the heat gained by the water.

    C. equilibrium temperature will be the same as before.

    D. change in temperature of the iron will have been equal to twice the change in the temperature of the water.

Questions 43 through 47 are **NOT** based on a descriptive passage.

43. Which of the following is not an integral part of the genetic code found in DNA?

    A. histone

    B. purine or pyrimidine base

    C. 5-carbon sugar

    D. a phosphate

44. Synthesis of proteins takes place in the:

    A. nucleolus.

    B. Golgi bodies.

    C. ribosomes.

    D. endoplasmic reticulum.

45. RNA base-pairing could be all of the following except:

    A. A – T

    B. G – C

    C. A – U

    D. C – G

46. Which of the following is a single substitution reaction?

    A. silver reacting with atmospheric oxygen

    B. sodium hydroxide reacting with hydrochloric acid

    C. copper reacting with silver nitrate

    D. hydrogen reacting with oxygen to form water

47. Which of the following would indicate an acid?

    A. $[H+] = 1 \times 10^7$ mol/L

    B. $[H+] = 1 \times 10^{-7}$ mol/L

    C. $[H+] = 1 \times 10^{-10}$ mol/L

    D. $[H+] = 1 \times 10^{-3}$ mol/L

PASSAGE 7

A beam of light traveling through air with index of refraction $n_1 = 1.00$ makes an angle of q_1 with the normal. It then travels through water with index of refraction $n_2 = 1.33$ and makes an angle of q_2 with the normal.

48. The speed of light through water is equal to:

A. 3.00×10^8 m/s.

B. 4.00×10^8 m/s.

C. 2.25×10^8 m/s.

D. 1.29×10^8 m/s.

49. As the angle of incidence q_1 increases to 90 degrees, the angle of refraction q_2:

A. increases to 90 degrees.

B. increases, but to an angle less than 90 degrees.

C. decreases to zero degrees.

D. decreases, but to an angle less than zero degrees.

50. If the angle of incidence $q_1 = 30$ degrees, then the angle of refraction q_2 is equal to:

A. 22.0 degrees.

B. 41.7 degrees.

C. 48.8 degrees.

D. 25.0 degrees.

51. If the index of refraction n_1 were increased slightly to 1.1 and the angle of incidence and the index of refraction n_2 were kept the same, the angle of refraction would:

A. increase, but not as much as the angle of incidence.

B. increase more than the angle of incidence.

C. decrease.

D. remain the same.

52. A beam of light is now traveling in the opposite direction from water into air. What is the critical angle for the water-air interface?

A. 48.6 degrees

B. 30.0 degrees

C. 90.0 degrees

D. 41.7 degrees

53. If the beam of light traveling from water to air struck the interface at an angle greater than the critical angle, then:

A. the angle of refraction would be 90 degrees.

B. the angle of refraction would be less than 90 degrees.

C. the angle of refraction would be zero degrees.

D. there would be no refraction, but total internal reflection.

PASSAGE 8

The term "mole" is a key concept in understanding many quantitative problems in chemistry. It has several definitions:

A. One mole of anything contains Avogadro's number (6.02×10^{23}) of particles.

B. One mole of an element contains Avogadro's number of atoms, and will have a mass equivalent to its atomic mass expressed in grams.

C. One mole of any compound will contain Avogadro's number of molecules, and will have a mass equivalent to its molecular mass expressed in grams.

D. One mole of any gas will contain Avogadro's number of particles and will occupy a volume of 22.4 liters at S.T.P. (Standard Temperature is 0 degrees Celsius or 273 degrees Kelvin and Standard Pressure is 760 torr or 1 atmosphere.)

Answer the following questions, which require a thorough knowledge of the mole concept with respect to Avogadro's number.

Note: Use the following molecular masses where needed:

calcium hydroxide =	74.0 grams/mole
magnesium phosphate =	262.0 grams/mole
sodium hydroxide =	40.0 grams/mole
oxygen =	32.0 grams/mole
magnesium hydroxide =	58.0 grams/mole
carbon dioxide =	44.0 grams/mole

54. 222.0 grams of calcium hydroxide will contain approximately how many oxygen atoms?

A. 6.0
B. 3.6×10^{23}
C. 3.6×10^{24}
D. 1.8×10^{24}

55. 3.2 moles of magnesium phosphate will contain approximately how many magnesium atoms?

A. 3.2×10^{23}
B. 1.04×10^{24}
C. 5.8×10^{24}
D. 9.6

56. 7.3×10^{24} molecules of sodium hydroxide will contain approximately how many total atoms?

A. 7.3×10^{24}
B. 1.5×10^{24}
C. 1.8×10^{24}
D. 2.2×10^{25}

57. Using the information in the previous questions, calculate the approximate *mass* of the sodium hydroxide.

A. 485.1 grams
B. 48.5 grams
C. 48.1 kg
D. 970.2 grams

58. 7.5×10^{23} atoms of oxygen gas will have what approximate mass?

A. 19.9 grams
B. 39.9 grams
C. 9.95 grams
D. 79.6 grams

59. How many *total* atoms can be found in 29.0 grams of magnesium hydroxide?

A. 5.0
B. 6.02×10^{23}
C. 3.01×10^{23}
D. 1.5×10^{24}

60. Using the information in the previous question, how many oxygen atoms would be found?

A. 6.02×10^{23}
B. 3.01×10^{23}
C. 1.5×10^{24}
D. 2.0

PASSAGE 9

Examine the data presented in the *reaction mechanism* graphs below.

Note: The ordinate is calibrated in kJ and is a measure of the energy of the reacting species, and the abscissa, the reaction coordinate.

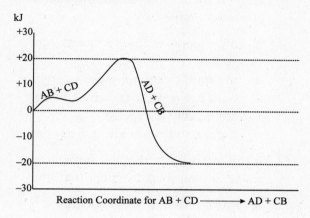

Reaction Coordinate for AB + CD ⟶ AD + CB

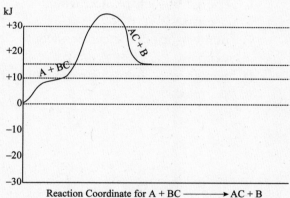

Reaction Coordinate for A + BC ⟶ AC + B

61. Based on graph A above, complete the following statement: "Graph A represents an _____ reaction, with an activation energy of approximately _____ kJ."

   A. endothermic, +40
   B. exothermic, +20
   C. endothermic, −20
   D. exothermic, +60

62. The ΔH (heat of reaction) for the reaction represented by graph A above is approximately _____ kJ.

   A. +20
   B. 0
   C. −20
   D. −40

63. The total amount of heat liberated by the equation represented by graph A above is approximately _____ kJ.

   A. 10
   B. 20
   C. 30
   D. 40

64. The reaction represented by graph B is an example of an _____ reaction, which has an activation energy of approximately _____ kJ.

   A. exothermic, 0
   B. endothermic, +35
   C. endothermic, +15
   D. exothermic, +10

65. The ΔH (heat of reaction) of the reaction represented by graph B is approximately _____ kJ.

   A. 35 kJ
   B. 20 kJ
   C. 15 kJ
   D. −15 kJ

66. The total amount of heat required for the reaction represented by equation B above is approximately _____ kJ.

   A. 10
   B. 15
   C. 20
   D. 40

PASSAGE 10

Photons of wavelength λ_1 = 500 nm impinge on a metal in a vacuum. It is noticed that photoelectrons emerge from the metal with a maximum energy of 1.48 electron volts. Another beam of photons with the same intensity as the first beam but with wavelength λ_2 = 400 nm impinges on the metal. A third beam of photons with λ = 600 nm and with a greater intensity than the second beam is then shined on the metal's surface.

67. Comparing the velocities of the three beams of light we can say that the:

- A. velocities of all three beams are equal.
- B. velocity of the first beam is greater than the other two.
- C. velocities of the second and third beams are equal and greater than the first beam.
- D. velocities of all three beams are different.

68. What is the frequency of the photons in the first beam?

- A. 6×10^{14} Hz
- B. 1.67×10^{-15} Hz
- C. 150 Hz
- D. 1.5×10^{11} Hz

69. The energy of a photon in the first beam is:

- A. 2.48 electron volts.
- B. 5×10^{-19} joules.
- C. greater than the energy of a photon in the second beam.
- D. equal to the energy of a photon in either the second or third beam.

70. What is the work function of the metal?

- A. 1.48 electron volts
- B. 1.00 electron volt
- C. 2.48 electron volts
- D. 3.11 electron volts

71. Compared to the photoelectrons emitted by the first beam, the photoelectrons emitted by:

- A. the second beam are more energetic.
- B. the third beam are more energetic.
- C. both the second and third beams are equally energetic.
- D. the second beam are less energetic.

72. If the intensity of the first beam were reduced, you would expect that the:

- A. work function would decrease.
- B. energy of each photon would decrease.
- C. number of photoelectrons would decrease.
- D. energy of a photoelectron would decrease.

Questions 73 through 77 are **NOT** based on a descriptive passage.

73. Two simple pendulums swing as shown in the accompanying figure. The shorter pendulum has a maximum swing of 40 degrees, while the longer has a maximum swing of 20 degrees. The period of the shorter pendulum is 0.5 seconds. What is the period of the longer pendulum?

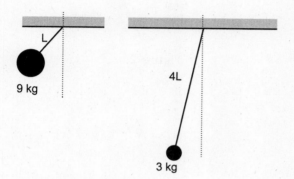

A. 0.5 seconds
B. 1.0 seconds
C. 10 seconds
D. 12 seconds

74. An isotope has a half-life of 3 years. If one starts with 80 grams of this isotope, how long will it take for the sample to decay so that only 10 grams are left?

A. 24 years
B. 12 years
C. 9 years
D. 6 years

75. Two liquids are tested by having a light ray traveling in the liquid impinge upon a block of glass. The results of two such measurements are sketched in the figure. Which material has the lowest index of refraction?

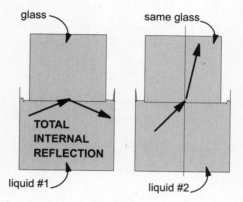

A. liquid #1
B. liquid #2
C. glass
D. Cannot be determined with data given.

76. A ball rolls off a horizontal table with initial velocity 5 m/sec, towards the right. It falls 1.2 meters to the floor. Just before it hits the floor, what are the vertical and horizontal components of its velocity?

A. 5 m/sec to the *right* and 4.85 m/sec *down*
B. 0 m/sec to the *right* and 5 m/sec *down*
C. 0 m/sec to the *right* and 11.76 m/sec *down*
D. 5 m/sec to the *right* and 11.76 m/sec *down*

77. An object is imaged by a concave mirror whose focal point is shown. Which of the diagrams in the figure is the correct ray diagram to locate the image?

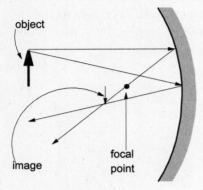

Figure 1

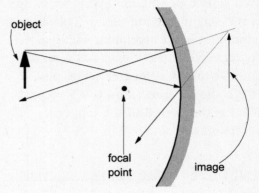

Figure 2

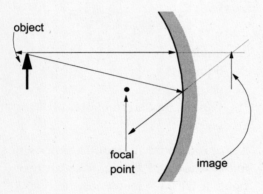

Figure 3

A. Figure 1
B. Figure 2
C. Figure 3
D. No true image is formed.

WRITING SAMPLE 1

In one's personal life, politics is a no-win situation.

Write a unified essay in which you perform the following tasks: explain what you think the statement means; describe specific situations in which politics invade one's personal life; discuss ways that the statement may not be true for those aspiring to a career in politics; provide evidence of what this means to today's society and the political ramifications therefrom; conclude with a justification of the positive or negative implications.

WRITING SAMPLE 2

Many authorities profess the opinion that a two-income family is really detrimental to the traditional home.

Write a unified essay in which you perform the following tasks: explain what you think the statement means; describe specific situations in which having both partners in a marriage employed may be detrimental to family life; discuss ways that the statement may not be proven; provide some evidence of what this means to today's society; conclude with a justification of the positive or negative implications.

Most questions in the Biological Sciences test are organized into groups, each preceded by a descriptive passage. After studying the passage, select the one best answer to each question in the group. Some questions are not based on a descriptive passage and are also independent of each other. You must also select the one best answer to these questions. If you are not certain of an answer, eliminate the alternatives that you know to be incorrect and then select an answer from the remaining alternatives.

PASSAGE 1 (QUESTIONS 1–5)

The interdependency of systems is most evident in the cardiovascular and respiratory systems of humans. The heart, our major organ of circulation, is intimately connected to all cells in the body and in particular, those of the respiratory system. Working in concert with each other, they harmoniously help the body get rid of carbon dioxide and take in oxygen to satisfy the demands of aerobic respiration.

1. In closed circulation systems:

   A. circulation stems from contractions of the dorsal vessel and body movements.
   B. relaxation of the dorsal vessel brings blood into the vessels.
   C. blood bathes internal organs while moving through the sinuses.
   D. contraction of the dorsal vessel sends blood into the vessels.

2. Veins carry:

   A. blood away from the heart.
   B. blood to the heart.
   C. oxygenated blood.
   D. deoxygenated blood.

3. The left ventricle pumps blood:

   A. to the body.
   B. to the lungs.
   C. from the lungs.
   D. from the body.

4. Gases in the alveoli are exchanged with gases in the pulmonary capillaries by:

   A. diffusion.
   B. osmosis.
   C. active transport.
   D. pinocytosis.

5. Air is moved into the human lungs:

   A. if the pressure gradient is equalized.
   B. when the diaphragm is relaxed.
   C. when the diaphragm is contracted.
   D. in between heart beats.

PASSAGE 2 (QUESTIONS 6–11)

You are working in a research laboratory where a senior scientist has just made a major breakthrough by determining the amino acid sequence of an important enzyme fraction. Your task is to verify his results. There are several methods available:

Acid hydrolysis—this will hydrolyze the peptide into its constituent amino acids, after which they can be identified and the ratios determined.

Cyanogen bromide treatment—cleaves the peptide bond on the C side of a methionine residue (molecule).

Trypsin digestion—cleaves on the C side of lysine and arginine residues.

Edman degradation—cleaves the N-terminal amino acid, which can be separated and identified. This process can be performed repeatedly.

You believe part of the peptide has the following amino acid sequence: Alanine-Lysine-Leucine-Serine-Glycine-Alanine-Lysine-Methionine-Methionine-Arginine. This sequence is normally written in the following abbreviated form:

Ala-Lys-Leu-Ser-Gly-Ala-Lys-Met-Met-Arg

6. The above peptide is processed and the following fragments isolated. Which methods were used?

   Ala-Lys-Leu-Ser-Gly-Ala-Lys-Met, Met, Arg

   A. cyanogen bromide treatment
   B. trypsin digestion
   C. both A and B
   D. neither A nor B

7. You obtain the following fragments. Which methods were used?

   Ala, Lys, Leu-Ser-Gly-Ala-Lys, Met-Met-Arg

   A. Edman degradation and trypsin digestion
   B. Trypsin digestion followed by acid hydrolysis
   C. Cyanogen bromide treatment
   D. None of the above.

8. Which of the following peptide fragments could have been produced from the parent peptide using the above methods?

   A. Ala, Leu-Ser-Gly-Ala-Lys-Met-Met-Arg, Leu
   B. Ala-Lys-Leu-Ser, Gly-Ala-Lys-Met, Arg, Met
   C. Ala-Lys, Leu-Ser-Gly-Ala-Lys-Met-Met-Arg
   D. Ala-Lys-Leu-Ser-Gly-Ala, Lys-Met, Met-Arg

9. You obtain the following fragments after cyanogen bromide and trypsin treatment:

   Ala-Lys, Leu-Ser-Gly-Ala-Lys, Met, Arg

   How would you determine if these data are consistent with your original hypothesis about the structure of the peptide?

   A. Perform an Edman treatment to determine if the Ala-Lys fragment is actually a part of the Leu-Ser-Gly-Ala-Lys fragment.
   B. These data are consistent with the original theory, and no further work is required.
   C. Perform acid hydrolysis, then determine the molar ratios of the individual amino acids.
   D. It cannot be determined.

10. Which of the following fragments cannot be obtained using the above methods alone or in sequence?

A. Ala, Lys-Leu, Ser-Gly-Ala-Lys-Met, Met, Arg

B. Ala, Lys, Leu, Ser-Gly-Ala-Lys-Met, Met, Arg

C. Ala, Lys, Leu-Ser-Gly-Ala-Lys, Met, Met, Arg

D. Ala, Gly, Lys, Leu, Ser, Met, Arg

11. Trypsin is normally secreted into the small intestine by the vertebrate pancreas. At what pH would optimum activity be expected?

A. 2
B. 4
C. 6
D. 8

PASSAGE 3 (QUESTIONS 12–18)

An important milestone in biology was the proposal of the operon model in 1961 by François Jacob and Jacques Monod. An operon is a group of adjacent genes controlled by a protein repressor molecule, as shown in this diagram of the lac operon:

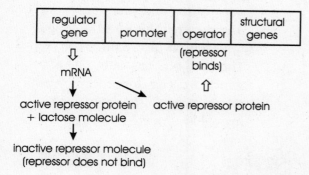

The structural genes are responsible for coding for the three enzymes produced when lactose is present.

12. The operon model explains gene regulation in:

A. eukaryotes.
B. prokaryotes.
C. all organisms.
D. only the bacterium Escherichia coli (E. coli).

13. Lactose is the _____ of the lac operon.

A. inducer
B. substrate
C. promoter
D. repressor

14. When lactose is present, the:

I. repressor molecule cannot bind to the operator.

II. structural genes that code for the enzymes are transcribed and mRNA is made.

III. active repressor molecule binds to lactose.

IV. cell can metabolize lactose.

Which of these statements are true?

A. I, II, and IV
B. I, II, and III
C. II, III, and IV
D. I, II, III, and IV

15. The enzyme genes in the lac operon are transcribed into mRNA when the cell:

A. needs lactate.
B. needs lactose.
C. has access to lactate.
D. has access to lactose.

16. The repressor molecule binds to the operator region and prevents transcription by:

A. preventing attachment of RNA polymerase.

B. blocking enzyme action through allosteric inhibition.

C. preventing attachment of DNA polymerase.

D. blocking the attachment of RNA polymerase at the regulator gene.

17. The trp operon is different from the lac operon in that the trp operon is:

A. inducible.

B. transcribed.

C. repressible.

D. suppressed.

18. The trp operon is repressed when:

A. lactose binds to the inactive repressor protein.

B. a tryptophan molecule binds to the operator region.

C. the inactive repressor protein is made active by binding to tryptophan.

D. the structural genes are being transcribed.

Questions 19–23 are **NOT** based on a descriptive passage.

19. True associations of the optic nerve of the eye are all of the following EXCEPT:

A. the ganglion cell layer fibers gather to form the optic nerve, CN II.

B. the optic disk is a blind spot on the retina.

C. fibers from the opposite optic nerve cross at the optic chiasm.

D. all of the above are true of the optic nerve.

20. The vestibular apparatus consists of all of the following EXCEPT:

A. saccule, macula, hairs of the sensory cell, and gelatinous otolithic.

B. saccule, macula, cochlea, gelatinous otolithic, and linear acceleration.

C. 3 semicircular canals, crista, and rotation.

D. utricle, macula, hairs of the sensory cell, and gelatinous otolithic.

21. The correct matches are in which one of the following?

A. incus, malleus, tensor tympani muscle, first pharyngeal arch, CN V

B. middle ear, inner surface eardrum, Eustachian tube, first pharyngeal arch

C. stapes, stapedius muscle, first pharyngeal arch, CN VII

D. external auditory canal, external surface eardrum, first pharyngeal arch

22. All but one of the following are true about the sense of taste:

A. The four basic tastes are sweet, salty, bitter, and sour.

B. Anterior two thirds of the tongue taste sensory nerve fiber CN V.

C. The taste bud has cells, one of which is a gustatory receptor cell.

D. Motor nerve to the tongue is the hypoglossal nerve (CN XII).

23. All but one of the following are true statements about the posterior pituitary:

A. A downgrowth from the brain forms the posterior lobe.
B. It secretes antidiuretic hormone and vasopressin.
C. Hypothalamus secretion by way of secretory neurons.
D. ADH makes the collecting ducts of the kidney more permeable to water.

PASSAGE 4 (QUESTIONS 24–30)

During glycolysis, the sugar glucose is converted into pyruvate (pyruvic acid) which is then fed into the Krebs cycle or turned into lactate or alcohol and carbon dioxide during fermentation. The process is summarized below. Use this diagram to help answer the questions.

GLUCOSE
1. ⇓
glucose-6-phosphate

STAGE I   2. ⇓
fructose-6-phosphate
3. ⇓
fructose-1, 6-diphosphate
4. ⇓
glyceraldehyde phosphate (2 molecules)

STAGE II   5. ⇓
1, 3-diphosphoglycerate (2 molecules)
6. ⇓
3-phosphoglycerate (2 molecules)
7. ⇓
2-phosphoglycerate (2 molecules)
8. ⇓
phosphoenol pyruvate (2 molecules)
9. ⇓
PYRUVATE (2 molecules)

24. How many moles of oxygen are used per mole of glucose during glycolysis?

A. 0
B. 1
C. 2
D. 4

25. At which steps (1–9) is ATP used?

A. 1 and 2
B. 1 and 3
C. 1, 3, and 5
D. 1 and 5

26. In summary, what is carried out in stages I and II of glycolysis?

I. In stage I, glucose is broken down into two three-carbon phosphate molecules, using ATP in the process.
II. In stage I, glucose is broken down into two three-carbon molecules, using ATP and NADH in the process.
III. In stage II, glyceraldehyde phosphate molecules are converted into pyruvate with the accompanying generation of ATP.
IV. In stage II, glyceraldehyde phosphate molecules are converted into pyruvate with the accompanying generation of ATP and NADH.
V. In stage II, glyceraldehyde phosphate molecules are converted into pyruvate using NADH, with the accompanying generation of ATP.

A. I and V
B. II and IV
C. I and IV
D. I and III

27. Are glyceraldehyde phosphate molecules oxidized or reduced during glycolysis?

A. The glyceraldehyde phosphate molecules are reduced, since they lose hydrogen atoms and electrons used to oxidize NAD+.

B. The glyceraldehyde phosphate molecules are oxidized, since they lose hydrogen atoms and electrons used to reduce NAD+.

C. The glyceraldehyde phosphate molecules are oxidized, since they lose hydrogen atoms and electrons used to oxidize NADH.

D. The glyceraldehyde phosphate molecules are reduced, since they lose hydrogen atoms and electrons used to oxidize NADH.

28. What is the correct empirical formula for glucose?

A. $C_{12}H_{22}O_5$
B. $C_6H_{12}O_6$
C. $C_3H_4O_3$
D. $C_6H_{12}O_6N_2$

29. ATP is made in glycolysis by:

A. chemiosmotic phosphorylation.
B. substrate-level phosphorylation.
C. photophosphorylation.
D. using ATPase.

30. Under anaerobic conditions in muscles, what is the end product of glycolysis?

A. pyruvate
B. acetyl-CoA
C. lactate
D. CO_2 and H_2O

PASSAGE 5 (QUESTIONS 31–36)

The most distinguishing characteristic of muscle tissue is its ability to convert chemical energy in the form of ATP into mechanical energy and in so doing, produce, exert, and direct forces. This provides the capacity for movement, both internally and externally. Three types of muscle tissue exist in the human body: cardiac, smooth, and striate (skeletal). Cardiac and smooth muscle are primarily responsible for the movement of matter through the body, such as the circulation of the blood or movement of food through the digestive tract. The skeletal muscle is responsible for movements of the body in the external environment, such as locomotion.

31. Two important contributions to the function of skeletal muscle produced by its associated connective tissue sheaths are the delivery of force to the origin and insertion of the muscle and the isolation of individual muscle fibers (cells). Which of the following is not a connective tissue sheath found in muscle?

A. periostium
B. perimysium
C. endomysium
D. epimysium

32. Which of the following best describes the characteristics of a skeletal muscle fiber?

   A. greatly elongated, multinucleate, has a striate appearance due to the bundles of myofibrils that fill the cell

   B. uninucleate or binucleate, often branched, contains intercalated discs, has irregular striations

   C. uninucleate, fusiform, has gap junctions, has no striations

   D. None of the above are correct.

33. Myofibrils of skeletal muscle fibers contain myofilaments which construct sarcomeres, the functional unit of a muscle cell. The two types of myofilaments are thick and thin. Which is not a component of thin myofilaments?

   A. globular actin

   B. troponin

   C. myosin

   D. tropomyosin

34. The function of transverse tubules (T-tubules) in muscle contraction is to:

   A. store glycogen.

   B. transmit the action (muscle) potential from the sarcolemma to the sarcoplasmic reticulum.

   C. store and release Ca^{++} ions.

   D. produce an anchor for the actin myofilaments.

35. The site of motor neuron activation of skeletal muscles occurs at the _____, which will contain _____.

   A. sarcomere, myofilaments

   B. T-tubule, Ca^{++}

   C. myoneural junction, chemically mediated Na^+ gates

   D. sarcolemma, voltage mediated Na^+ gates

36. What is a tetanic contraction?

   A. a single muscle twitch

   B. increases in muscle tension due to summation

   C. the absence of shortening

   D. a smooth, sustained contraction due to rapid stimulation

PASSAGE 6 (QUESTIONS 37–41)

Tissues are defined as groups of cells with common structure and function. There are four main categories: connective, epithelial, muscle, and nervous. Within each type of tissue, there are specialized levels of cells forming specialized "sub-tissues" such as skeletal, visceral, and cardiac tissue in the system of muscle tissues.

37. Which of the following is *not* a type of connective tissue?

   A. bone and blood

   B. loose

   C. adipose

   D. squamous

38. Tissue that contains cells capable of contraction is:

   A. nervous tissue.

   B. muscle tissue.

   C. epithelial tissue.

   D. connective tissue.

39. In all but the simplest of animals, tissues are organized into:

   A. systems.

   B. organs.

   C. cells.

   D. organisms.

40. The ability to secrete as well as absorb is most likely associated with which tissue?

   A. adipose
   B. visceral
   C. fibrous connective
   D. epithelial

41. Which of the following is most true about organ systems?

   A. They are interdependent and part of an organism that is greater than the sum of its parts.
   B. They are suspended by sheets of connective tissues.
   C. Several organs with separate functions act in coordinated ways.
   D. All of the above.

Questions 42–46 are **NOT** based on a descriptive passage.

42. All but one of the following are true statements about the anterior pituitary:

   A. Growth hormone or somatostatin is from the pituitary anterior lobe.
   B. GH effect is through an acceleration of protein synthesis.
   C. It stimulates the mobilization of stored fats and glycogen into glucose.
   D. Adult excess of GH causes the characteristic appearance of acromegaly.

43. The following are true associations of the thyroid gland except:

   A. When the thyroid underfunctions, hypothyroidism results.
   B. The thyroid responds to a surplus of thyroxin, forming a goiter.
   C. Thyroxin acts in the body to increase the rate of metabolism.
   D. Hypothyroidism at birth results in cretinism, the failure to grow normally.

44. The endocrine activity of glucagon includes all but one of the following:

   A. gluconeogenesis in the liver.
   B. increases the metabolic rate, increases ketogenesis, and is lipolytic.
   C. glycogenolysis in muscle.
   D. glucagon deficiency causes hypoglycemia.

45. All but one of the following are true statements about insulin:

   A. Insulin is secreted into fenestrated capillaries leading to the portal vein.
   B. Insulin is packaged by the Golgi apparatus and secreted by exocytosis.
   C. Insulin rapidly causes increased metabolism of glucose.
   D. Insulin rapidly causes increased facilitated transport of glucose into the cell.

46. All but one of the following are true statements about the adrenal medulla:

   A. Adrenal medulla is necessary for life.
   B. Medulla develops from ectodermal cells from the neural crest.
   C. Medulla cells secrete when stimulated by the preganglionic fibers.
   D. All of the above are true.

PASSAGE 7 (QUESTIONS 47–51)

Most animals are bulk feeders, ingesting relatively large pieces of food. The process by which they break down food into smaller pieces is known as digestion. The mammalian digestive system includes not only the main tube or alimentary canal, but also glands not directly in the path of food that secrete juices into the canal through ducts. These juices aid digestion.

47. Which of the following is the name given to the process that pushes food along in the alimentary canal?

    A. pinocytosis
    B. facilitated diffusion
    C. active transport
    D. peristalsis

48. True digestion does not begin until food enters the:

    A. alimentary canal.
    B. stomach.
    C. pancreas.
    D. intestine.

49. Which of the following is NOT a function of HCl in the stomach?

    A. denatures proteins
    B. hydrolyzes starch
    C. inactivates salivary amylase
    D. kills most bacteria

50. Which of the following accessory organs does NOT contribute to digestion?

    A. salivary glands
    B. pancreas
    C. appendix
    D. liver

51. Which of the following is NOT true of amino acids?

    A. Adult humans can only produce 12.
    B. There are 20 kinds needed for protein synthesis.
    C. They are stored in the ribosomes.
    D. Protein deficiency occurs when 1 or more essential amino acids is lacking in the diet.

PASSAGE 8 (QUESTIONS 52–59)

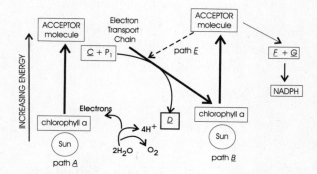

Photosynthesis is used by green plants and other organisms to turn solar energy, water, and carbon dioxide into carbohydrate and other compounds. The process may be conveniently divided into two parts: (1) the light dependent reactions and (2) the light-independent reactions (Calvin-Benson Cycle). In the light-dependent reactions (see the Z-Scheme energy profile diagram), energy from sunlight (captured by pigments) and protons from water are incorporated into organic molecules, which are then used in the light-independent reactions where carbon dioxide is fixed and reduced.

52. In the Z-scheme (above), the item labeled "path A" is:

   A. Photosystem I (PS I).
   B. Photosystem II (PS II).
   C. carbon dioxide fixation reactions.
   D. None of the above is correct.

53. In the same diagram, "path E" represents:

   A. Photosystem I (PS I).
   B. Photosystem II (PS II).
   C. cyclic photophosphorylation.
   D. non-cyclic photophosphorylation.

54. Solar energy is used to convert "C " and Pi to "D" in the diagram. "C" and "D" are, respectively:

   A. NAD+, NADH.
   B. NADP+, NADPH.
   C. ADP, ATP.
   D. ATP.

55. Items "F" and "G" in the diagram are, respectively:

   A. NAD+, NADH.
   B. NADP+, NADPH.
   C. NADP+, H+.
   D. NADPH, H+.

56. What two products of the light-dependent reactions are used in the independent reactions?

   A. ATP, NADH
   B. ADP, NADP+
   C. ADP, NADH
   D. ATP, NADPH

57. Which is the older photosystem, PS I or PS II (i.e., which evolved first)?

   A. PS I
   B. PS II
   C. Both are of the same age.
   D. Cannot be determined by any means known today.

58. In what part of the chloroplast do the light-dependent reactions occur?

   A. in the matrix
   B. in the stroma
   C. on or in the thylakoid
   D. on the cristae

59. The independent reactions used to be known as the "dark reactions." Why is the former the preferred name?

   A. These reactions can't happen in the dark.
   B. The independent reactions are just that—they are independent of light but can occur in the light or dark.
   C. These reactions require darkness only to make the final carbohydrate product.
   D. Carbon dioxide can't be fixed by RuBP unless it is dark, but the other reaction can happen with or without light.

PASSAGE 9 (QUESTIONS 60–65)

Eukaryotes and prokaryotes reflect a fundamental division among organisms. Prokaryotic cells first appeared between 3 and 4 billion years ago and are today represented by only the bacteria and cyanobacteria (formerly the blue-green algae). Eukaryotes appeared about 1.5 billion years ago and include the fungi, protists, plants, and animals. Eukaryotic cells are larger than prokaryotic cells by a factor of about 10 and show an almost bewildering range of diversity in terms of form and function. Unlike prokaryotes, they have a well-developed system of internal membranes and membrane-bound organelles. Other contrasts between prokaryotes and eukaryotes abound. Prokaryotes are often anaerobic, rarely multicellular, small, usually asexual, and have a single circular DNA molecule; eukaryotes are almost all aerobic, many are multicellular, sexual and asexual reproduction are both commonly found, and nuclear DNA is complexed with histones as (usually multiple) chromosomes. They represent two very different but very successful approaches to life.

60. The nominal (naming) difference between eukaryotes and prokaryotes is:

  A. prokaryotes have a membrane-bound nucleus and eukaryotes do not.
  B. eukaryotes have a membrane-bound nucleus and prokaryotes do not.
  C. prokaryotes lack an internal (endo-) membrane system.
  D. unlike prokaryotes, eukaryotes have true, membrane-bound organelles.

61. If typical prokaryotic cells range from 1–10 μm in diameter, what is the size range for most eukaryotic cells?

  A. 10–20 μm
  B. 1–100 μm
  C. 10–100 μm
  D. 100–1000 μm

62. Which of the following structures are present in eukaryotic cells but not in prokaryotic cells?

  I.   flagella made up of flagellin protein
  II. mitochondria
  III. chloroplasts
  IV. microtubules
  V.   Golgi bodies

  A. None of these are structures found in both types of cells.
  B. II, III, IV, and V are found in eukaryotic cells but not prokaryotic cells.
  C. II and III are found in eukaryotic cells but not prokaryotic cells.
  D. I, II, III, and V are found in eukaryotic cells but not prokaryotic cells.

63. Which of these are found in the eukaryotic cell nucleus?

  I.   RNA
  II. DNA
  III. proteins
  IV. histones

  A. I, II, and III are found in the eukaryotic nucleus.
  B. I and II are found in the eukaryotic nucleus.
  C. I, II, and IV are found in the eukaryotic nucleus.
  D. All are found in the eukaryotic nucleus.

64. Is all DNA in the eukaryotic cell restricted to the nucleus?

  A. Yes.
  B. No, DNA is also found in the mitochondria and, in cells that possess them, in the chloroplasts.
  C. No, DNA is found in mitochondria (mDNA) as well as in the nucleus.
  D. No, DNA is also found in the mitochondria and, in cells that possess them, in the chloroplasts, and free in the cytoplasm in short segments.

65. Which eukaryotic cell organelles most resemble prokaryotes?

  I.   ribosomes
  II. mitochondria
  III. microbodies
  IV. chloroplasts
  V.   Golgi bodies

  A. I, II, and IV
  B. II, III
  C. III, IV, and V
  D. II and IV

PASSAGE 10 (QUESTIONS 66–72)

All living organisms are cellular in nature, whether they exist as single or multicelled organisms. In multicellular organisms, such as humans, the individual cells become very specialized in structure and function. Unlike single-celled organisms, which must perform all the necessary physiological processes proficiently, multicellularity allows an organism to utilize the cooperative and coordinated action of various cells specialized for particular processes. Despite the specialization evident in human cells, certain structural and functional characteristics are common to all cells.

66. Which of the following concepts is not a component of cell theory?

A. The continuity of life has a cellular basis.

B. The activity of an organism is dependent upon both the individual and collective activities of its cells.

C. The activity of subcellular structures varies from cell to cell.

D. The cell is the basic structural and functional unit of life.

67. The fluid mosaic model of the cell plasma membrane includes which of the following structures?

 I. a phospholipid bilayer with integral proteins

 II. a glycocalyx composed primarily of complex carbohydrates

 III. integral and peripheral proteins

 IV. cholesterol molecules associated with phospholipids to increase stability

A. I only

B. I and III only

C. II and III only

D. All of the above are correct.

68. Interactions between cells must occur across their plasma membranes. While some cells move unfettered through the body, many are tightly bound together. Which of the following are not examples of the specialized membrane junctions between cells?

A. tight junctions

B. microvilli

C. desmosomes

D. gap junctions

69. Movement across cell membranes is necessary for the entry of nutrients and the removal of wastes, as well as the secretion of special products. Which of the following is not an example of passive transport across plasma membranes?

A. simple diffusion

B. pinocytosis

C. facilitated diffusion

D. osmosis

70. Mitochondria are organelles that might best be described by the following statement:

A. a membrane-bound cylindrical structure filled primarily with microtubules.

B. a membrane-bound structure with an additional inner membrane folded to form cristae; the site of aerobic ATP production.

C. a membrane-bound vesicle typically filled with digestive enzymes.

D. a membrane-bound structure with an additional inner membrane folded to form cristae; the site of protein synthesis.

71. An organelle of human cells that appears as a group of flattened membranous sacs associated with many tiny vesicles and is involved with the modification, concentration, packaging and shipping of proteins is the:

    A. endoplasmic reticulum.
    B. peroxisome.
    C. Golgi apparatus.
    D. centriole.

72. Which of the following is not true of the nucleus of the cell?

    A. It is bound by a single-layer membrane called the nuclear envelope.
    B. It contains dark staining, spherical bodies called nucleoli, which are primarily areas of RNA production.
    C. It contains DNA.
    D. It contains histone proteins.

Questions 73–77 are **NOT** based on a descriptive passage.

73. The period of cell growth following cell division is known as what stage of the cell cycle?

    A. G_1
    B. G_2
    C. S
    D. mitosis

74. A unique feature of sponges is that they are:

    A. sessile.
    B. heterotrophic.
    C. photosynthetic autotrophs.
    D. composed of cells, with a cell wall to give the sponge shape.

75. The gap between one neuron and another is called a _____. In response to membrane depolarization, _____ is/are released from vesicles in one neuron and _____ to the other neuron.

    A. synaptic cleft, insulin, diffuse
    B. synaptic cleft, neurotransmitters, are actively transported
    C. gap junction, neurotransmitters, diffuse
    D. synaptic cleft, neurotransmitters, diffuse

76. In the mammalian reproductive tract, where does fertilization usually occur?

    A. vagina
    B. uterus
    C. oviduct (Fallopian tube)
    D. ovary

77. Which one of the following statements is not true of enzymes?

    A. Enzyme activity always increases as temperature increases.
    B. An enzyme functions best within a particular range of pH values.
    C. In almost all instances, enzymes are proteins.
    D. An enzyme is specific for a particular substrate.

QUICK-SCORE ANSWERS

ANSWERS FOR PRACTICE TEST 2

Verbal Reasoning

1. D	23. B	45. D
2. D	24. C	46. D
3. B	25. C	47. B
4. D	26. C	48. A
5. A	27. D	49. D
6. D	28. A	50. D
7. C	29. B	51. D
8. C	30. A	52. B
9. D	31. C	53. C
10. D	32. D	54. D
11. B	33. C	55. D
12. D	34. B	56. C
13. A	35. C	57. A
14. C	36. A	58. B
15. D	37. D	59. D
16. C	38. D	60. D
17. D	39. B	61. D
18. B	40. A	62. A
19. B	41. D	63. D
20. D	42. C	64. C
21. A	43. B	65. D
22. A	44. D	

Physical Sciences

1. C	27. B	53. D
2. B	28. B	54. C
3. A	29. D	55. C
4. B	30. C	56. D
5. C	31. D	57. A
6. D	32. B	58. A
7. B	33. C	59. C
8. B	34. C	60. A
9. C	35. C	61. B
10. A	36. B	62. C
11. B	37. B	63. B
12. C	38. A	64. B
13. C	39. B	65. C
14. D	40. D	66. B
15. A	41. A	67. A
16. B	42. B	68. A
17. C	43. A	69. A
18. B	44. C	70. B
19. B	45. A	71. A
20. C	46. C	72. C
21. A	47. D	73. B
22. D	48. C	74. C
23. C	49. B	75. B
24. A	50. A	76. A
25. C	51. A	77. A
26. A	52. A	

Biological Sciences

1. D	27. B	53. C
2. B	28. B	54. C
3. A	29. B	55. C
4. A	30. C	56. D
5. C	31. A	57. A
6. A	32. A	58. C
7. B	33. C	59. B
8. A	34. B	60. B
9. C	35. C	61. C
10. A	36. D	62. B
11. D	37. D	63. D
12. B	38. B	64. B
13. A	39. B	65. D
14. D	40. D	66. C
15. D	41. D	67. D
16. A	42. A	68. B
17. C	43. B	69. B
18. C	44. C	70. B
19. D	45. C	71. C
20. B	46. A	72. A
21. C	47. D	73. A
22. B	48. A	74. A
23. B	49. B	75. D
24. A	50. C	76. C
25. B	51. C	77. A
26. D	52. B	

EXPLANATORY ANSWERS FOR PRACTICE TEST 2

VERBAL REASONING

PASSAGE 1

1. The correct answer is (D). The author makes the point that challenges have occurred in 34 percent of the communities compared to 30 percent five years earlier. Answer (A) is incorrect. Although young-adult literature strives to deal with honest subjects, censorship of books still continues into the 1990s. Answer (B) is incorrect. The opposite is true: students want to focus upon issues appropriate to them. Answer (C) is incorrect. While there may be some communities that are doing this, there is no evidence to support it as a real factor.

2. The correct answer is (D). The two titles mentioned are familiar ones from movie titles as well as bestselling novels. Answers (A) and (C) are incorrect; there is no evidence of the author's attempts to urge the avoidance of any works. Answer (B) is incorrect. Although this may be a true statement, it is not a part of the selection.

3. The correct answer is (B). The author makes the point that the problems and interests of young people are represented in the works that are being censored. Answer (A) is incorrect. Although there may be some truth here, there is nothing in the article to support this argument. Answer (C) is incorrect. While on the surface, this seems to be true, the reader must realize that there is no indicator of the need to watch the subject matter. Answer (D) is incorrect. The point is made that parents DO have a voice in these choices.

4. The correct answer is (D). The selection indicates a growth of 4 percent in a five-year period and indicates other censorship concerns. Answer (A) is incorrect. There is no evidence of this; in fact, the choice is given to the censors. Answer (B) is incorrect. The point is made that parents and community leaders do have a choice. Answer (C) is incorrect. Again, the point made is the opposite of this choice.

5. The correct answer is (A). The selection points out that students can carry the books in a purse or pocket. Answer (B) is incorrect. While the dubious beginning is inferred, it is not the author's purpose. Answer (C) is incorrect. Again, while there is some evidence, the premise is not supported. Answer (D) is incorrect. There is no evidence that this is true.

6. The correct answer is (D). The selection clearly states that drug and alcohol issues together with divorce, suicide, and prejudice, formulate the plots of young-adult novels. Answer (D) is incorrect. There is no mention of adoption. Answers (B) and (C) are incorrect because each is only partly correct.

7. The correct answer is (C). The author states that, while all the novels were "hardly great or honest, a surprising number were." Answer (A) is incorrect. The point is made that today's young-adult novels are not the "good-old-pure" ones of yesterday. Answer (B) is incorrect; there is no mention of the works as forthright. Answer (D) is incorrect; the word superficial is used to describe the paperback books that predate the young-adult novel.

8. The correct answer is (C). To have the books made available would challenge the priority of censorship. Answer (A) is incorrect. If the books were available, this would agree with the statement of answer (C). Answer (B) is incorrect. There is no mention of censorship as a popular trend in education. Answer (D) is incorrect. While this may be true, the article does not state this as a certainty.

9. The correct answer is (D). "Pedagogy" means art of teaching; therefore, the books were lacking in material that was teachable. Answer (A) is incorrect; the point is made that there was a lack of intellectual appeal. Answer (C) is incorrect; while there may be truth in the statement, it is not borne out in this article.

10. The correct answer is (D). The author lists the subjects with which today's paperback young-adult novels deal and relates them to life. Answer (A) is incorrect. There is no mention of titles as unattractive. Answer (B) is incorrect. No authors are described by the author as questionable. Answer (C) is incorrect. The cheap price of the book is referred to as a positive factor but not in relation to the construction.

PASSAGE 2

11. The correct answer is (B). The author makes the point that cognitive competence does result in consistently high grades. Answer (A) is incorrect. Students do not become informed about life's wider purposes. Answer (C) is incorrect. While students do learn to postpone many of life's experiences and demands until later in life, this is not necessarily a virtue. Answer (D) is incorrect. While pressures are anti-emotional, this is not a virtue, according to the author.

12. The correct answer is (D). The author dwells upon the achievement of all other areas, but notes the lack of practical application. Therefore, answers (A), (B), and (C) are incorrect.

13. The correct answer is (A). The author points out in the first paragraph the importance of the "baby boomers" to academic requirements. Answer (B) is incorrect. While the standards of private schools may be rising, the author makes the point that primary and secondary school standards are rising. There is no mention of "private schools." Answer (C) is incorrect. The article states that colleges are "slowly" expanding. Answer (D) is incorrect because it includes the erroneous statement of (B).

14. The correct answer is (C). The author is detached only in that he states information solely but does not embrace one specific idea concerning the subject. Answer (A) is incorrect. To be melancholy, one must have longings or memories that stir. There is no evidence of melancholia in this article. Answer (B) is incorrect. There is no evidence of authorial involvement at all. Note the absence of the pronoun I. Answer (D) is incorrect. To be sentimental, the author would have to illustrate deep emotional attachment; there is no evidence of such feeling.

15. The correct answer is (D). The author indicates that simple intelligence (cognitive awareness) is inadequate and must be balanced with choices about values. Answer (A) is incorrect. There is no indication of guidance for choosing a profession. Answer (B) is incorrect. There is no mention of personal goals and their relation to profession. Answer (C) is incorrect. The author infers that successful completion of a college education does not always ensure financial security.

16. Answer (C) is the correct answer. The author indicates that what matters ". . . is the kind of ability that enables a student to do well on college boards, graduate records, and other admission tests." Answer (A) is incorrect; while desirable, the author indicates that this philosophy is not yet being accepted by admissions officers. Answer (B) is incorrect. The author does not mention the importance of "grades" as such for academic admission. Answer (D) is incorrect; there is no mention of health records or personal information.

17. The correct answer is (D). The author makes this statement: "Not only have academic pressures mounted in the past generation, but these pressures have become more and more cognitive. . ." Answer (A) is incorrect. The author carefully points out that social pressures take a backseat to the cognitive ones. Answer (B) is incorrect for the same reason. Answer (C) is incorrect. There is no mention of energizing the student.

18. The correct answer is (B). The author makes the point that focusing upon high performance academically robs the student of exposure to other areas of life. Answer (A) is incorrect. There is an allusion to cognitive dependence being helpful in certain areas of admission into educational programs, but not in one subject. Answer (C) is incorrect. The author leaves the impression that with cognitive dependence comes an absence of the belief that all of life depends upon who one really is. Answer (D) is incorrect. This is contradicted by the article in question.

PASSAGE 3

19. The correct answer is (B). The author clearly states that: "the normal capacity to defend oneself against undue stimulations and inner excitation is exaggerated and automatized, so that it not only protects, but walls off the individual from inner and outer experience." Answers (A), (C), and (D) are incorrect. While each of these may be a true fact, there is not an indicator of this factor in this selection.

20. The correct answer is (D). All of the answers are correct. Answer (A) is repeatedly illustrated to show that we take things for granted with continued exposure. Answer (B) is true of the cadaver experience. Answer (C) is correct because the medical student learns not to think about the cadaver.

21. The correct answer is (A). Those external forces or objects of which we become aware stimulate us to learn new identities or skills, thereby becoming our stimuli. Answer (B) is incorrect. While this may be true of many of the stimuli in life, the author does not make that point. Answer (C) is incorrect. While a stimuli may cause us to react sharply, that is not the only indicator. Answer (D) is incorrect. A stimulus is what makes us feel, not that which we allow to affect us willingly.

22. The correct answer is (A). The author explains that overexposure to the same stimuli for a lengthy period of time can numb one. Answer (B) is incorrect; there is no indicator of this as being a numbing factor. Answer (C) is incorrect; bland subjects are not mentioned. Answer (D) is incorrect. Underexposure would create no stimuli.

23. The correct answer is (B). The author states depression, fatigue, and let-down, which are synonymous with the choices here. Answer (A) is incorrect. The author indicates that the numbness might come from overexposure, but there is not a mention of boredom. The same is true for answers (C) and (D) which are also incorrect.

24. The correct answer is (C). The author speaks of the one numbed as being overly-enamored. Answer (A) is incorrect; while there is a sense of immobilization, there is no indicator of lack of talking. Answer (B) is incorrect. One might infer immobilization and silence, but there is not the open mention. Answer (D) is incorrect. Again, while there is an inference, there is no indicator of communications.

PASSAGE 4

25. The correct answer is (C). The last paragraph makes this statement. Answer (A) is incorrect. According to paragraph one, exercise does not stop the aging process but helps to control it. Answer (B) is incorrect. The author clearly states that physical development ends at about age twenty-two. Answer (D) is incorrect; weight loss or gain is a byproduct of physical exercise, not its purpose.

26. The correct answer is (C). According to paragraph 3, ". . . cardiovascular system particularly." Answers (A) and (B) are not mentioned by the author. Since (A) and (B) are incorrect, answer (D) must be incorrect.

27. The correct answer is (D). Answer (A) is incorrect; while this may be a consideration, it is not the main concern. Answer (B) is incorrect. While this may be true for a given individual, the author does not mention this as a concern. Answer (C) is incorrect. While some activities might require a partner, this is not the main concern.

28. The correct answer is (A). Paragraph one states that brain power can be increased or sustained by physical activity. Answer (B) is incorrect; there is no mention of fewer chronic illnesses. Answer (C) is incorrect; there is no mention of less need for vitamins or other medication. Answer (D) is incorrect. While this may be very true, the author does not make this point.

29. The correct answer is (B). The author makes the statement throughout the article that continued physical activity will produce a longer life, increased brain power, muscle toning, and body system functioning. Answer (A) is incorrect. There is no mention of sustained sexual potency in later life. Answer (C) is incorrect; there is no mention of the regeneration of skin cells to prohibit drying. Answer (D) is incorrect; while this may be true, the author only mentions that thinness may be overcome by physical activity.

30. The correct answer is (A). The activities of golf, bowling, and individual exercise would all fit into the parameters established by the author and could be carried on throughout one's lifetime. Answer (B) is incorrect; the author states that one should select an activity that requires minimal search for a partner, and baseball requires a team and would not fit this description. Answer (C) is incorrect; while swimming and diving are options, the activity of surfing, while an appropriate physical exercise, would not fit the author's criteria. Answer (D) is incorrect; ice skating and golf would be appropriate activities if the climate and conditions were appropriate; however, scuba diving would require the site and partner search that would place it outside the author's recommendations.

31. The correct answer is (C). The author states: "It is considerably more difficult to control premature biological aging when it has already set in." Answer (A) is incorrect. The thrust of the author's argument is that there is an activity for everyone. Answer (B) is incorrect; the author infers that equipment is not a primary factor in finding a suitable physical exercise. Answer (D) is incorrect; the author downplays the use of a gym as a factor.

32. The correct answer is (D). The author clearly states in paragraph four: "A program that would overdevelop specific muscles would be unhealthy for males or females. Answer (A) is incorrect; the author infers that exercise is important for all. Answers (B) and (C) are incorrect. The difficulty of exercise by gender is not discussed.

33. The correct answer is (C). The author makes the paramount point that one's interest is important as well as a consideration for one's age, and implies that location and finances must play a minor part. Answers (A), (B), and (D) are incorrect. Gender is not mentioned as a factor.

34. The correct answer is (B). The author states in paragraph four: "Contrary to some common thought" physical exercise does not build bulky muscles. Answer (A) is incorrect. While physical exercise may help to control weight, this is not the primary intent. Answers (C) and (D) are incorrect. The author states that the opposite is true.

PASSAGE 5

35. The correct answer is (C). The author points out the magnitude of some of the explosions and likens them to an equivalent amount of dynamite. Answer (A) is incorrect. While there might be validity, this is not inferred from the article at hand. Answer (B) is incorrect; there is no mention of other planets, nor the possibility of life on other planets. Answer (D) is incorrect. There is no mention of density nor changes in activity, even though this might be a by-product.

36. The correct answer is (A). The first sentence of the article provides the foundation for this inference. Answer (B) is incorrect. There is no evidence to support this data although it might be correct. Answer (C) is incorrect; there is no mention of danger associated with the flashes. Answer (D) is incorrect. The article infers that scientists were interested but that this was not the purpose of the material.

37. The correct answer is (D). Paragraphs one and three contain the material to indicate that the equipment is able to accomplish items (A), (B), and (C).

38. The correct answer is (D). Without specifically voicing support, the author indicates ways to make the recording a reality which indicates his support of the project. Answer (A) is incorrect. The author makes a case for knowing the data, indicating that there is a purpose. Answer (B) is incorrect; while the premise is correct, there is no mention of "hastening peace." Answer (C) is incorrect; the author does not discuss the use of satellites for military reasons but mentions that that is their function.

39. The correct answer is (B). The article states: "Most of the explosions seen so far have occurred at altitudes of 18 to 31." Answer (A) is incorrect. The allusion is that there is no regularity to the explosions. Answers (C) and (D) are incorrect; there is nothing in the article to support either of these two assumptions.

40. The correct answer is (A). The last sentence of paragraph five indicates that "many more asteroids are crossing the earth's path than once believed—perhaps ten or even 100 times more. Answer (B) is incorrect. The author carefully makes a case for the use of satellites for military purposes and underscores it in the conclusion of the selection. Answers (C) and (D) are incorrect; there is no support for either of these statements in the article.

41. The correct answer is (D). In paragraph three, the writer alludes to data recorded between 1975 and 1992, making answer (A) correct. The same paragraph reports the comparison with the atomic bomb making answer (B) correct. Answer (C) is correct, since the author reports that 136 records are recorded. Therefore, answer (D) is correct.

PASSAGE 6

42. The correct answer is (C). The author points out ways in which English vocabulary changed during that time. Answer (A) is incorrect. Certain words are explained to make a point but this is not the focus. Answer (B) is incorrect. Although there is an allusion to the difficulty of learning the language, it is not the point. Answer (D) is incorrect. The opposite is true. The language is not static.

43. The correct answer is (B). The author makes no mention or allusion to taking words from one language to another, or "borrowing." Answer (A) is incorrect; pronunciation differences are mentioned in paragraph one. Answer (C) is incorrect. Most of the examples are from poetry. Answer (D) is incorrect. Paragraph three illustrates the "coining," or making up, of words.

44. The correct answer is (D). The author states in paragraph two that "Many new philosophic and scientific names" were added. Answer (A) is incorrect. The field of philosophy is mentioned as one that introduced terms into the language not philosophic differences. Answer (B) is incorrect. There is no evidence to support this theory. Answer (C) is incorrect. Syllabification increase is not mentioned as a factor.

45. The correct answer is (D). Paragraph one supports this argument. Answer (A) is incorrect. There is no evidence to support making English the official language of business. Answer (B) is incorrect; there is no evidence to support that more people speak and read English than any other language. Answer (C) is incorrect. There is no evidence to support that English is an inferior language.

46. The correct answer is (D). Answers (A) and (B) are correct—paragraph two indicates both of these. Answer (C) is correct. The end of paragraph two indicates this. Therefore, answer (D) is correct.

47. The correct answer is (B). Paragraph three states: "In their search for color, the Romantics use . . ." many variations of the language. Answer (A) is incorrect. While this may be true, the author does not make that point. Answers (C) and (D) are incorrect. Again, there is no evidence to support either of these statements.

PASSAGE 7

48. The correct answer is (A). The author is attempting to inform the reader of the effects and growth of drug use. Answer (B) is incorrect. Little effort is made to describe either the effect or growth of drug use. Answer (C) is incorrect. No effort is made to narrate an incident of growth. Answer (D) is incorrect. There is no effort to tempt readers to use drugs.

49. The correct answer is (D). The statement assumes that mankind has the potential for a life of order and sanity that is outmoded with the use of drugs. Answer (A) is incorrect. While there are drugs that are valuable in society, the doctor's statement does not allude to those positive uses. Answer (B) is incorrect. Again, while there may be drugs that can make the life of an individual better, the doctor is not referring to those drugs. Answer (C) is incorrect. There is a place for drugs in society, but not the misuse of them, which is the doctor's point.

50. The correct answer is (D). The author is making the point that while Americans use alcohol without realizing that it is a drug, such use is increasing and has the potential for addiction. Answers (A), (B), and (C) are incorrect; while these may be true statements in some ways, the author does not support these statements.

51. The correct answer is (D). Paragraph two states all of the answers, which are fragmented into answers (A), (B), and (C).

52. The correct answer is (B). In the last paragraph, the author makes this point. Answer (A) is incorrect. The evidence used by the author does not bear this out. Answer (C) is incorrect; the illustration of alcohol is not intended for this purpose. Answer (D) is incorrect; the author makes the point that the reverse is almost true.

53. The correct answer is (C). The author makes the statement that there will be increased drug use in the following decade. Answer (A) is incorrect. While this may be true, the author does not indicate a more permissive attitude about drug use. Answer (B) is incorrect. While this may be true, the author does not indicate a less permissive attitude about drug use. Answer (D) is incorrect; the author predicts the opposite.

PASSAGE 8

54. The correct answer is (D). The author points out that using those who "pretend" or pose as doctors but who do it for money is futile—useless and frustrating. Answer (A) is incorrect. There are allusions to cancer and possible cures but that is not the focus. Answer (B) is incorrect. The search by a patient for less expensive treatment is mentioned, but not as a focus. Answer (C) is incorrect. Alternative medicines may be sought or secured, but the focus is not on them.

55. The correct answer is (D). The author makes the point that quackery is widespread when he discusses its many forms. So answer (A) is correct. Answer (B) is correct because the author points out how quacks rise to take advantage of what is most prevalent at the moment. Answer (C) is correct; the author makes this point. Because all of these choices are true, answer (D) is the correct selection.

56. The correct answer is (C). Using the services and products of a nondoctor puts all the responsibility on the patient. Answer (A) is incorrect; while the treatment may be unique in its form, the unique treatment is not designed for the patient's well-being. Answer (B) is incorrect; the patient usually has less chance for successful treatment. Answer (D) is incorrect; while this may be a true statement, there is no support for it in this article.

57. The correct answer is (A). In paragraph one, the author makes this definition and spends the rest of the article illustrating it. Answer (B) is incorrect. While the doctor in the illustration is a chiropractor, there is no evidence that he represents all practitioners of chiropractic. Answer (C) is incorrect. There is no support for this statement in the article. Answer (D) is incorrect; while this may be true, there is no evidence in the article to suggest that this statement is to be inferred.

58. The correct answer is (B). The author gives the definition of a quack and how one works, then provides an illustration of one to indicate the importance of wise choices. Answer (A) is incorrect. The author implies that quacks are prevalent today. Answers (C) and (D) are incorrect. There is no evidence of either of these conclusions.

59. The correct answer is (D). In paragraph three, the author implies that officials are attempting to control cancer quackery. Answer (A) is incorrect; there is no evidence that the government wants to license those who are promising more than they can deliver. Answer (B) is incorrect. There is no evidence that there are efforts to test and market the drugs used as alternative medicines. Answer (C) is incorrect. The government agencies are not mentioned in connection with treatment costs.

PASSAGE 9

60. The correct answer is (D). In the last paragraph, the author points out the effects of early training on intelligence. Answer (A) is incorrect. While the author does point out the importance of state funding for early education, this is not the focus of the selection. Answer (B) is incorrect. Again, while the author does point out the importance of federal government in education, this is not the focus. Answer (C) is incorrect. The author points out that there has been a decade of change, not of degeneration.

61. The correct answer is (D). Paragraph five states: ". . . All areas—social, emotional, intellectual and physical— are equally important." Therefore, answers (A), (B), and (C) are all correct.

62. The correct answer is (A). In the last paragraph, the author points out that control of environment can raise the IQ. Answer (B) is incorrect; the effect is as much as twenty points. Answer (C) is incorrect. While the purist educator might agree with this statement, there is no evidence in this selection to support it. Answer (D) is incorrect. According to the last paragraph, modifying one's environment can change the IQ.

63. The correct answer is (D). Child development centers offer an environment conducive to intellectual, emotional, physical, and social growth. Answer (A) is incorrect. There may be differences so insignificant that they are inconsequential, but the mission of a child-development center is significant. Answer (B) is incorrect. The personnel have no bearing on the naming of the center. Answer (C) is incorrect. There is a distinctive difference in the types of facilities.

64. The correct answer is (C). The author states that the increased number of women employed has led to a rise in the need for child care. Answer (A) is incorrect; while there is a socializing influence in early education, this is not the primary factor. Answer (B) is incorrect. There is no evidence in this article of the popularity of educating at an early age. Answer (D) is incorrect; while this may be true, there is no evidence of this in this selection.

65. The correct answer is (D). The inference is that child development prepares students for the first grade by stressing skills that their environment might not include. Answer (A) is incorrect. The author's inference is that with so many mothers employed, there is not an opportunity for young children to learn at home what they need to know. Answer (B) is incorrect. There is evidence in this article that parents are not able to accept this responsibility. Answer (C) is incorrect. There is no evidence to indicate that this is possible.

PHYSICAL SCIENCES

PASSAGE 1

1. The correct answer is (C). Proton count *always* equals the atomic number (13). The atomic mass is the *sum* of the number of protons and neutrons (27).
   Physics 12, 12.2, 12.4

2. The correct answer is (B). An ion is an "electrically charged particle" created by either electron loss or gain. Since the symbol indicates a +2 charge, there must be 2 more positive components (protons) than negative components (electrons). Since there are 56 protons listed in the table, there must be 54 electrons. *General Chemistry 1.6, 3.1, 5.2*

3. The correct answer is (A). Atomic number [15] *always* is the same as the number of protons, which is listed in the table as [15]. From your periodic table, [P] is the symbol for the element with the atomic number of 15, and since the atomic mass (the sum of the protons and neutrons) is listed on the table as 31.0, the number of neutrons is [16]. 31.0 − 15 = 16 *Physics 12, 12.2, 12.4*

4. The correct answer is (B). The number of protons is *always* equal to the atomic number. *Physics 12.2*

5. The correct answer is (C). Since the atomic number is listed in the table as 12, checking in a periodic table indicates that the element in question is magnesium [Mg]. However, the table also shows an *unequal* number of protons (12) and electrons (10). Therefore, this species has an overall electric charge of +2. The correct symbol that represents this imbalance is Mg^{+2}. *General Chemistry 1.6; Physics 12.2*

6. The correct answer is (D). The −1 charge in this problem has no effect on the atomic mass. The atomic mass is the sum of the number of protons and neutrons. The number of protons *always* equals the atomic number (in this case 9). Therefore, protons [9] + neutrons [10] = 19.0 *Physics 12.2*

7. The correct answer is (B). The two particles with charges are electrons (-) and protons (+); therefore, to be electrically neutral, electrons must equal protons. *Physics 12.1*

PASSAGE 2

8. The correct answer is (B). Although the fired shell is moving very fast horizontally, it is not moving in the vertical direction at all until it leaves the cannon and starts to free fall.
   Physics 2.5, 2.6

9. The correct answer is (C). Both shells have the same initial vertical velocity, acceleration, and displacement, and therefore will hit the ground at the same time: $S = V_0 t + \frac{1}{2}at^2$
   Physics 2.5, 2.6

10. The correct answer is (A). Although both shells will hit the ground with identical, vertical velocities, the shell fired from the cannon will also have a horizontal component; therefore, its overall velocity will be greater than the shell dropped off the edge of the cliff.
    Physics 2.5, 2.6, 5.3

---

* For more information, refer to this section in Peterson's *Gold Standard MCAT.*

11. The correct answer is (B). The initial vertical velocity $V_{0y} = V_0 \sin q$, where q is the muzzle angle relative to the ground. The greater the angle, the greater the initial vertical velocity and the greater the amount of time spent in the air, according to the vector equation: $S = V_0 t + \frac{1}{2}at^2$.
Physics 1.5, 1.6, 2.6

12. The correct answer is (C). The maximum range occurs at an angle of $45°$. As the angle increases, the range increases until $45°$ and then decreases from there on. *Physics 2.6*

13. The correct answer is (C). The kinetic energies of the two shells are equal because they both had identical initial kinetic energies, and they both dropped through the same gravitational potential. *Physics 2.6, 5.3, 5.5*

Passage 3

14. The correct answer is (D). The equation does not need to be balanced to answer the question; however, the reaction must be completed.

$$NaCl + Al(NO_3)_3 \rightarrow NaNO_3 + AlCl_3$$
General Chemistry 1.5, 1.5.1, 3.1, 5.2

15. The correct answer is (A). The correctly balanced equation will appear as:

$$3Ca + 2H_3PO_4 \rightarrow Ca_3(PO_4)_2 + 3H_2$$

Note: In a balanced chemical equation, if no number appears before a chemical, the number 1 is understood.
General Chemistry 1.5, 1.5.1, 3.1, 5.2, 6.1

16. The correct answer is (B). The correctly balanced equation will appear as:

$$3Mg(OH)_2 + 2FeCl_3 \rightarrow 3MgCl_2 + 2Fe(OH)_3$$
General Chemistry 1.5, 1.5.1, 3.1, 5.2

17. The correct answer is (C). See the balanced equation in the previous answer. *General Chemistry 1.5, 1.5.1, 3.1, 5.2*

18. The correct answer is (B). The correctly balanced equation will appear as:

$$C_3H_8 + 5O_2 \rightarrow 3CO_2 + 4H_2O$$
General Chemistry 1.5, Organic Chemistry 3.2.1

19. The correct answer is (B). The correctly balanced equation will appear as:

$$2H_3PO_3 + 3Ca(OH)_2 \rightarrow Ca_3(PO_3)_2 + 6HOH$$

Note: As a help in balancing equations involving hydroxides and water, it is often easier to "visualize" the equation by expressing water as HOH rather than H_2O. (It makes the balancing of the OH^- "easier to see.")
General Chemistry 1.5, 1.5.1, 3.1, 5.2, 6.1

20. The correct answer is (C). The correctly balanced equation will appear as:

$$XeF_6 \rightarrow Xe + 3F_2$$

Note: It is important to remember that fluorine is *diatomic* (F_2) when it appears as an element in an equation.
General Chemistry 3.3

21. The correct answer is (A). The buoyant force by a fluid is equal to the weight of the fluid displaced, $m_{displaced}g$. Since the mass of the displaced fluid is the density of the fluid multiplied by the volume displaced, the buoyant force is:

$$F_{buoyant} = (80m^3)(1\frac{kg}{m^3})(10\frac{m}{sec^2}) = 800 \ Newtons$$
Physics 6.1.2

---

* For more information, refer to this section in Peterson's *Gold Standard MCAT.*

22. The correct answer is (D). Since heat is removed from the liquid tea to provide the latent heat necessary to evaporate the 0.1 mole to gas, the temperature of the remaining tea decreases. The heat required to vaporize 0.1 mole is:

$$Q =$$

$$(0.1 \text{ mole})(9000 \times \frac{cal}{mole \; Kelvin})(900 \; cal)$$

Removal of this amount of heat is associated with a temperature change in the liquid via the specific heat capacity:

$$Q = -900cal =$$

$$(6 \text{ mole})(15 \times \frac{cal}{mole \; Kelvin}) \times (\Delta T)$$

where the (−) sign represents heat removed from the liquid, and ΔT is the change in temperature. This is solved for a temperature change of $\Delta T = -10 Kelvin$.

General Chemistry 8.7

23. The correct answer is (C). Ohm's law relates current, I; potential difference, V; and resistance, R, by $V = IR$.

　　If Ohm's law is obeyed, a plot of V versus I is a straight line, with slope R. Device 1 obeys Ohm's law, although it was not tested for negative current. Device 2 does not obey, because the graph is not a straight line. Device 3 obeys. Device 4 has two different slopes; one for negative current and one for positive, and thus does not obey Ohm's law.　*Physics 10.1, 10.3*

24. The correct answer is (A). The (RMS) effective current is $I_{effective} = I_{RMS} =$

$$\frac{I_{max}}{\sqrt{2}}$$

The (RMS) effective voltage is:

$$V_{effective} = V_{RMS} = \frac{V_{max}}{\sqrt{2}}$$

The average power is

$$I_{RMS}V_{RMS} = \frac{I_{max}V_{max}}{2} \; Watts$$

Physics 10.5

25. The correct answer is (C). If no work is done by friction, energy is conserved: total energy at bottom of hill = total energy at top of path:

$$\frac{1}{2}mv^2_{bottom} + mgh_{bottom} = \frac{1}{2}mv^2_{top} + mgh_{top}$$

Since the velocity is zero at the top of this path, we can solve for the height difference:

$$\frac{1}{2}(30m/sec)^2 = gh_{top} - gh_{bottom}$$

$$h_{top} - h_{bottom} = \frac{900m^2/sec^2}{2x9.8m/sec^2} = 46m$$

Physics 5.5, 5.5.1

PASSAGE 4

26. The correct answer is (A). Potassium chlorate and oxygen are in a 2:3 ratio in the balanced equation. Therefore, using 3.4 moles in the ratio in place of the 2 sets up a stoichiometric relationship of $\frac{3.4}{2}$ (potassium chlorate) as $\frac{X}{3}$ (oxygen), X=5.1 moles, which converts to 163.2 grams.　*General Chemistry 1.4, 1.5*

---

* For more information, refer to this section in Peterson's *Gold Standard MCAT*.

27. The correct answer is (B). Ethene and oxygen are in a 2:7 ratio in the balanced equation. Therefore, if 2 moles of ethene react with 7 moles of oxygen, 4 moles of ethene will react with 14 moles of oxygen. Fourteen moles of oxygen have a mass of 448.0 grams (14 mol × 32 g/mol).
  * *General Chemistry 1.3, 1.5*

28. The correct answer is (B). Sodium hydroxide and sodium chloride are in a 2:2 (or 1:1) ratio. 58.5 grams of sodium chloride = 1 mole. Therefore, 1 mole of sodium hydroxide will be needed. 1 mole of NaOH has a mass of 40.0 grams.   * *General Chemistry 1.3, 1.5*

29. The correct answer is (D). Based on the balanced equation, aluminum and hydrogen are in a 2:3 stoichiometric (mole) ratio. First convert 100 grams of aluminum to moles ($\frac{100}{27}$ = 3.7 moles). Now establish the ratio $\frac{3.7}{2}$ (aluminum) as $\frac{X}{3}$ (hydrogen), X = 5.55 moles.
  * *General Chemistry 1.3, 1.5*

30. The correct answer is (C). To solve this problem, it is necessary to remember one of the basic definitions of a mole. One mole of *any gas* will occupy a volume of 22.4 liters at S.T.P. (Standard Temperature and Pressure—0 degrees C and 1 atmosphere pressure). Since we found 5.55 moles of hydrogen in the previous answer, (5.55 × 22.4) = 124.32 liters.   * *General Chemistry 4.1.1*

31. The correct answer is (D). To solve this problem, you essentially have to create two stoichiometric situations. Situation A assumes 75 grams of calcium and an unlimited supply of chlorine. Situation B assumes the opposite, 75 grams of chlorine and an unlimited supply of calcium. All of the chemicals are in a 1:1 mole ratio. In situation A, 75 grams of calcium is 1.875 moles, which would produce 1.875 moles of calcium chloride. In situation B, 75 grams of chlorine is 1.06 moles, which would produce 1.06 moles of calcium chloride. In these "double stoichiometry situations" the *smaller value* is the correct answer: 1.06 moles of calcium chloride = 117.66 grams (1.06 moles 111.0 g/mol). Chlorine is the "limiting reagent."   * *General Chemistry 1.3, 1.5*

PASSAGE 5

32. The correct answer is (B). If two objects collide, stick together, and move off as a single unit, they have undergone an inelastic collision.
  * *Physics 4.4*

33. The correct answer is (C). The momentum of the system before they collide is the vector sum of the momenta of the two blocks, $m_1v_1 + m_2v_2$. (10 kg)(10 m/s) + (40kg)(0 m/s) = 100 kg m/s. The momentum of the system after the two blocks collide and stick together is $(m_1 + m_2)$ V, (10kg + 40kg) V. This must be equal to the momentum before they collide, 100 kg m/s. Therefore, V = 2 m/s.
  * *Physics 4.4, 4.4.1*

34. The correct answer is (C).
  * *Physics 4.4, 4.4.1*

35. The correct answer is (C). In any isolated system, the total momentum is always conserved. Momentum is a vector, and its magnitude and direction are the same before and after the collision.   * *Physics 4.4*

---

* For more information, refer to this section in Peterson's *Gold Standard MCAT.*

36. The correct answer is (B). In an elastic collision, both the momentum and kinetic energy of the system are conserved.   *Physics 4.4*

PASSAGE 6

37. The correct answer is (B). Heat always flows from higher to lower temperature. The iron will lose heat and its temperature will decrease, and the ice will gain heat and its temperature will increase. Since the ice was initially below its melting point, its temperature will increase until it reaches its melting point at which time a phase change takes place.
   General Chemistry 7.1, 7.2, 8.8, 8.9

38. The correct answer is (A). All things being equal, substances with a higher specific heat will undergo smaller temperature changes than those with lower specific heat.
   General Chemistry 8.7

39. The correct answer is (B). The ice gains heat and its temperature increases until it reaches its melting point, and then a phase change occurs. As long as the ice is melting, its temperature remains constant.   *General Chemistry 8.7*

40. The correct answer is (D). All systems in contact eventually come to the same temperature. The heat lost by one part of the system equals the heat gained by the other part.
   General Chemistry 7.1, 7.2, 8.7, 8.8, 8.9

41. The correct answer is (A). When a phase change occurs, the temperature of that substance does not change. The temperature of the iron continues to decrease because it is at a higher temperature and it is not undergoing a phase change.
   General Chemistry 8.7

42. The correct answer is (B). The heat lost by one part of the system is always equal to the heat gained by the other part, provided the system is completely insulated.
   General Chemistry 7.1, 7.2, 8.7, 8.8, 8.9

43. The correct answer is (A). Histone is a protective molecule that surrounds the DNA.   *Biology 1.2.2; Organic Chemistry 12.5*

44. The correct answer is (C). While the synthesis of proteins does take place in the ribosomes, and these are on the endoplasmic reticulum, proteins are primarily made in the ribosomes.
   Biology 1.2.1, 3

45. The correct answer is (A). A–T base-pairing occurs only in DNA.
   Biology 1.2.2

46. The correct answer is (C). The copper replaces the silver in the nitrate.
   General Chemistry 1.5.1

47. The correct answer is (D). pH is the negative log of the hydrogen ion concentration, and acids are below a pH of 7.   *General Chemistry 6.5*

PASSAGE 7

48. The correct answer is (C). The speed of light in a medium is equal to the speed of light in a vacuum (3.0×10^8 m/s) divided by its index of refraction.
   Physics 11.4

49. The correct answer is (B). In this case, light is traveling into a medium with a greater index of refraction; therefore, it will be bent toward the normal, and the angle of refraction will be less than the angle of incidence.   *Physics 11.4*

---

* For more information, refer to this section in Peterson's *Gold Standard MCAT.*

50. The correct answer is (A). This is determined by using Snell's law

$$n_1\sin\theta_1 = n_2\sin\theta_2$$
Physics 11.4

51. The correct answer is (A). By Snell's law, the left side of the equation becomes larger with an increase in n1, therefore, $\sin\theta_2$ must increase. The angle of refraction will still be smaller than the angle of incidence, however, because n_2 remains greater than n_1.
Physics 11.4

52. The correct answer is (A). The critical angle occurs when the angle of refraction is 90 degrees. This only occurs when light travels from a medium with a greater index of refraction to a medium with a lesser index. The angle is given by:

$$\sin\theta_c = \frac{n_1}{n_2}$$
Physics 11.4

53. The correct answer is (D). When the angle of incidence is greater than the critical angle there is no refraction, but total internal reflection.   *Physics 11.4*

PASSAGE 8

54. The correct answer is (C). Convert grams to moles: $\frac{222.0}{74}$ = 3 moles. Then multiply moles (3) Avogadro's number to get the total number of molecules (1.81×10^{24}), and this answer is then multiplied by 2 because there are 2 atoms of oxygen in each molecule of calcium hydroxide {$Ca(OH)_2$}.
General Chemistry 1.3

55. The correct answer is (C). Multiply 3.2 × Avogadro's number to get the total number of molecules (1.93×10^{24}), and then this answer is multiplied by 3 because there are 3 atoms of magnesium in each molecule of magnesium phosphate {$Mg_3(PO_4)_2$}.
General Chemistry 1.3, 3.1, 5.2

56. The correct answer is (D). There are 3 atoms total in a molecule of NaOH. Multiply Avogadro's number × 3 to get the total number of atoms.
General Chemistry 1.3, 3.1, 5.2

57. The correct answer is (A). Divide the 7.3×10^{24} molecules given in the problem by Avogadro's number to get the number of moles. Then multiply by the molecular mass of sodium hydroxide (40 grams/mole) to get the correct answer (485.1 grams).   *General Chemistry 1.3*

58. The correct answer is (A). Remember that oxygen gas is *diatomic* {O_2}. Therefore, 7.5×10^{23} atoms represents only 3.75×10^{23} molecules. Dividing this molecule total by Avogadro's number results in the number of moles of oxygen molecules, and then multiplying by the molecular mass (32.0 grams/mole) results in the correct answer (19.9 grams).
General Chemistry 1.3, 3.3

59. The correct answer is (D). Convert grams to moles first by dividing 29.0 by the molecular mass of $Mg(OH)_2$, which is 58 grams/mole. Multiply now by Avogadro's number to convert to total number of molecules, and then multiply by 5 because there are 5 individual atoms in each molecule.
General Chemistry 1.3, 3.1, 5.2

60. The correct answer is (A). From your work in the previous answer, take the total number of molecules found (3.01×10^{23}) and multiply by 2, because there are 2 oxygen atoms in each molecule of $Mg(OH)_2$.
General Chemistry 1.3

---

* For more information, refer to this section in Peterson's *Gold Standard MCAT.*

PASSAGE 9

61. The correct answer is (B). This is a graph of an exothermic reaction. 20 kJ of energy are needed to successfully complete the reaction (activation energy), and the total amount of energy released is 20 kJ (the difference in energy between the reactants and products). The ΔH for *exothermic* reactions is expressed as a (−) negative number.

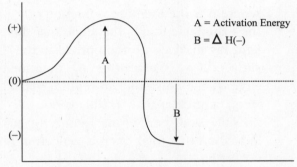

General Chemistry 9.5

62. The correct answer is (C). (See explanation above.) *General Chemistry 9.5*

63. The correct answer is (B). The total amount of heat liberated is equal to the exothermicity. *General Chemistry 9.5*

64. The correct answer is (B). This is a graph of an endothermic reaction. Approximately 35 kJ of energy are needed to successfully complete the reaction, and the net reaction requires +15 kJ. The ΔH for *endothermic* reactions is expressed as a (+) positive number.

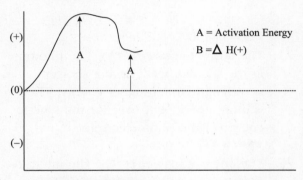

General Chemistry 9.5

65. The correct answer is (C). (See explanation for the previous question.)
General Chemistry 9.5

66. The correct answer is (B). The total amount of heat required is equal to the endothermicity. *General Chemistry 9.5*

PASSAGE 10

67. The correct answer is (A). Photons always travel at the speed of light, $c = 3 \times 10^8$ m/s in a vacuum.
Physics 11.4

68. The correct answer is (A). $c = \lambda f$, c is the speed of light, λ is the wavelength, and f is the frequency. *Physics 7.1.2, 11.4*

69. The correct answer is (A). The energy of a photon in joules is given by E=hf. Planck's constant $h = 6.63 \times 10^{-34}$ J*s. To convert from joules to electron-volts, divide the number of joules by 1.6×10^{-19}. *Physics 12.5; Appendix B2*

---

* For more information, refer to this section in Peterson's *Gold Standard MCAT.*

70. The correct answer is (B). The energy of the photoelectrons is equal to the energy of the incoming photon minus the work function of the metal.

Energy of incoming photon	=	work function	+	kinetic energy of photoelectron
hf	=	ϕ	+	$\frac{1}{2}mv^2$
2.48ev	=	ϕ	+	1.48ev

Physics 5.3, 12.5

71. The correct answer is (A). The photons in the second beam have a shorter wavelength and a higher energy. There is more energy left over for the kinetic energy of the photoelectrons.
Physics 7.1.2, 12.5

72. The correct answer is (C). The intensity of the beam can be defined as the number of photons in the beam. The energy of each photon depends on the frequency of the photon, not on the intensity of the beam. Since there are fewer photons, there will be fewer photoelectrons, although the kinetic energy of the photoelectrons will be the same. *Physics 8.3, 9.2.4*

73. The correct answer is (B). The period of a simple pendulum depends only on the gravitational field, g, and the length of the pendulum, L:

$$T = 2\pi\sqrt{\frac{L}{g}}$$

The longer pendulum has a period that is $\sqrt{4} = 2$ longer than the period of the short pendulum. *Physics 7.2.2, 7.2.3*

74. The correct answer is (C). It takes three years to reduce the sample from 80 grams to 40 grams; three more to reduce from 40 grams to 20 grams; and three more to reduce from 20 grams to 10 grams, for a total of 9 years.
Physics 12.4

75. The correct answer is (B). Snell's law for refraction as light moves across a boundary between two materials, called "A" and "B," is:

$$n_A\sin\theta_A = n_B\sin\theta_B$$

where n is the index of refraction of the material, and q is the angle that the light ray makes with the normal to the surface. If n_A is larger than n_B, then for large q_A the equation can require that $\sin q_B$ be greater than 1. This is not possible, and the "wrong" answer is an indication that total internal reflection is occurring.

From the figure with liquid #1, the presence of total internal reflection in the liquid makes it clear that the index of refraction of the liquid #1 must be greater than the index for the glass. In the figure with liquid #2, the angle in the glass is smaller than the angle in the liquid. This means that the index of refraction in the glass must be greater than that in the liquid in order to make the equation balance. Thus liquid #2 has the lowest index of refraction.
Physics 11.4

---

* For more information, refer to this section in Peterson's *Gold Standard MCAT.*

76. The correct answer is (A). The horizontal component of the acceleration is zero, so the horizontal component of the velocity does not change. It remains 5 m/sec as it was at the start. The vertical component of the motion is accelerated downward at 9.8 m/sec^2. If we choose up to be plus, this acceleration is $a_y = -9.8$ m/sec^2. The equations of motion for the vertical component are:

$$y = y_0 + v_{0y}t + \frac{1}{2}at^2 \text{ and } v_y = v_{0y} + a_y t$$

We can find the velocity must before it hits, provided we know the time when it hits. We can find that time from the position equation, because we know how far it falls. We choose $y = 0$ at the floor, so the $y_0 = 1.2$ meter. Call the particular time when the ball hits the floor "t_1." Now the equations of motion for the time t_1 are:

$$0 = 1.2m + 0 + \frac{1}{2}\left(-9.8\frac{m}{sec^2}\right)t_1{}^2 \text{ and}$$

$$v_y = 0 + \left(-9.8\frac{m}{sec^2}\right)t_1$$

Notice that $v_{0y} = 0$:

Initially the vertical component of the velocity is zero.

Solving the left equation for t_1 gives:

$$t_1 = \sqrt{2\left(\frac{-1.2m}{-9.8\frac{m}{sec^2}}\right)} = 0.49 \text{ sec}$$

Plugging this time into the right equation gives:

$$v_y = 0 + \left(9.8\frac{m}{sec^2}\right)(0.49sec)$$

$$= -4.85\frac{m}{sec^2}$$

or 4.85 m/sec^2 *down.*
 Physics 1.5, 1.6, 2.6

77. The correct answer is (A). The ray parallel to the optic axis reflects through the focal point. The ray that strikes the mirror where the optic axis meets the mirror makes an equal angle with the optic axis when it leaves the mirror. *Physics 11.3*

---

* For more information, refer to this section in Peterson's *Gold Standard MCAT.*

BIOLOGICAL SCIENCE

PASSAGE 1

1. The correct answer is (D). In a closed system, which the term suggests, circulation is entirely within vessels. Contraction of the heart [dorsal vessel] sends blood into vessels called arteries, which move blood out from the heart to the capillaries and back to the heart through vessels called veins. The other choices refer to open systems similar to those found in insects. *Biology 7.1*

2. The correct answer is (B). Veins carry blood back to the heart. Those coming from the body carry deoxygenated blood, but those coming from the lungs carry oxygenated blood. Therefore one cannot make the blanket statement that veins carry blood that is either high or low in oxygen. Arteries carry blood away from the heart. *Biology 7.2, 7.3*

3. The correct answer is (A). When blood is delivered to the left ventricle, it has just come from the lungs and is high in oxygen. Therefore, the next stop is to be delivered to the cells of the body. The right ventricle pumps blood to the lungs and blood arrives at the heart from various places through arteries. *Biology 7.2*

4. The correct answer is (A). Osmosis is the diffusion of water only and therefore is not an exchange mechanism. Active transport is a means of facilitated transport, i.e., requires far too much energy to be the mechanism for exchanging gases in the lungs. Pinocytosis involves movement of macromolecules into cells. Simple diffusion accounts for the exchange of gases in the lungs. *Biology 7.3, 12.3*

5. The correct answer is (C). When the diaphragm is contracted, it creates a downward pull on the tissues of the lungs, thus expanding the lungs and causing the atmosphere to push air into the lungs. If the pressure gradient is equalized, gases will not move in large enough quantities to satisfy the need for an oxygen-carbon dioxide exchange. When we relax the diaphragm it reduces the volume of the lungs forcing air out of the lungs. In between heart beats would mean we would inhale at the rate of 70–90 beats a minute on average. The average number of inhalations is 15–20 per minute. *Biology 12.4*

PASSAGE 2

6. The correct answer is (A). The fragments obtained indicate a cleaving of methionine. Arginine was cleaved, but not on the C side as was methionine consistently. *Biology 3; Organic Chemistry 12.1, 12.2*

7. The correct answer is (B). Clearly, there has been cleavage on the C side of lysine indicating trypsin digestion followed by acid hydrolysis, we can assume, from the isolated Ala at the beginning of the peptide. The cleavage at the Lys and Met junction contradicts Edmund degradation, but supports trypsin digestion. Methionine has not been cleaved on the C side, arguing against cyanogen bromide treatment. *Biology 3; Organic Chemistry 12.1, 12.2*

---

* For more information, refer to this section in Peterson's *Gold Standard MCAT*.

8. The correct answer is (A). The alanine would have been cleaved using the Edman degradation, then Edman degradation could have been performed on the other fragment cleaving the new N-terminal amino acid. The other fragments are not consistent with the other processes presented.

Biology 3; Organic Chemistry 1.1, 1.2

9. The correct answer is (C). The molar ratio of methionine to serine or glycine should be 2:1. With an already isolated Ala-Lys fragment, the results of an Edman treatment might be misleading and the data are not consistent, a fact which can be determined with the original theory since only one Met is presented here.

Biology 3; Organic Chemistry 12.1, 12.2

10. The correct answer is (A). The available methods do not permit specific C-terminal cleavage of leucine. The fragments in (B) can be obtained using cyanogen bromide cleavage and repeated Edman treatments. The fragments in (C) can be obtained using cyanogen bromide treatment, trypsin digestion, and cyanogen bromide treatment. The fragments in (D) can be obtained using acid hydrolysis.

Biology 3; Organic Chemistry 12.1, 12.2

11. The correct answer is (D). The pH of the small intestine is alkaline (> pH 7).

Biology 9.4.2

PASSAGE 3

12. The correct answer is (B). The lac operon model was based on research done with E. coli but is considered a general model for prokaryotic gene regulation and not a special feature unique to that particular organism.

Biology 2.2

13. The correct answer is (A). In the presence of lactose, the structural genes are expressed and enzymes are made; lactose is termed the inducer since it induces the production of the enzymes. The entire unit is called an inducible operon. *Biology 15.1, 15.3*

14. The correct answer is (D). All of the statements are true.

15. The correct answer is (D). Lactate has nothing to do with the lac operon's expression. The genes are expressed only when lactose is actually present.

16. The correct answer is (A). The repressor molecule is coded for by the regulator gene. When lactose is not present, the repressor binds to the operator and prevents attachment of RNA polymerase, precluding transcription of the structural genes.

Biology 3

17. The correct answer is (C). A lac operon is normally switched off (genes are not being transcribed) and becomes active only in the presence of lactose. The trp operon is normally on (genes are being transcribed) and is only switched off in the presence of tryptophan, and this operon is termed repressible since tryptophan represses the expression of the genes.

18. The correct answer is (C). Tryptophan binds to the inactive form of the repressor molecule, which cannot bind to the operator region. This interaction modifies the shape of the repressor molecule and allows it to bind to the operator region, blocking transcription.

---

* For more information, refer to this section in Peterson's *Gold Standard MCAT*.

19. The correct answer is (D). The axons of the ganglion layer gather to form the optic nerve, CN II, and exit the retina at the optic disk, which is a blind spot on the retina because it has no rods or cones. The optic nerve travels posteriorly out the back of the eyeball and bony orbit to cross some fibers with the opposite optic nerve at the optic chiasm.   *Biology 6.1, 6.2.4*

20. The correct answer is (B). The macula is a structure in the utricle and in the saccule that functions in a manner very similar to the crista.
Biology 6.2.3

21. The correct answer is (C). The stapes ossicle bone and the stapedius muscle are derived from the second pharyngeal arch (hyoid arch), and the muscle is supplied by its nerve (cranial nerve seven).   *Biology 6.2.3*

22. The correct answer is (B). Not taste, but general sensation, pain, cold, for the anterior two thirds of the tongue is the lingual branch of the trigeminal nerve (cranial nerve five).
Biology 6.1, 6.2.2

23. The correct answer is (B). The neural posterior lobe, the neurohypophysis, communicates with the hypothalamus by way of secretory neurons, which secrete oxytocin and vasopressin (or antidiuretic hormone, ADH) into the posterior lobe. Oxytocin acts primarily on the breasts and uterus.
Biology 6.3.1

Passage 4

24. The correct answer is (A). Glycolysis is an anaerobic process and uses no oxygen.   *Biology 4.4, 4.5*

25. The correct answer is (B). Phosphate is added at step 5, but it is not derived from ATP.   *Biology 4.5, 4.6*

26. The correct answer is (D). In stage I the six-carbon glucose molecule is phosphorylated by ATP and turned into fructose-6-phosphate (an isomer of glucose-6-phosphate) and finally split into two glyceraldehyde phosphate molecules. ATP is required at two points, unless the starting point is glycogen and not glucose, since glucose derived from glycogen can be phosphorylated directly and does not require ATP at that step. In stage two, the glyceraldehyde phosphate molecules are made into three-carbon pyruvate molecules, with the generation of ATP and NADH.
Biology 4.5, 4.6

27. The correct answer is (B). The hydrogen atoms and electrons are used to reduce the oxidized form of NADH, that is, NAD+. Recall what is oxidized and what is reduced by this mnemonic: *LEO* the lion says *GER—Lose Electrons Oxidized, Gain Electrons Reduced.*
Biology 4.5, 4.6, 4.7, 4.10

28. The correct answer is (B). Glucose is a six-carbon sugar, so the answer must be either (B) or (D). (A) is sucrose, (C) is pyruvate, and (D) is nothing—glucose does not contain any nitrogen.
Organic Chemistry 12.3.1, 12.3.2

29. The correct answer is (B). The chemiosmotic method of ATP synthesis is used in the mitochondrion. Photophosphorylation would apply to photosynthesis, and ATPase breaks down and does not synthesize ATP.   *Biology 4.6*

30. The correct answer is (C). Lactate is produced by fermentation in muscles under conditions where free oxygen is lacking. (In plants and yeast, carbon dioxide and alcohol are the end products of fermentation.) The lactate can be used in the Krebs cycle in some cells such as liver, kidney, and heart muscle. Otherwise it can be reprocessed to make glucose. *Biology 4.4, 4.5*

Passage 5

31. The correct answer is (A). Periostium is the connective tissue sheath found around bones. *Biology 5.4.4*

32. The correct answer is (A). (B) is a description of cardiac muscle, (C) is a description of smooth muscle. *Biology 5.2*

33. The correct answer is (C). Myosin makes up the thick myofilaments. *Biology 5.2*

34. The correct answer is (B). The T-tubule is an invagination of the sarcolemma which provides for the excitation occurring along the sarcolemma to be delivered into the muscle fiber. *Biology 5.2*

35. The correct answer is (C). Motor neurons activate skeletal muscle fibers by the release of a chemical neurotransmitter, acetylcholine. The myoneural junction must contain chemically mediated gates for a response. The propagation of the impulse along the sarcolemma will utilized voltage mediated gates. *Biology 5.1, 5.1.1, 5.1.2, 5.1.3, 5.2*

36. The correct answer is (D). All are characteristics of muscle fiber contraction, but tetanus occurs due to the rapidly delivered stimulus. *Biology 11.2*

Passage 6

37. The correct answer is (D). Bone, blood, loose, and adipose tissue are all types of connective tissue. Squamous is a cell shape found mainly in epithelial tissue. *Biology 5.3, 5.4*

38. The correct answer is (B). The only cells on the list that are long and excitable as well as capable of changing shape by elongation and contraction are muscle tissues. *Biology 5.2*

39. The correct answer is (B). Systems (also called organ systems) are the level of organization one step above organs. Organisms are one step above systems, and cells are one step below tissues. Therefore, organs are defined as being composed of different kinds of tissues organized to contribute to a common function.

40. The correct answer is (D). Epithelial tissue is capable of secretion. While material passes into and out of the other three types of tissue, that material is not designed for an effect at a target cell, as is the definition of a secretion and therefore mainly the function of certain epithelial cells. *Biology 5.3*

41. The correct answer is (D). All three statements are true of organ systems. *Biology 5.4*

42. The correct answer is (A). GHRH, growth hormone releasing hormone, releases GH, growth hormone or somatostatin, from the anterior lobe. *Biology 6.3.1*

43. The correct answer is (B). In the adult, the thyroid responds to a lack of thyroxin by increasing the size of the thyroid gland tissue itself, forming a goiter. *Biology 6.3.3*

---

* For more information, refer to this section in Peterson's *Gold Standard MCAT.*

44. The correct answer is (C). Glucagon increases gluconeogenesis in the liver, increases the metabolic rate, increases ketogenesis, and is lipolytic   ** Biology 6.3.4.*

45. The correct answer is (C). Insulin rapidly causes increased facilitated transport of glucose into the cell by increasing the number of transporters available. Once glucose is inside the cell, other hormones regulate the rate of phosphorylation of glucose.
* Biology 6.3.4

46. The correct answer is (A). The medulla is not necessary for life as is the cortex, but it helps prepare the body for emergencies.   ** Biology 6.3.2*

PASSAGE 7

47. The correct answer is (D). Choices (A), (B), and (C) are all means by which materials move into and out of cells. Peristalsis is the series of smooth muscle contractions that pushes food through the digestive system.
* Biology 9.2

48. The correct answer is (A). The tricky word here is true. Since digestion is the breakdown, both physical and chemical, of food in the digestive system, the moment it enters the alimentary canal by way of the mouth, digestion, both physical and chemical, begins. Food never enters the pancreas. After the mouth comes the stomach, followed by the intestine(s).   ** Biology 9.1, 9.2*

49. The correct answer is (B). The HCl contributes in one way or another to all of the processes listed except the hydrolyzing of starch. Saliva in the mouth does this, breaking starch down into smaller polysaccharides.   ** Biology 9.2, 9.3*

50. The correct answer is (C). By the time the treated food reaches the appendix, it has been completely digested; absorption is now taking place. More importantly, however, the appendix is composed of lymphoid tissue with no digestive function. The salivary glands secrete a carbohydrate digesting enzyme, the pancreas secretes several digestion enzymes, and the liver produces bile, a fat emulsifier. All of these have digestive functions.
* Biology 9.1, 9.2, 9.4.1, 9.4.2, 9.5

51. The correct answer is (C). The human body cannot store essential amino acids—the ones not capable of being made by humans. There are 20 kinds we need, 12 of which we can make. If we lack even one of the essential amino acids, we suffer protein deficiency, often referred to by the African word, *kwashiorkor*.
* Biology 3; Organic Chemistry 12.1

PASSAGE 8

52. The correct answer is (B). The younger of the two photosystems (PS II) is, in a sense, "piggy-backed" on the older PS I.

53. The correct answer is (C). The process of cyclic photophosphorylation recycles electrons and uses energy derived from PS I ("path B" in the diagram) to make ATP from ADP and inorganic phosphate.

54. The correct answer is (C). Inorganic phosphate is combined with ADP and energy to manufacture ATP.

---

* For more information, refer to this section in Peterson's *Gold Standard MCAT.*

55. The correct answer is (C). Electrons leaving the light-dependent reactions are channeled into combining with NADP+ and H+ to make NADPH, a source of reducing power in the light-independent reactions.

56. The correct answer is (D). ATP is used as a source of energy and NADPH as a source of reducing power in the reduction of carbon dioxide to carbohydrate.

57. The correct answer is (A). PS I is the older of the two photosystems, that is, it appeared earlier than PS II in the evolution of photosynthesis.

58. The correct answer is (C). The pigment complexes, which capture photons of light are located on the thylakoid membrane, as are the molecules which comprise the electron transport system. ATP is synthesized across the membrane. The light-independent reactions occur in the stroma. "Cristae" and "matrix" are features of the mitochondrion, not the chloroplast.

59. The correct answer is (B). The term "dark reactions" was considered too misleading, since these reactions happen independently of the presence of light, that is, regardless of whether or not light is present.

PASSAGE 9

60. The correct answer is (B). This is the difference that gives the two groups their names. Choices (C) and (D) are true, but are not the nominal differences between the two groups.
   Biology 2.2, 2.3

61. The correct answer is (C). As stated in the passage, as a generalization, eukaryotic cells are typically about ten times larger than prokaryotic cells.

62. The correct answer is (B). II through V are found in eukaryotic but not prokaryotic cells. Eukaryotic flagella are made up of tubulin and other proteins, but not flagellin, which is unique to prokaryotes. *Biology 1.2, 2.2*

63. The correct answer is (D). Histones are proteins complexed with DNA in eukaryotic chromosomes. *Biology 1.2.1*

64. The correct answer is (B). Both mitochondria and chloroplasts contain DNA (mDNA and cDNA). This is one point of evidence for the endosymbiotic theory of the origin of these organelles from once free-living prokaryotes. *Biology 1.2.1*

65. The correct answer is (D). Mitochondria and chloroplasts both have a double-membrane structure, have their own unique DNA, and are about the same size as most prokaryotes.

PASSAGE 10

66. The correct answer is (C). The activity of subcellular structures is remarkably consistent between cells (complementarity). *Biology 1.2, 1.2.1*

67. The correct answer is (D). All are characteristics of plasma membranes. *Biology 1.1; Organic Chemistry 12.3.3*

68. The correct answer is (B). Microvilli are membrane specializations, but not involved in cell membrane junctions. *Biology 1.2*

69. The correct answer is (B). Pinocytosis is an active transport process. *Biology 1.1.1, 1.1.2, 1.1.3*

---

* For more information, refer to this section in Peterson's *Gold Standard MCAT*.

70. The correct answer is (B). (A) does not exist, (C) describes a lysosome, (D) describes a mitochondria but gives an inappropriate function.
  Biology 1.2.1, 4.8

71. The correct answer is (C). Rough ER is involved with synthesis of protein, but not its "handling". Peroxisomes are involved with free-radical oxygen processing and centrioles are involved with the control of certain structures of the cytoskeleton.   *Biology 1.2.1*

72. The correct answer is (A). The envelope of the nucleus is called a nuclear membrane, but it is a double membrane (phospholipid bilayer).   *Biology 1.2.1*

73. The correct answer is (A).   *Biology 1.3*

74. The correct answer is (A). All animals are heterotrophs, but no animals are photosynthetic autotrophs or have cell walls.

75. The correct answer is (D). At the end of the axon the action potential causes chemicals (neurotransmitters) to be released from membrane-bound vesicles in the axon. The chemicals diffuse across the gap (synaptic gap) to excite another neuron, or a muscle cell. Depending on the circumstances, the action can be inhibitory or excitatory. The former works against depolarization of the membrane, while the excitatory action depolarizes the membrane. Mixed signals can be received, and the sum total of the effects determines the integrated response of the neuron or cell.   *Biology 5.1*

76. The correct answer is (C). Fertilization normally occurs in the oviduct. The fertilized egg normally descends into the uterus; if it does not, an ectopic, or more specifically, a tubal pregnancy, may result.   *Biology 14.5*

77. The correct answer is (A). Enzymes work best with a specific temperature range. Enzyme activity reaches a maximum at a point of optimum temperature and falls off as the temperature rises above or falls below this point. If the temperature rises high enough, the enzyme will be denatured and no longer function as a catalyst.
  Biology 4.1, 4.3

---

* For more information, refer to this section in Peterson's *Gold Standard MCAT.*

Paying for School—Financing Your Graduate Education

Support for graduate study can take many forms, depending upon the field of study and program you pursue. For example, some 60 percent of doctoral students receive support in the form of either grants/fellowships or assistantships, whereas most students in master's programs rely on loans to pay for their graduate study. In addition, doctoral candidates are more likely to receive grants/fellowships and assistantships than master's degree students, and students in the sciences are more likely to receive aid than those in the arts and humanities.

For those of you who have applied for financial aid as an undergraduate, there are some differences for graduate students you'll notice right away. For one, aid to undergraduates is based primarily on need (although the number of colleges that now offer undergraduate merit-based aid is increasing), but graduate aid is often based on academic merit. Second, as a graduate student, you are automatically declared "independent" for federal financial aid purposes, meaning your parents' income and asset information is not required in assessing your need for federal aid. Third, at some graduate schools, the awarding of aid may be administered by the academic departments or the graduate school itself, not the financial aid office. That means that at some schools, you may be involved with as many as three offices: a central financial aid office, the graduate school, *and* your academic department.

Be Prepared

Being prepared for graduate school means you have to put together a financial plan. So, before you enter graduate school, you should have answers to these questions:

- What should I be doing now to prepare for the cost of my graduate education?

- What can I do to minimize my costs once I arrive on campus?

- What financial aid programs are available at each of the schools to which I am applying?

- What financial aid programs are available outside the university, at the federal, state, or private level?

- What financing options do I have if I cannot pay the full cost from my own resources and those of my family?

- What should I know about the loans I am being offered?

- What impact will these loans have on me when I complete my program?

You'll find your answers in three guiding principles: think ahead, live within your means, and keep your head above water.

Think Ahead

The first step to putting together your financial plan comes from thinking about the future: the loss of your income while you're attending school, your projected income after you graduate, the annual rate of inflation, additional expenses you will incur as a student and after you graduate, and any loss of income you may experience later on from unintentional periods of unemployment, pregnancy, or disability. The cornerstone of thinking ahead is following a step-by-step process.

1. *Set your goals.* Decide what and where you want to study, whether you will go full- or part-time, whether you'll work while attending, and what an appropriate level of debt would be. Consider whether you would attend full-time if you had enough financial aid or whether keeping your full-time job is an important priority in your life. Keep in mind that many employers have tuition reimbursement plans for full-time employees.

2. *Take inventory.* Collect your financial information and add up your assets—bank accounts, stocks, bonds, real estate, business and personal property. Then subtract your liabilities—money owed on your assets, including credit card debt and car loans—to yield your net worth.

3. *Calculate your need.* Compare your net worth with the costs at the schools you are considering to get a rough estimate of how much of your assets you can use for your schooling.

4. *Create an action plan.* Determine how much you'll earn while in school, how much you think you will receive in grants and scholarships, and how much you plan to borrow. Don't forget to consider inflation and possible life changes that could affect your overall financial plan.

5. *Review your plan regularly.* Measure the progress of your plan every year and make adjustments for such things as increases in salary or other changes in your goals or circumstances.

Live Within Your Means

The second step in being prepared is knowing how much you spend now so you can determine how much you'll spend when you're in school. Use the standard cost of attendance budget published by your school as a guide, but don't be surprised if your estimated budget is higher than the one the school provides, especially if you've been out of school for a while. Once you've figured out your budget, see if you can pare down your current costs and financial obligations so the lean years of graduate school don't come as too large a shock.

Keep Your Head Above Water

Finally, the third step is managing the debt you'll accrue as a graduate student. Debt is manageable only when considered in terms of five things:

1. Your future income

2. The amount of time it takes to repay the loan

3. The interest rate you are being charged

4. Your personal lifestyle and expenses after graduation

5. Unexpected circumstances that change your income or your ability to repay what you owe

To make sure your educational debt is manageable, you should borrow an amount that requires payments of no more than 8 percent of your starting salary.

The approximate monthly installments for repaying borrowed principal at 5, 8-10, 12, and 14 percent are indicated below.

Estimated Loan Repayment Schedule Monthly Payments for Every $1,000 Borrowed

Rate	5 years	10 years	15 years	20 years	25 years
5%	$18.87	$10.61	$ 7.91	$ 6.60	$ 5.85
8%	20.28	12.13	9.56	8.36	7.72
9%	20.76	12.67	10.14	9.00	8.39
10%	21.74	13.77	10.75	9.65	9.09
12%	22.24	14.35	12.00	11.01	10.53
14%	23.27	15.53	13.32	12.44	12.04

You can use this table to estimate your monthly payments on a loan for any of the five repayment periods (5, 10, 15, 20, and 25 years). The amounts listed are the monthly payments for a $1,000 loan for each of the interest rates. To estimate your monthly payment, choose the closest interest rate and multiply the amount of the payment listed by the total amount of your loan and then divide by 1,000. For example, for a total loan of $15,000 at 9 percent to be paid back over 10 years, multiply $12.67 times 15,000 (190,050), divided by 1,000. This yields $190.05 per month.

If you're wondering just how much of a loan payment you can afford monthly without running into payment problems, consult the following chart.

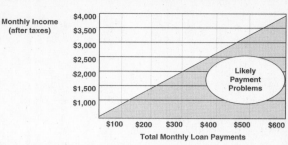

How Much Can You Afford to Repay?

This graph shows the monthly cash-flow outlook based on your total monthly loan payments in comparison with your monthly income earned after taxes. Ideally, to eliminate likely payment problems, your monthly loan payment should be less than 15% of your monthly income.

Of course, the best way to manage your debt is to borrow less. While cutting your personal budget may be one option, there are a few others you may want to consider:

- *Ask Your Family for Help:* Although the federal government considers you "independent," your parents and family may still be willing and able to help pay for your graduate education. If your family is not open to just giving you money, they may be open to making a low-interest (or deferred-interest) loan. Family loans usually have more attractive interest rates and repayment terms than commercial loans. They may also have tax consequences, so you may want to check with a tax adviser.

- *Push to Graduate Early:* It's possible to reduce your total indebtedness by completing your program ahead of schedule. You can either take more courses per semester or during the summer. Keep in mind, though, that these options reduce the time you have available to work.

- *Work More, Attend Less:* Another alternative is to enroll part-time, leaving more time to work. Remember, though, to qualify for aid, you must be enrolled at least half-time, which is usually considered six credits per term. And if you're enrolled less than half-time, you'll have to start repaying your loans once the grace period has expired.

ROLL YOUR LOANS INTO ONE

There's a good chance that as a graduate student you will have two or more loans included in your aid package, plus any money you borrowed as an undergraduate. That means when you start repaying, you could be making loan payments to several different lenders. Not only can the recordkeeping be a nightmare, but with each loan having a minimum payment, your total monthly payments may be more than you can handle. If you owe more than $7,500 in federal loans, you can combine your loans into one consolidated loan at either a flat 9 percent interest rate or a weighted average of the rates on the loans consolidated. Your repayment can also be extended to up to thirty years, depending on the total amount you borrow, which will make your monthly payments lower (of course, you'll also be paying more total interest). With a consolidated loan, some lenders offer graduated or income-sensitive repayment options. Consult with your lender about the types of consolidation provisions offered.

CREDIT: DON'T LET YOUR PAST HAUNT YOU

Many schools will check your credit history before they process any private educational loans for you. To make sure your credit rating is accurate, you may want to request a copy of your credit report before you start graduate school. You can get a copy of your report by sending a signed, written request to one of the three national credit reporting agencies at the address listed below. Include your full name, social security number, current address, any previous addresses for the past five years, date of birth, and daytime phone number. Call the agency before you request your report so you know whether there is a fee for this report. Note that you are entitled to a free copy of your credit report if you have been denied credit within the last sixty days.

Credit criteria used to review and approve student loans can include the following:

- Absence of negative credit

- No bankruptcies, foreclosures, repossessions, charge-offs, or open judgments

---

CREDIT REPORTING AGENCIES

Experian National Assistance Center
P.O. Box 9530
Allen, Texas 75013
888-397-3742

Equifax
P.O. Box 105873
Atlanta, Georgia 30348
800-685-1111

CSC Credit Services
Consumer Assistance Center
P.O. Box 674402
Houston, Texas 77267-4402
800-759-5979

Trans Union Corporation
P.O. Box 390
Springfield, Pennsylvania 19064-0390
800-888-4213

- No prior educational loan defaults, unless paid in full or making satisfactory repayments

- Absence of excessive past due accounts; that is, no 30-, 60-, or 90-day delinquencies on consumer loans or revolving charge accounts within the past two years

TYPES OF AID AVAILABLE

There are three types of aid: money given to you (grants, scholarships, and fellowships), money you earn through work, and loans.

Grants, Scholarships, and Fellowships

Most grants, scholarships, and fellowships are outright awards that require no service in return. Often they provide the cost of tuition and fees plus a stipend to cover living expenses. Some are based exclusively on financial need, some exclusively on academic merit, and some on a combination of need and merit. As a rule, grants are awarded to those with financial need, although they may require the recipient to have expertise in a certain field. Fellowships and scholarships often connote selectivity based on ability—financial need is usually not a factor.

Federal Support

Several federal agencies fund fellowship and trainee programs for graduate and professional students. The amounts and types of assistance offered vary considerably by field of study. The following are programs available for those studying engineering and applied sciences:

National Science Foundation. Graduate Research Program Fellowships include tuition and fees plus a $14,000 stipend and a $1,000 total allowance for three years of graduate study in engineering, mathematics, the natural sciences, the social sciences, and the history and philosophy of science. The application deadline is in early November. For more information, write to the National Science Foundation at Oak Ridge Associated Universities, P.O. Box 3010, Oak Ridge, Tennessee 37831-3010 or call 423-241-4300.

National Institutes of Health (NIH). NIH sponsors many different fellowship opportunities. For example, it offers training grants administered through schools' research departments. Training grants provide tuition plus a twelve-month stipend of $11,496. For more information, call 301-435-0714.

Veterans' Benefits. Veterans may use their educational benefits for training at the graduate and professional levels. Contact your regional office of the Veterans Administration for more details.

State Support

Many states offer grants for graduate study, with California, Michigan, New York, North Carolina, Texas, and Virginia offering the largest programs. Due to fiscal constraints, however, some states have had to reduce or eliminate their financial aid programs for graduate study. To qualify for a particular state's aid you must be a resident of that state. Residency is established in most states after you have lived there for at least twelve consecutive months prior to enrolling in school. Many states provide funds for in-state students only; that is, funds are not transferable out of state. Contact your state scholarship office to determine what aid it offers.

Institutional Aid

Educational institutions using their own funds provide more than $3 billion in graduate assistance in the form of fellowships, tuition waivers, and assistantships. Consult each school's catalog for information about aid programs.

Corporate Aid

Many corporations provide graduate student support as part of the employee benefits package. Most employees who receive aid study at the master's level or take courses without enrolling in a particular degree program.

Aid from Foundations

Most foundations provide support in areas of interest to them. The Foundation Center of New York City publishes several reference books on foundation support for graduate study. They also have a computerized databank called Grant Guides that, for a fee, will produce a listing of grant possibilities in a variety of fields. For more information call 212-620-4230.

Financial Aid for Minorities and Women

Patricia Roberts Harris Fellowships. This federal award provides support for minorities and women. Awards are made to schools, and the schools decide who receives these funds. Fellows receive a stipend of $14,400 for up to four years, and their institutions receive up to $9493 per year. Consult the graduate school for more information. No fund is guaranteed beyond the 1998 fiscal year.

Bureau of Indian Affairs. The Bureau of Indian Affairs (BIA) offers aid to students who are at least one quarter American Indian or native Alaskan and from a federally recognized tribe. Contact your tribal education officer, BIA area office, or call the Bureau of Indian Affairs at 202-208-3710.

The Ford Foundation Doctoral Fellowship for Minorities. The Ford Foundation provides three-year doctoral fellowships and one-year dissertation fellowships. Predoctoral fellowships include an annual stipend of $14,000 to the fellow and an annual institutional grant of $7500 to the fellowship institution in lieu of tuition and fees. Dissertation fellows receive a stipend of $18,000 for a twelve-month period. Applications are due in early November. For more information contact the Fellowship Office, National Research Council at 202-334-2872, or visit their Website at www.4. nationalacademies.org/losep/fo.nsf

National Consortium for Graduate Degrees in Engineering and Science (GEM). GEM was founded in 1976 to help minority men and women pursue graduate study in engineering and science by helping them obtain practical experience through summer internships at consortium work sites and finance graduate study toward a master's or Ph.D. degree. GEM administers the following programs:

Ph.D. Fellowship Program. The Ph.D. Science Fellowship and the Engineering Fellowship programs provide opportunities for minority students to obtain a Ph.D. in the natural sciences or in engineering through a program of paid summer research internships and financial support. Open to U.S. citizens who belong to one of the ethnic groups underrepresented in the natural sciences and engineering, GEM fellowships are awarded for a twelve-month period. Fellowships are tenable at universities participating in the GEM science or engineering Ph.D. programs. Awards include tuition, fees, and a $12,000 stipend. After the first year of study fellows are supported completely by their respective universities and support may include teaching or research assistantships. Forty fellowships are awarded annually in each program. The application deadline is December. Contact: GEM, Box 537, Notre Dame, Indiana 46556 or call 219-287-1097.

National Physical Sciences Consortium. Graduate fellowships are available in astronomy, chemistry, computer science, geology, materials science, mathematics, and physics for women and Black, Hispanic, and Native American students. These fellowships are available only at member universities. Awards may vary by year in school; the application deadline is November 1. Fellows receive tuition plus a stipend between $10,000 and $15,000. Contact National Physical Sciences Consortium, c/o New Mexico State University, O'Loughlin House, P.O. Box 30001, Department 3NPS, Las Cruces, New Mexico 88033-0001 or call 505-646-6037.

In addition, below are some books available that describe financial aid opportunities for women and minorities.

The Directory of Financial Aids for Women, 5th ed., by Gail Ann Schlachter (Reference Service Press, 1991), lists sources of support and identifies foundations and other organizations interested in helping women secure funding for graduate study.

The Association for Women in Science publishes *Grants-at-a-Glance,* a booklet highlighting fellowships for women in science. It can be ordered by calling 202-326-8940.

Books such as the *Directory of Special Programs for Minority Group Members,* 5th ed. (Garrett Park, Md: Garrett Park Press, 1990) describe financial aid opportunities for minority students. If you register with the *Minority Graduate Student Locator Service* sponsored by the Educational Testing Service, you will be contacted by schools interested in increasing their minority student enrollment. Such schools may have funds designated for minority students.

Students with disabilities are eligible to receive aid from a number of organizations. *Financial Aid for the Disabled and Their Families, 1992-94* (Reference Service Press) lists aid opportunities for disabled students. The Vocational Rehabilitation Services in your home state can also provide information.

Researching Grants and Fellowships

The books listed below are good sources of information on grant and fellowship support for graduate education and should be consulted before you resort to borrowing. Keep in mind that grant support varies dramatically from field to field.

Annual Register of Grant Support: A Directory of Funding Sources, Wilmette, Ill.: National Register Publishing Co. This is a comprehensive guide to grants and awards from government agencies, foundations, and business and professional organizations.

Corporate Foundation Profiles, 8th ed. New York: Foundation Center, 1994. This is an in-depth, analytical profile of 250 of the largest company-sponsored foundations in the United States. Brief descriptions of all 700 company-sponsored foundations are also included. There is an index of subjects, types of support, and geographical locations.

The Foundation Directory, 16th ed. Edited by Stan Olsen. New York: Foundation Center, 1994. This directory, with a supplement, gives detailed information on U.S. foundations with brief descriptions of the purpose and activities of each.

The Grants Register 1998, 16th ed. Edited by Lisa Williams. New York: St. Martin's, 1998. This lists grant agencies alphabetically and gives information on awards available to graduate students, young professionals, and scholars for study and research.

Peterson's Grants for Graduate and Postdoctoral Study, 5th ed. Princeton: Peterson's Guides, 1998. This book includes information on more than 1,400 grants, scholarships, awards, fellowships, and prizes. Originally compiled by the office of Research Affairs at the Graduate School of the University of Massachusetts Amherst.

Graduate schools sometimes publish listings of support sources in their catalogs, and some provide separate publications, such as the *Graduate Guide to Grants,* compiled by the Harvard Graduate School of Arts and Sciences. For more information, call 617-495-1814.

The Internet as a Source of Funding Information

If you have not explored the financial resources on the Internet, your research is not complete. Now available on the Web is a wealth of information ranging from loan and entrance applications to minority grants and scholarships.

University-Specific Information on the Web

Many universities have Web financial aid directories. Florida, Virginia Tech, Massachusetts, Emory, and Georgetown are just a few. Applications of admission can now be downloaded from the Web to start the graduate process. After that, detailed information can be obtained on financial aid processes, forms, and deadlines. University-specific grant and scholarship information can also be found, and more may be learned about financing by using the Web than by an actual visit. Questions can be asked on-line.

Scholarships on the Web

When searching for scholarship opportunities, one can search the Web. Many benefactors and other scholarship donors have pages on the Web listing pertinent information with regard to their specific scholarship. You can reach this information through a variety of methods. For example, you can find a directory listing minority scholarships, quickly look at the information on-line, decide if it applies to you, and then move on. New scholarship pages are being added to the Web daily.

The Web also lists many services that will look for scholarships for you. Some of these services cost money and advertise more scholarships per dollar than any other service. While some of these might be helpful, beware. Check references to make sure a bonafide service is being offered. Your best bet initially is to surf the Web and use the traditional library resources on available scholarships.

Bank and Loan Information on the Web

Banks and loan servicing centers have pages on the Web, making it easier to access loan information. Having the information on screen in front of you instantaneously is more convenient than being put on hold on the phone. Any loan information such as interest rate variations, descriptions of loans, loan consolidation programs, and repayment charts can all be found on the Web.

Work Programs

Certain types of support, such as teaching, research, and administrative assistantships, require recipients to provide service to the university in exchange for a salary or stipend; sometimes tuition is also provided or waived.

Teaching Assistantships

Because the physical sciences and engineering classes are taught at the undergraduate level, you stand a good chance of securing a teaching assistantship. These positions usually involve conducting small classes, delivering lectures, correcting class work, grading papers, counseling students, and supervising laboratory groups. Usually about 20 hours of work are required each week.

Teaching assistantships provide excellent educational experience as well as financial support. TAs generally receive a salary (now considered taxable income). Sometimes tuition is provided or waived as well. In addition, at some schools, teaching assistants can be declared state residents, qualifying them for the in-state tuition rates. Appointments are based on academic qualifications and are subject to the availability of funds within a department. If you are interested in a teaching assistantship, contact the academic department. Ordinarily you are not considered for such positions until you have been admitted to the graduate school.

Research Assistantships

Research assistantships usually require that you assist in the research activities of a faculty member. Appointments are ordinarily made for the academic year. They are rarely offered to first-year students. Contact the academic department, describing your particular research interests. As is the case with teaching assistantships, research assistantships provide excellent academic training as well as practical experience and financial support.

Administrative Assistantships

These positions usually require 10 to 20 hours of work each week in an administrative office of the university. For example, those seeking a graduate degree in education may work in the admissions, financial aid, student affairs, or placement office of the school they are attending. Some administrative assistantships provide a tuition waiver, others a salary. Details concerning these positions can be found in the school catalog or by contacting the academic department directly.

Federal Work-Study Program (FWS)

This federally funded program provides eligible students with employment opportunities, usually in public and private nonprofit organizations. Federal funds pay up to 75 percent of the wages, with the remainder paid by the employing agency. FWS is available to graduate students who demonstrate financial need. Not all schools have these funds, and some only award undergraduates. Each school sets its application deadline and work-study earnings limits. Wages vary and are related to the type of work done.

Additional Employment Opportunities

Many schools provide on-campus employment opportunities that do not require demonstrated financial need. The student employment office on most campuses assists students in securing jobs both on and off the campus.

Loans

Most needy graduate students, except those pursuing Ph.D.'s in certain fields, borrow to finance their graduate programs. There are two sources of student loans—the federal government and private loan programs. You should read and understand the terms of these loan programs before submitting your loan application.

Federal Loans

Federal Stafford Loans. Federal Stafford Loans are low-interest loans made to students by a private lender such as a bank. For Subsidized Federal Stafford Loans, interest is paid by the federal government while you are in school. Eligibility is determined by the school's financial aid office from the information you provide on the financial aid application.

Eligible borrowers may borrow up to $8,500 per year, up to a maximum of $65,500 in total loans, including undergraduate borrowing. The interest rate depends on whether you have borrowed previously. For those who have borrowed in the past, the rate is 7, 8, or 9 percent, depending on the date of previous loans. The rate for first-time borrowers varies annually and is set every July. It is based on the 91-day U.S. Treasury Bill rate plus 2.5 percent, capped at 8.25 percent. The 2001–02 rate is 6.39%. However, the interest rate may soon be based on the ten-year Treasury Bill, pending current legislation. There is a 4 percent fee that is deducted from the proceeds.

Unsubsidized Federal Stafford Loans. Graduate students may also apply for Unsubsidized Federal Stafford Loans through participating banks. These loans are available regardless of income although lenders usually check your creditworthiness before making the loan. The federal government guarantees these loans but does not pay the interest while you are in school. In fact, some lenders may require that some payments be made even while you are in school, although, generally, lenders will allow students to defer payments and will add the accrued interest to the loan balance. The interest rate is set annually at the 91-day U.S. Treasury Bill rate plus 2.5 percent, capped at 8.25 percent. You may borrow up to the cost of the school in which you are enrolled or will attend, minus estimated financial assistance from other federal, state, and private sources. There is a 4 percent fee that is deducted from the loan proceeds.

Although Unsubsidized Federal Stafford Loans may not be as desirable as Subsidized Federal Stafford Student Loans, they are a useful source of support for those who may not qualify for the lower-interest loans or who need additional financial assistance.

Federal Direct Loans

Some schools are opting to join the Department of Education's new Direct Lending Program instead of offering Federal Stafford Loans. The two programs are essentially the same except that with Direct Loans, schools themselves originate the loans with funds provided from the Treasury Department. Terms and interest rates are virtually the same except that there are a few more repayment options with Federal Direct Loans.

Federal Perkins Loans

The Federal Perkins Loan is a long-term loan available to students demonstrating financial need and is administered directly by the school. Not all schools have these funds, and some may award them to undergraduates only. Eligibility is determined from the information you provide on the FAFSA.

You may borrow up to $5000 per year, to a maximum of $30,000, including undergraduate borrowing (even if your previous Perkins Loans have been repaid). Each school sets its own application deadline, and it's important to apply as early as possible. The school will notify you of your eligibility.

Repayment begins nine months after you graduate, leave school, or drop below half-time status. Repayment can be arranged over a ten-year period, depending upon the size of your debt, but usually you must pay at least $50 per month.

Private Loans

Several alternative loan programs have been developed to supplement the various federal loan programs and to provide borrowing opportunities for students who do not qualify for federal loans. It is advisable to contact private lenders directly for the most recent information on their loan programs. Financial aid administrators can also advise you about which loans best suit your needs.

GradSHARE and GradEXCEL. The New England Education Loan Marketing Association (Nellie Mae) offers two privately funded graduate loan programs—GradSHARE and GradEXCEL. GradSHARE loans are available to students attending any of the thirty-two member schools of the Consortium on Financing Higher Education (COFHE); GradEXCEL loans are available to students attending any accredited, degree-granting college or university in the United States. Eligibility is based on creditworthiness, not need. Students borrowing through GradSHARE or GradEXCEL can choose either a monthly variable interest rate or a one-year renewable interest rate. There is a guarantee fee of 8 percent for GradEXCEL (6 percent for GradEXCEL with a co-borrower) and 6 percent for GradSHARE loans. For more information, call 888-2TUITION.

INTERNATIONAL EDUCATION AND STUDY ABROAD

A variety of funding sources are offered for study abroad and for foreign nationals studying in the United States. The Institute of International Education in New York assists students in locating such aid. It publishes *Funding for U.S. Study—A Guide for Foreign Nationals* and *Financial Resources for International Study,* a guide to organizations offering awards for overseas study. The Council on International Educational Exchange in New York publishes the *Student Travel Catalogue,* which lists fellowship sources and explains the council's services both for United States students traveling abroad and for foreign students coming to the United States.

The U.S. Department of Education administers programs that support fellowships related to international education. Foreign Language and Area Studies Fellowships and Fulbright-Hays Doctoral Dissertation Awards were established to promote knowledge and understanding of other countries and cultures. They offer support to graduate students interested in foreign languages and international relations. Discuss these and other foreign study opportunities with the financial aid officer or someone in the graduate school dean's office at the school you will attend.

HOW TO APPLY

All applicants for federal aid must complete the Free Application for Federal Student Aid (FAFSA). This application must be completed *after* January 1 preceding enrollment in the fall. On this form you report your income and asset information for the preceding calendar year and specify which schools will receive the data. Two to four weeks later you'll receive an acknowledgment on which you can make any corrections. The schools you've designated will also receive the information and may begin asking you to send them documents, usually your U.S. income tax return, verifying what you reported.

APPLICATION DEADLINES

Application deadlines vary. Some schools require you to apply for aid when applying for admission; others require that you be admitted before applying for aid. Aid application instructions and deadlines should be clearly stated in each school's application material. The FAFSA must be filed after January 1 of the year you are applying for aid but the Financial Aid PROFILE should be completed earlier, in October or November.

Some graduate schools want additional information and will ask you to complete a new form, the CSS Financial Aid PROFILE. Schools requiring this form are listed in the PROFILE Registration form available in college financial aid offices. Other schools use their own supplemental application. Check with your financial aid office to confirm which forms they require.

If you have already filed your federal income tax for the year, it will be much easier for you to complete these forms. If not, use estimates, but be certain to notify the financial aid office if your estimated figures differ from the actual ones once you have calculated them.

DETERMINING FINANCIAL NEED

Eligibility for need-based financial aid is based on your income during the calendar year prior to the academic year in which you apply for aid. Prior-year income is used because it is a good predictor of current-year income and is verifiable. If you have a significant reduction in income or assets after your aid application is completed, consult a financial aid counselor. If, for example, you are returning to school after working, you should let the financial aid counselor know your projected income for the year you will be in school. Aid counselors may use their "professional judgment" to revise your financial need, based on the actual income you will earn while you are in graduate school.

Need is determined by examining the difference between the cost of attendance at a given institution and the financial resources you bring to the table. Eligibility for aid is calculated by subtracting your resources from the total cost of attendance budget. These standard student budgets are generally on the low side of the norm. So if your expenses are higher because of medical bills, higher research travel, or more costly books, for example, a financial aid counselor can make an adjustment. Of course, you'll have to document any unusual expenses. Also, keep in mind that with limited grant and scholarship aid, a higher budget will probably mean either more loan or more working hours for you.

TAX ISSUES

Since the passage of the Tax Reform Act of 1986, grants, scholarships, and fellowships may be considered taxable income. That portion of the grant used for payment of tuition and course-required fees, books, supplies, and equipment is excludable from taxable income. Grant support for living expenses is taxable. A good rule of thumb for determining the tax liability for grants and scholarships is to view anything that exceeds the actual cost of tuition, required fees, books, supplies related to courses, and required equipment as taxable.

- If you are employed by an educational institution or other organization that gives tuition reimbursement, you must pay tax on the value that exceeds $5250 until 12/31/01, when tuition benefits will no longer be taxable.

- If your tuition is waived in exchange for working at the institution, the tuition waiver is taxable. This includes waivers that come with teaching or research assistantships.

- Other student support, such as stipends and wages paid to research assistants and teaching assistants, is also taxable income. Student loans, however, are not taxable.

- If you are an international student you may or may not owe taxes depending upon the agreement the U.S. has negotiated with your home country. The United States has tax treaties with over forty countries. You are responsible for making sure that the school you attend follows the terms of the tax treaty. If your country does not have a tax treaty with the U.S., you may have as much as 14 percent withheld from your paycheck.

A FINAL NOTE

While amounts and eligibility criteria vary from field to field as well as from year to year, with thorough research you can uncover many opportunities for graduate financial assistance. If you are interested in graduate study, discuss your plans with faculty members and advisers. Explore all options. Plan ahead, complete forms on time, and be tenacious in your search for support. No matter what your financial situation, if you are academically qualified and knowledgeable about the different sources of aid, you should be able to attend the graduate school of your choice.

Patricia McWade
Dean of Student Financial Services
Georgetown University

NOTES

NOTES

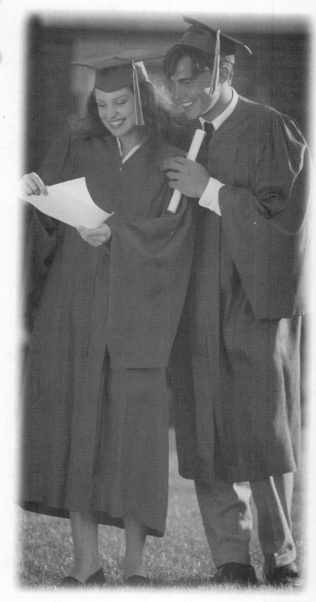
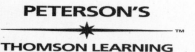

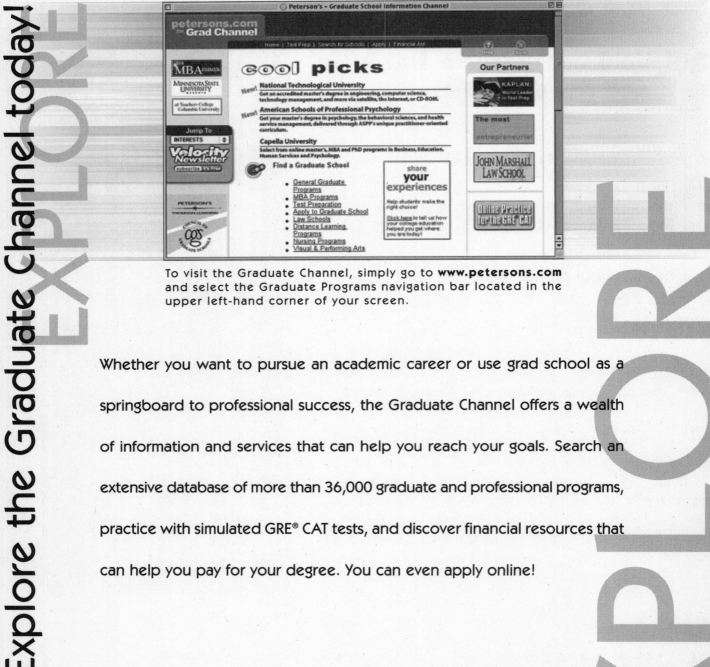